Advance praise

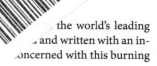

'This extraordinary book summarizes the resear⌐ ⌐the world's leading scientists dealing with health inequalities. Based on r⌐ ⌐and written with an inspired and critical mind, the book will be a vital resour⌐ ⌐oncerned with this burning public health problem.'

Johannes Siegrist,
Senior Professor of Medical Sociology,
Heinrich Heine University Düsseldorf, Germany

'Health inequalities are on the rise, even in the advanced welfare states of Western Europe. In his new and timely book, Mackenbach is able to unfold this and other paradoxes of public health in a way which brings new clarity to one of the biggest challenges of public health. I would recommend the book for scholars and students in both the medical and social sciences, and for all others, including policy makers searching for new and effective tools in their strive to reduce social inequalities in health.'

Terje Andreas Eikemo,
Editor-in-Chief,
Scandinavian Journal of Public Health

'This book comes at an important moment. A decade after the WHO report on Social Determinants of Health and with inequalities in health *growing* in many advanced industrialized nations, solutions are hard to come by. Mackenbach offers us scientific insights, new approaches to evaluating programs to reduce health inequities, and ultimately some sound solutions for countries around the world to adopt. A sobering look at where we are and where we need to go.'

Lisa Berkman,
Cabot Professor of Epidemiology and Public Policy,
Harvard TH Chan School of Public Health, USA

'One might have expected a tour de force based on Mackenbach's extensive and rigorous comparative research on health inequalities, and here it is. But here also is a much deeper theoretical and philosophical treatment that will take both the scientific and policy debates forward.'

Mel Bartley,
Professor Emeritus of Medical Sociology,
University College London, UK

Health inequalities
Persistence and change in European welfare states

Johan P. Mackenbach
Professor of Public Health, Department of Public Health, Erasmus MC,
University Medical Center Rotterdam, Netherlands

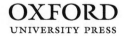

OXFORD
UNIVERSITY PRESS

OXFORD
UNIVERSITY PRESS

Great Clarendon Street, Oxford, OX2 6DP,
United Kingdom

Oxford University Press is a department of the University of Oxford.
It furthers the University's objective of excellence in research, scholarship,
and education by publishing worldwide. Oxford is a registered trade mark of
Oxford University Press in the UK and in certain other countries

Published in the United States of America by Oxford University Press
198 Madison Avenue, New York, NY 10016, United States of America

British Library Cataloguing in Publication Data

Data available

Library of Congress Control Number: 2019946587

ISBN 978–0–19–883141–9

Preface

The world we live in is hugely unequal. When you happen to be born in the global North, you are much more likely to live a relatively comfortable life than if you are born in the global South—regardless of how talented you are and how hard you work. And while the gap in material living conditions *between* countries has gradually become smaller over time, the last decades have witnessed a serious widening of the gap in income and wealth *within* many countries.

Mirroring these social inequalities there are stark health inequalities too, both between and within countries. Better socioeconomic conditions are generally associated with better health and a longer life—not only in the poorer parts of the world but also in the richest countries, including the advanced welfare states of Western Europe. Health inequalities within rich countries even seem to be on the rise, thereby aggravating the challenge that social inequality poses to public policy.

In this book I explore the connections between social inequalities and health inequalities. Why are health inequalities—systematically higher rates of disease, disability, and premature death among people with a lower level of education, occupation, or income—so persistent? The persistence of health inequalities in the advanced welfare states of Western Europe is a paradox that is difficult to explain. This is unfortunate, because a lack of understanding of this paradox may foster naïve expectations on the impact of public policy on health inequalities.

This lack of understanding is not due to a lack of research *per se*. On the contrary, hundreds of epidemiological, sociological, and other studies from Europe and other parts of the world have provided detailed insights into the specific living conditions and behavioural, psychological, and biological factors underlying health inequalities within a particular population at a particular point in time. This is important, but in order to explain the paradox that we observe at the macro-level it is necessary to take a broader comparative view, and to study the evolution of health inequalities over time in different countries. This will help us to identify their 'upstream' economic, cultural, policy, and political determinants, and to see health inequalities in the context of the evolution of other aspects of social inequality. That is what this book does.

It comes at an important moment. Around the world there is a strong momentum to address health inequalities. Starting with the publication of the British Black report in 1980, this momentum has purposely been built using national research programmes, dissemination of research findings among policymakers, think-tank reports, government committees and experiments with policy interventions in several European countries. This has culminated in the World Health Organization's Commission on Social Determinants of Health report 'Closing the gap in a generation', published in 2008, which is still percolating into national and local efforts to tackle health inequalities worldwide.

However, since the publication of this landmark report, there is also an undercurrent of doubt fed by inconsistencies in the evidence-base on health inequalities. One such inconsistency was mentioned above—how can we expect to be able to substantially reduce health inequalities when they persist even in the advanced welfare states of Europe? Another inconsistency, which will be discussed in this book, is that it has been surprisingly difficult to find convincing scientific evidence for a causal effect of socioeconomic disadvantage on health. And a third disturbing fact: how to explain that the only large-scale and well-resourced policy programme to reduce health inequalities, pursued by the English government between 1997 and 2010, seems not to have had a measurable impact on health inequalities?

After almost 40 years of research we therefore need to step back and think again, and this book is an attempt to deconstruct and then reassemble the available evidence. Reader, be warned that some of the conclusions of this book are sobering. For example, taking a broader view makes clear that health inequalities are partly driven by forces—such as changes in the structure of society and differences in the pace of health improvement—that are very difficult to counteract.

On the other hand, the book also brings some good news to those—such as its author—who see compelling reasons to continue to try to reduce health inequalities. Variations in the magnitude of health inequalities between countries and over time show that there is enormous scope for reducing health inequalities. And we can reduce health inequalities, at least as measured on an absolute scale, if we ensure that interventions and policies that improve average population health also provide sufficient benefit to lower socioeconomic groups.

Acknowledgements

This book is partly based on a series of comparative studies of health inequalities listening to strange names like 'SEdHA', 'Eurothine', 'EURO-GBD-SE', 'DEMETRIQ', and 'LIFEPATH', that would not have been possible without financial support from the European Commission. I had the good fortune to collaborate with many bright and kind colleagues who joined me in Rotterdam for shorter or longer periods of time to work on these projects: Anton Kunst, Feikje Groenhof, Adriënne Cavelaars, Irina Stirbu, Martijn Huisman, Vivian Bos, Mauricio Avendaño, Caspar Looman, Gerard Borsboom, Alyson van Raalte, Terje Eikemo, Ivana Kulhánová, Marlen Toch-Marquardt, Margarete Kulik, Gwenn Menvielle, Olof Ostergren, Rasmus Hoffmann, Iris Plug, Rianne de Gelder, Yannan Hu, Frank van Lenthe, Kristina Hoffmann, Giorgia Gregoraci, Blin Nagavci, Wilma Nusselder, José Rubio Valverde, Marlies Baars, Line Ullits, Bibiana Perez, Hiro Tanaka, and Chiara Di Girolamo. Many of the data that I analyse in this book were originally prepared by Rianne de Gelder, Yannan Hu, Wilma Nusselder, and José Rubio Valverde. Most of the tables and graphs are based on mortality and survey data collected and harmonized in the DEMETRIQ study (European Commission grant number FP7-CP-FP grant no. 278511) and the LIFEPATH study (Horizon 2020 grant number 633666).

In addition, many international collaborators contributed to this work by providing and analysing national data, and by helping in the interpretation of the results for their country: Barbara Artnik (Slovenia), Matthias Bopp (Switzerland), Henrik Brønnum-Hansen (Denmark), Carme Borrell (Spain (Catalonia)), Bo Burström (Sweden), Giuseppe Costa (Italy), Patrick Deboosere (Belgium), Dagmar Dzúrová (Czech Republic), Ola Ekholm (Denmark), Santi Esnaola (Spain (Basque Country)), Domantas Jasilionis (Germany and Lithuania), Ken Judge (United Kingdom), Ramune Kalediene (Lithuania), Johannes Klotz (Austria), Jurate Klumbiene (Lithuania), Katalin Kovács (Hungary), Eero Lahelma (Helsinki), Richard Layte (Ireland), Mall Leinsalu (Estonia and Sweden), Olle Lundberg (Sweden), Pekka Martikainen (Finland), Steve Platt (United Kingdom), Remigijus Prochorskas (Lithuania), Enrique Regidor (Spain (Madrid)), Jitka Rychtaříková (Czech Republic), Maica Rodríguez-Sanz (Spain (Catalonia)), Paula Santana (Portugal), Teresa Spadea (Italy), Bjørn Heine Strand (Norway), and Bogdan Wojtyniak (Poland).

A few special words of thanks go to Christiaan Monden (who hosted me at Nuffield College, Oxford, to help me better understand social mobility), Peter Schroeder Back (who helped me in understanding what 'solidarity' is), Katalin Kovács (who helped me in interpreting long-term trends in health inequalities in Hungary), Bjørn Heine Strand and Tord Vinne Vedøy (who helped me in understanding trends in smoking in Norway), Johan Fritzell (who helped me to understand the Swedish welfare state), and Joost Oude Groeniger (who helped me in setting up the analyses reported in Chapter 4).

A first crude draft of this book was written during a residency at the *Fondation Brocher* in Hermance (Switzerland) in April 2017. I am grateful to the *Fondation* for their generous support, and for the lovely and quiet surroundings which allowed me to work like a zombie without feeling like a zombie. More than a year later, a much more developed draft version was read by Mel Bartley, Matthias Bopp, Inez de Beaufort, Tanja Houweling, Frank van Lenthe, Hafez Ismaili

M'Hamdi, Joost Oude Groeniger, and Johannes Siegrist, whose comments helped me to bring more balance in the text and to repair some obvious (to them) errors and omissions.

Parts of this book have been based on the following papers that I wrote for scientific journals:

- 'The persistence of health inequalities in modern welfare states: the explanation of a paradox' (*Social Science & Medicine* 2012;75:761–9)
- 'Persistence of social inequalities in modern welfare states: Explanation of a paradox' (*Scandinavian Journal of Public Health* 2017;45:113–20)
- 'Can we reduce health inequalities? An analysis of the English strategy (1997–2010)' (*Journal of Epidemiology and Community Health* 2011;65:568–75)
- 'Nordic paradox, Southern miracle, Eastern disaster: persistence of inequalities in mortality in Europe' (*European Journal of Public Health* 2017;27 suppl. 4:14–17)
- '"Fundamental causes" of inequalities in mortality: an empirical test of the theory in 20 European populations' (*Sociology of Health and Illness* 2017;39:1117–33)
- I originally wrote parts of Chapter 3 as a discussion paper for the FEAM/ALLEA Committee on Health Inequalities ('Health inequalities; an interdisciplinary exploration of socioeconomic position, health and causality', Amsterdam: Koninklijke Nederlandse Academie van Wetenschappen, 2018)

Let me end by expressing my sincere hope that this book, in spite of (or perhaps precisely because of) its sobering conclusions will contribute to a better world, in which the prospects for a long and healthy life are shared more equally than is currently the case.

Rotterdam, August 2018
Johan Mackenbach

Contents

Chapter 1

Introduction

1.1 More illness within shorter lives

Flat, flatter, flattest

The Netherlands, the country where I live and work, is among the flattest of all European countries. This does not only apply to its physical geography—most of the country is completely flat—but also to its social geography. Income inequalities are smaller than in most other European countries, and our Prime Minister aptly illustrates the Dutch distaste for social hierarchy by going to work on a bicycle. The unemployed and disabled are protected from poverty by relatively generous social security benefits, and out-of-pocket payments for health care access are among the lowest in the world.[i]

Nevertheless, life expectancy differs substantially between different population groups—not only between men and women, and between the married and non-married, but also between richer and poorer people, between those with professional and manual occupations, and between people with a higher and a lower level of education. These inequalities are amazingly large for such a flat country (Figure 1.1): Dutch men in the highest income group live seven years longer than men in the lowest income group. They also live many more years in good health: on average, men in the highest income group are 14 years older when they start having disabilities, and 18 years older when they start perceiving their health as less than 'good'. As a result, men with a high income spend only six years of their longer lives with disability, against 11 years for the shorter living men with a low income. Among women, inequalities in total life expectancy are somewhat smaller, but inequalities in life expectancy free of disability are even larger than among men.

These are the 'health inequalities' that this book is about: systematic differences in health within a country between people with a lower and higher socioeconomic position, as indicated by their level of education, occupational class, or income. Often, these inequalities manifest themselves as a gradient, in the sense that average health deteriorates gradually with every step down the social ladder, as in Figure 1.1.

The reason why this book's focus is on socioeconomic inequalities in health, as opposed to inequalities by marital status or other social distinctions, is that socioeconomic inequalities in health are seen by many as unfair—unlike similarly systematic differences in health between married and unmarried people, inequalities between groups of people defined in socioeconomic terms are often perceived as contradicting basic notions of justice. Why should people who are less well off in terms of housing, working conditions, financial security, and many other living conditions, also live shorter lives, and within those shorter lives spend more years with disability?

An old problem

Historical evidence suggests that socioeconomic inequalities in health are not a recent phenomenon. Data from parish registers of baptisms and burials show that substantial differences in mortality rates between persons with higher and lower social ranks were already present in the seventeenth and eighteenth centuries, at least in European urban areas.[1,2]

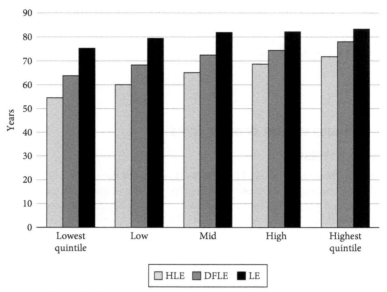

Figure 1.1 Inequalities in health expectancy by income in the Netherlands

Notes: HLE = life expectancy in good self- assessed health. DFLE = disability-free life expectancy. LE = life expectancy. Income in quintiles of equivalized net household income. Life expectancy etc. from birth. Men; women similar. Data for 2011–14.

Source: data from Statistics Netherlands (http://statline.cbs.nl/StatWeb/, accessed 26 February 2018).

It is not certain whether socioeconomic inequalities in mortality also existed before that time. Some believe that these inequalities emerged only when the large epidemics started to recede and when the first improvements in nutrition, housing, and individual and public hygiene began to have an impact.[3,4] A study of the British peerage suggests that the life expectancy of this upper-class group was no different from that of the general population until it began to diverge after the middle of the eighteenth century.[5,6]

It is, however, difficult to believe that in earlier centuries higher placed persons did indeed have the same survival chances as the majority of the population. Earlier times had seen frequent mortality crises, arising from three interlinked causes: war, pestilence, and famine. Famine was certainly unequally distributed within the population, and reports of health commissions in plague-ridden towns often mentioned that there were large differences in mortality between rich and poor.[7]

In any case, it was only during the nineteenth century that socioeconomic inequalities in health were really 'discovered'. Before that time, health inequalities simply went unrecognized by contemporaries because of lack of information. In the nineteenth century the founding fathers of public health, such as Villermé in France, Chadwick in England, and Virchow in Germany, devoted a large part of their work to studying health inequalities.[8–10] This was facilitated by the creation of national population statistics, which permitted the calculation of mortality rates by occupation or by city district.

French physician Louis René Villermé (1782–1863), for example, analysed inequalities in mortality between *arrondissements* in Paris in 1817–21. He showed that poorer districts tended to have systematically higher mortality rates than more well-to-do neighbourhoods. He concluded

that life and death are not primarily biological phenomena, but are closely linked to social circumstances.[9] German pathologist and public health physician Rudolf Virchow (1821–1902) went
even further in his famous statement that 'medicine is a social science, and politics nothing but
medicine at a larger scale'.[11]

Since the nineteenth century, there has been a marked decline in mortality in all European
countries, leading to a doubling of average life expectancy at birth. As a result, some inequalities
in mortality have declined as well, but this is far from a generalized phenomenon. For example,
in England and Wales, the only European country where long time-series about occupational
class differences in mortality are available, inequalities in infant mortality declined substantially
between the 1920s and 1970s, but over the same period inequalities in adult mortality remained
largely stable in absolute terms, and even increased in relative terms.[12]

1.2 **The great paradox of public health**

Welfare typologies

It is certain that health inequalities have not disappeared, despite the advent of the welfare state.
In the course of the twentieth century all high-income countries have become 'welfare states' that
redistribute income from the rich to the poor (e.g. by progressive taxation and social security
arrangements) and offer a range of collectively financed services (e.g. public housing, education,
health care, access to culture, and leisure facilities), in order to create some degree of equality in
material and other living conditions.[13,14]

Countries differ substantially in the way in which, and the degree to which, this has been
achieved. Various typologies of these welfare arrangements have been proposed, such as the three
'welfare regimes' of Danish sociologist Gøsta Esping-Andersen:[15]

a 'social-democratic' regime, which is based on the principle of 'universalism' (i.e. granting
access to benefits and services to all citizens), is usually financed through taxes, and has a high
degree of 'decommodification' in which supply and demand of services are removed from the
market;

a 'Christian-democratic' or conservative regime, which is based on the principle of subsidi-
arity (i.e. limiting the role of the state to what others cannot offer), is usually financed through
'Bismarckian' social insurance schemes, and has a medium degree of decommodification;

and a 'liberal' model, which is based on the principles of market dominance and private pro-
vision, with the state intervening only to alleviate poverty and provide for basic needs on a
'means-tested' basis, and with a very limited degree of decommodification.

Esping-Andersen's typology originally covered Western Europe and North America only. Others
have proposed slightly different typologies and have added a fourth and fifth regime to include
Mediterranean and Central and Eastern European countries, respectively. The 'Mediterranean'
regime shares characteristics with the 'Christian-democratic' regime, but has peaks of generosity
(e.g. with regard to pensions) combined with serious gaps in coverage due to its reliance on the
family as first pillar of support.[16] Post-communist countries in Central and Eastern Europe have
hybrid and rapidly changing systems based on remnants from the Bismarckian systems of the
Habsburg empire, mixed with remnants from the service-based systems of state socialism.[17]

In reality, very few countries fit neatly into one of these ideal types, and single countries have
been classified in different regimes by different authors.[18] For example, the Netherlands was
classified by Esping-Andersen as having a 'social-democratic' regime, but as its main financing
mechanism is based on social insurance rather than taxes, others have classified it as having a

Table 1.1 A classification of European countries by 'welfare regime'

	Welfare regime				
	Social-democratic	**Christian-democratic**	**Liberal**	**Mediterranean**	**Post-communist**
Main characteristics	Universal, high levels of benefits, tax funded	Selective, high levels of benefits, insurance funded	Means-tested, low levels of benefits, tax funded	Subsidiarity with family, varying levels of benefits, fragmented funding	Hybrid, in flux, little commonality
Countries	Finland, Sweden, Norway, Denmark	Netherlands, Belgium, Luxembourg, Germany, Austria, Switzerland, France	United Kingdom, Ireland	Spain, Portugal, Italy, Greece	Slovenia, Czech Rep., Slovakia Hungary, Poland, Bulgaria, Romania, Lithuania, Latvia, Estonia

'Christian-democratic' regime. Table 1.1 gives a possible classification of European countries based on various sources, without attempting to be consistent with any specific typology.

A paradox

The 'rediscovery' of health inequalities

In the 1960s and 1970s it was widely believed that the modern welfare state had not only reduced poverty and inequalities in access to education, health care, and other services, but had also reduced health inequalities to almost non-existence. This illusion was, however, shattered by the publication in 1980 of the Black Report in the United Kingdom, and shortly thereafter by reports in other countries, such as a study of inequalities in mortality between neighbourhoods in the city of Amsterdam in the Netherlands published in 1981.[19] The Black Report clearly showed that, despite overall improvements in population health, mortality and morbidity were still much higher in the lower occupational classes.[20]

The 'rediscovery' of health inequalities in the United Kingdom was facilitated by the availability since the early twentieth century of a continuous series of 'occupational mortality statistics'. These had shown that mortality from ischemic heart disease had become progressively more common in working-class men and women than in the middle and upper classes.[21] British epidemiologists, including Michael Marmot whom we will encounter again in later chapters in this book, had already taken steps in the 1970s to study the determinants of health inequalities by setting up cohort studies such as the famous 'Whitehall' studies, in which London civil servants in lower and higher 'grades' were followed up for morbidity and mortality.[22]

Paradox, puzzle, conundrum, ...

The persistence of socioeconomic inequalities in health is a major disappointment, and at the same time a large 'paradox'[14] or 'puzzle'.[23] It is difficult to accept, but also difficult to understand, that the welfare state has not eliminated these inequalities. This conundrum is made even more puzzling by the fact that there appears to be no association between the extent or intensity of welfare policies in a country and the magnitude of its health inequalities.

Within Europe, there are substantial differences in welfare spending, for example, as illustrated in Figure 1.2. The Nordic countries, with their social-democratic welfare regimes, spend the most, followed by some continental-European countries, with their Christian-democratic welfare regimes. The two countries with a liberal regime, United Kingdom and Ireland, spend less, as do most Mediterranean countries. Countries in Central and Eastern Europe spend the least, both in relative terms (as a proportion of GDP) and of course, because of their lower GDP, in absolute terms.[24]

Before the results of the first systematic comparison of the magnitude of health inequalities between European countries was published, it was believed that Sweden had smaller inequalities in mortality than the United Kingdom.[25] This proved to be an illusion when the data were duly corrected for the fact that these countries differed in the proportion of economically inactive men who had been excluded from the analysis in previous, less rigorously conducted comparisons.[26]

As will be illustrated in Chapter 2, despite their universal and generous welfare arrangements the Nordic countries do not have smaller health inequalities than other European countries.[27–29,30] There is good evidence that welfare policies have contributed to a reduction of inequalities in income, and also that not all welfare regimes have been equally effective in reducing inequality in material living conditions. For example, countries with a social-democratic welfare regime have been more effective in reducing poverty than those with a Christian-democratic or liberal regime.[13,31] Countries with more generous welfare spending also have better average health outcomes.[32] But why are health inequalities not smaller in countries with more generous welfare spending? Is welfare spending unimportant for health? Are there counteracting mechanisms which undo the effect of welfare spending?

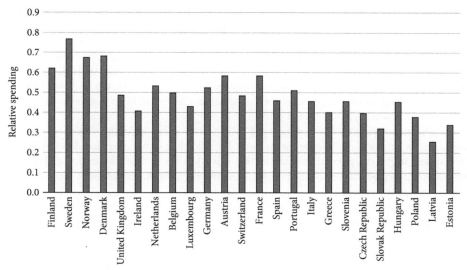

Figure 1.2 Social spending in European countries

Notes: Relative spending calculated as % of Gross Domestic Product spent on social benefits (cash benefits, social services, and tax breaks), divided by % of population not in paid employment.

Source: data from OECD (2007). *Social Expenditure Database (SOCX)*. (http://www.oecd.org/social/expenditure.htm, accessed 20 February 2018).

A 'macroscopic' view

In this book I will explore the explanation of this paradox. What explains the persistence of socioeconomic inequalities in health in highly developed welfare states? The sudden awareness, in the 1980s, that health inequalities had not disappeared has given rise to substantial research efforts, particularly in a small number of Western European countries, such as the United Kingdom, Sweden, Finland, and the Netherlands. This research, which will be summarized in Chapter 3, has given us a detailed understanding of the way inequalities in behavioural risk factors, occupational hazards, psychosocial conditions, and many other determinants contribute to inequalities in health outcomes—all measured at the individual level.

These 'microscopic' studies can, however, not adequately address the more fundamental question why these inequalities in exposure to various health risks exist, and persist, in the first place. This conundrum can only be resolved by taking a 'macroscopic view', in which we 'zoom out' to study the contextual determinants of inequalities in health and health determinants. In this book I will therefore exploit between-country and intertemporal variations in health inequalities and their determinants to find out what makes health inequalities larger or smaller.

1.3 **The need for a broader picture**

Social inequality

Persistence of social inequality

Such a macroscopic view also makes it easier to put health inequalities into a broader perspective, for example, that of social inequality *per se*. Health is not the only valuable thing that is distributed unequally in society, and any explanation for the persistence of health inequalities in modern welfare states must take into account what we know about the stubborn persistence of inequalities in other things. Why is social inequality so persistent, despite a century of struggle to create a fairer distribution of living conditions, through welfare arrangements and other policies?

The welfare state has reduced inequalities in material living conditions, but it has certainly not eliminated them, and inequalities in non-material factors, including child raising patterns, health literacy, social connections, job control, visits to the opera, personality traits, dietary habits, leisure time activities, political influence, etc. etc. are still enormous. It should be clear to even the most casual observer of modern societies that social inequality has never gone away, and that it still permeates all areas of life. Why is this?

In order to answer that question we need to delve into sociological theories of where social inequality in a more generic sense comes from. The discipline of sociology has developed partly in response to the sharp social inequalities that existed in the nineteenth century, and offers us several sophisticated theories of the processes and mechanisms that make social inequality such a persistent phenomenon.

Some theories argue that social stratification benefits society as a whole because it gives monetary and non-monetary rewards to those who are most useful to society. Sociologists in this 'functionalist' tradition also regard social inequality as at least partly arising from differences between individuals in properties that make them useful for society.[33,34] A second, more 'radical' tradition of sociological theorizing on the origins of social inequality suggests that competition or conflict over scarce resources is the root cause of social inequality. For example, classical Marxism focuses on the exploitative nature of capitalism: those who own the means of production exploit those who are dependent on selling their labour in the labour market.[35]

These sociological theories also suggest very different explanations for the persistence of health inequalities. Functionalist theories imply that the persistence of social inequality is partly due to the persistence of differences between individuals in talent—suggesting that the persistence of health inequalities is governed by the persistence of differences between individuals in cognitive ability and other personal characteristics that help them to avoid health risks. On the other hand, conflict-oriented theories suggest that the persistence of health inequalities is due to the persistence of differences in power over scarce resources—an idea with rather different policy implications.

Rising income inequality

The relevance of a broader scope is underlined by current concerns over rising inequalities in income and wealth. Inequality in material living conditions has not only persisted, but new empirical evidence shows that, after a period of shrinking inequalities in income and wealth around the middle of the twentieth century, these inequalities have risen again to levels resembling those at the beginning of the twentieth century. In Western Europe and North America, over the past few decades the incomes of the rich have continued to increase, whereas the incomes of the poor have often stagnated, probably due to globalization and displacement of industries to emerging economies in Asia.[36]

French economist Thomas Piketty has argued that the rise of inequalities in wealth is due to the fact that the rate of return on capital is always greater than the rate of economic growth, and that during the course of the twentieth century the rise of wealth inequalities has only been stopped by wars (which destroyed capital) and taxation (which redistributed money from the rich to the poor). Decades of peace combined with a neoliberal distaste for redistribution have conspired to let wealth inequalities rise again to very high levels.[37] This has even led to the uncomfortable thought that in the absence of a democratic mandate for redistribution, the only way in which these trends will be reversed is war.[38]

In any case, growing inequalities in income and wealth within high-income countries have given rise to considerable concern, not only among those on the political left but also among economists, because these inequalities may have a range of negative effects, including reduced social mobility, high rates of crime, and political instability.[39] Did they perhaps also contribute to the persistence, or even widening, of health inequalities over the past decades, or is this a coincidence?

British social epidemiologist Richard Wilkinson, in a series of very influential publications, has drawn attention to the possible effect of rising income inequality on average population health. In an early paper, published in the *British Medical Journal* in 1992, he showed that countries with higher income inequality tended to have lower life expectancies at birth.[40] In later work, he showed many other correlations as well, ranging from homicide to teenage births and from obesity to lack of social mobility.[41] Despite the fact that the empirical basis for some of these findings has been disputed,[42] they do raise important questions about the link between income inequality and health inequalities. Wilkinson argues that greater income inequality harms everyone, by increasing competition and uncertainty, but does it also lead to greater health inequalities?

The moral significance of inequality

In this book I will use the term 'health inequalities' in a purely descriptive sense, without necessarily claiming that the differences we see are unfair. The English language is not entirely unambiguous in this respect—it is almost impossible to use the term 'inequality' without automatically implying that this is an undesirable state of affairs, and that 'equality' would be better. However, because this term is widely used in Europe we will also use it in this book and refrain from using the term 'health disparities', which was introduced in the United States as a morally more neutral term. For health inequalities that are also unfair we will reserve the term 'health inequities'.

Despite the intended neutrality of the term, interest in health inequalities among public health researchers and policymakers is closely linked to their intuitive conviction that these inequalities are, to a large extent, unfair. This probably also applies to most readers of this book. Is not the fact that people who have less of most things in life also live shorter lives, simply unfair? Well, finding a good answer to that question is not as simple as it may seem, and here again we will benefit from broadening the scope from health inequalities to social inequalities in a more general sense.

The most widely used framework for the normative assessment of health inequalities, published in 1992 by British public health scientist Margaret Whitehead, defines health inequity as 'differences in health that are unnecessary, avoidable, unfair and unjust'. It lists a number of criteria to determine which health differences would fall within this definition, focusing on whether or not the health effects of certain living conditions or behaviours could be avoided by the individuals involved.[43] We will discuss this framework, as well as other approaches, in more detail in Chapter 5, section 5.3, 'Health inequalities and social justice'.

This framework has proven to be very useful, but surprisingly it does not explicitly take into account whether the differences in health are generated by social inequality, that is, inequalities in access to resources along socioeconomic lines, or by differences along some other social dimension, such as gender, marital status, migrant status, urban versus rural location, etc. Does it not matter that we are dealing with health differences along a socioeconomic dimension?[44]

If it does matter, the unfairness of health inequalities will partly depend on whether the broader social inequalities generating them are considered unfair. This then implies that when deciding about the unfairness of health inequalities we cannot avoid political ideology. Discussions about the acceptability of social inequality have a very long history, not only within the scientific discipline of sociology, but also in politics. The choice between acceptance and rejection of social inequality has for a long time been the major fault-line between left and right in politics.

French historian Pierre Rosanvallon has traced the history of this discussion, highlighting the origin of 'egalitarianism' in the decades preceding the French and American revolutions in the eighteenth century, with their rejection of autocratic forms of government and call for *liberté, égalité, fraternité*. This period was followed by the re-emergence of stark social inequalities in the nineteenth century as a result of industrialization and capitalism, which not only produced a new proletariat but also strong disagreements on how to deal with these inequalities. Whereas conservatives and liberals tended to legitimize inequality by referring to the 'immorality' of the proletariat and their 'natural' inferiority, socialists and communists pointed to heritable advantage and cruel exploitation as the root causes of social inequality.[45]

Although over-politicization of the issue of health inequalities may be counterproductive, it will be necessary to analyse how the moral significance of health inequalities is affected by its being part of the broader phenomenon of social inequality.

The crisis of the welfare state

While researchers are still scratching their heads over why health inequalities persist despite the welfare state, many other reasons to reconsider the welfare state have arisen, and according to some the welfare state is even in a severe crisis.

Ideas about the welfare state were first articulated in the late nineteenth century, mainly as collective insurance against the risks of the labour market, and many European countries had already implemented rudimentary welfare arrangements before World War II. The experience of increased social cohesion during World War II, and the necessity to fight off communism in the post–World War II years, led to the 'Golden Age' of the welfare state, exemplified by the creation of the National Health Service in the United Kingdom, and different but often similarly generous arrangements elsewhere in Europe.[17]

However, since the 1970s the welfare state has come under pressure everywhere, initially because of the perceived necessity of reducing public expenditure and improving economic competitiveness, but later also because of the rise of neoliberal ideas. Since the 1980s, many countries have made substantial changes to their welfare arrangements.[17] According to some, if ideal types like those proposed by Esping-Andersen ever existed they certainly no longer do.[13]

Here again, the broader picture helps us to raise more specific questions. Has welfare reform—sometimes called 'welfare retrenchment', because of the reductions of eligibility and benefits that have been carried through—contributed to the persistence or even widening of health inequalities since the 1980s? Or, perhaps more fundamentally, can the persistence of health inequalities be seen as a sign of the failure of the welfare state, and another reason for welfare reform? If health inequalities signal a failure of the welfare state, how should the welfare state be reformed to tackle health inequalities more effectively?

1.4 Preview: this book's main conclusions

Why health inequalities persist in modern welfare states

Drawing upon a unique series of studies covering 30 European countries and more than three decades of quantitative observations on socioeconomic inequalities in morbidity, mortality, and risk factors for morbidity and mortality, this book shows that although health inequalities are ubiquitous and persistent, they are also highly variable between countries *and* change dynamically over time. These variations and trends are important for two reasons: they suggest that health inequalities are potentially remediable, and they provide opportunities for studying the determinants of health inequalities. The latter is what we do in a number of in-depth analyses in this book. We summarize the main conclusions in this section—the arguments will be given in more detail later, so do not expect to be convinced already.

While the analyses confirm that health inequalities are potentially remediable, they also show that health inequalities are partly driven by autonomous forces that are difficult to counteract, or that we may not even want to counteract. First, the nature of social inequality has changed in such a way that new mechanisms linking social inequality to health inequalities have arisen. The most important of these changes relates to education, which has become a more important stratification variable than half a century ago. This has strengthened the association between socioeconomic position and cognitive ability and other personal characteristics that do not only partly determine a person's educational achievements, but also his or her health in later life. Societies have also become more 'fluid', in the sense that a person's socioeconomic position has become less dependent on his or her parents' socioeconomic position, but this has also created more opportunities for selection into lower and higher socioeconomic groups on the basis of health and health determinants.

Second, population health has dramatically improved in many countries, but for various reasons (such as dependence of health improvement on behaviour change, and thus on health literacy) these improvements have almost always been smaller in proportional terms in lower socioeconomic groups. This is almost inevitable, but as a result relative inequalities in health outcomes invariably go up, even if lower socioeconomic groups share in the benefits of health improvement, as they have done in many European countries. Also, when population health deteriorates, as it sometimes does when new health hazards arise, it takes time before these new hazards can effectively be tackled collectively, and in the meantime those with higher education or income will usually be better able to protect themselves.

Third, despite the welfare state people in lower socioeconomic groups still have less access to a range of both material and non-material resources that are important for their health. Even in the most generous welfare states, inequalities in material resources have only partly been removed, and inequalities in non-material resources such as social and cultural capital may not have been reduced at all. As a result, there are social inequalities in practically all health determinants, including for the chronic conditions that currently dominate the health profile of high-income countries. It is this third mechanism driving health inequalities that we definitely want to counteract, but sociological theories about the explanation of social inequality warn against optimism for our possibilities to eliminate these inequalities.

These three mechanisms—remodelling plus persistence of social inequality, in interaction with a rapidly changing health landscape—have counteracted the beneficial effects of the European welfare state. These mechanisms also explain the 'Nordic paradox', that is, the fact that countries with more highly developed welfare arrangements do not necessarily have smaller health inequalities, and may even sometimes have larger health inequalities than other countries. For example, countries with more advanced welfare systems also tend to be more advanced in economic and cultural terms, which implies that they are often also ahead of other countries in, for example, shifts in educational distribution of the population and the progression of the smoking epidemic.

A broader perspective

When we broaden the perspective to social inequality *per se*, we do find evidence that widening income inequalities have played a role in widening health inequalities, particularly in Central and Eastern Europe. However, widening health inequalities cannot simply be seen as a product of widening social inequality, and more generally health inequalities cannot simply be seen as a product of social inequality. Other mechanisms—such as selection during social mobility—are involved as well. At the same time, even where health inequalities are not caused by social inequality, they aggravate other social inequalities, which heightens their salience for public policy.

When we relate health inequalities and the mechanisms generating them to various theories of justice, it becomes clear that health inequalities cannot integrally be labelled 'inequitable', first because there is not one single, commonly accepted conception of justice, and second because in practically all conceptions of justice at least some mechanisms underlying health inequalities are *not* 'inequitable'. However, there are other compelling reasons for reducing health inequalities, such as widespread feelings of solidarity with those who are less lucky in life, and the substantial costs to society induced by health inequalities.

We conclude that the persistence of health inequalities is an argument for strengthening and reforming the welfare state, and cannot be used to legitimize reducing the welfare state. Without the welfare state health inequalities would probably be larger than they currently are. Current initiatives to reform the welfare state, for example, by putting more emphasis on getting people into paid work, offer new opportunities for reducing health inequalities. Also, the success of pension reforms will depend on our ability to raise life expectancy in good health of lower socioeconomic groups to the proposed future pension age.

Policy implications

Over the past decades, several European countries have made efforts to reduce health inequalities, building on the rapidly accumulating results of research in this area. Unfortunately, as we will see these attempts have been largely unsuccessful, due to a combination of insufficient scale of the efforts as compared to the massive nature of health inequalities, and insufficient knowledge of the effectiveness of interventions and policies to reduce health inequalities.

While this implies that we should avoid setting our goals for reducing health inequalities too highly, the experience of the past decades also shows that it is feasible to reduce health inequalities, but more so when measured on an absolute scale than when measured on a relative scale. When overall health improves, it is very difficult to reduce relative health inequalities (measured by, e.g. a *percentage* excess of mortality in lower as compared to higher socioeconomic groups), and much easier to reduce absolute health inequalities (measured by, e.g. an excess *number* of deaths in lower as compared to higher socioeconomic groups). The good news is that a reduction of absolute health inequalities can be achieved by making sure that lower socioeconomic groups derive sufficient benefit from interventions and policies aiming to improve average population health.

This book

This book is rather different from other books on health inequalities, of which there are quite a few. I mention two, to indicate the place of this book within the available literature.

The best theoretical introduction to health inequalities is Mel Bartley's 'Health inequality: an introduction to concepts, theories and methods', of which a second edition was published in 2017. This is a systematic account of what social inequalities in health are, and how they might be explained—integrating sociological and epidemiological insights. It describes and criticizes various theories of health inequalities: behavioural, psychosocial, materialist, and macrosocial theories.[46] Although its conclusions on the relative merits of these theories differ from those in this book—particularly when it comes to the causal role of socioeconomic factors in generating health and ill-health—readers will benefit greatly from the theoretical and empirical rigor with which the theories are approached.

Michael Marmot's 'The health gap: the challenge of an unequal world', published in 2015, is a completely different kind of book. It is an account of how the author, who chaired the WHO Commission on Social Determinants of Health as well as policy advisory committees in the United Kingdom and Europe, came to his radical views on the causes of, and remedies for, health inequalities. It is inspiring, because it is personal, humorous, and rhetorically strong, and based on interesting exchanges with bureaucrats, economists, fire-fighters, and many others around the world. Although it is not written in a systematic way, it does dig deeply, for example when the author explains the philosophical basis for his conviction that 'social injustice is killing on a large scale'.[47] The European experience that we will study in this book sometimes suggests differently, but readers will certainly appreciate the author's breadth of vision.

The book you are now reading is unique not only in its 'macroscopic' view, and reliance on international-comparative studies, but also in its more critical—as compared to Bartley's and Marmot's books—assessment of the scientific evidence. For example, Marmot complains that '[m]ore or less every time I have given a lecture and someone has asked if I have considered the possibility that everything that I have said is wrong, […] that someone has been an economist'.[47] (p. 108) As we will see in this book, it is true that health economists have challenged some widely held views about the causes of health inequalities, but I think they should be taken seriously—and may well be right.

Chapter 2 sets the scene with a description of patterns of health inequalities in a wide range of European countries, and Chapter 3 then summarizes explanatory insights, based on the abundant results from micro-level studies of the determinants of health inequalities carried out over the past decades. Chapter 4 reports on a number of analyses especially conducted for this book, and zooms out to the macro-level to look at the determinants of population level health inequalities. Chapter 5 puts these findings in a broader perspective, and Chapter 6 focuses on policy implications.

Key points

- Health is unevenly distributed within society: people in a lower socioeconomic position live shorter lives, and within those shorter lives they spend more years with disability and other health problems.

- Health inequalities have existed for many years, and have not disappeared with the build-up of the welfare state. Health inequalities are also not smaller in countries with more advanced welfare states. This paradox is what this book aims to explain.

- Research into the determinants of health inequalities as measured at the individual level has produced many important insights, but this book takes a macro-view by comparing health inequalities between countries and over time.

- This macroscopic view also makes it easier to put health inequalities into the broader perspectives of social inequality *per se*, crisis and reform of the welfare state, and the requirements of social justice.

- Chapter 1 ends with a preview of the main conclusions of this book, which are based on a more-critical-than-usual assessment of the available evidence, and therefore challenge some of the received wisdoms in this area.

Chapter 2

Patterns of health inequalities

2.1 Measurement issues

Three steps

Studying health inequalities without quantifying them is impossible—how can we otherwise know that poor people have more illness within their shorter lives? Quantifying the magnitude of health inequalities goes in three steps: (i) determining people's socioeconomic position and creating groups of people with a similar socioeconomic position, (ii) determining the rate at which health problems in each group occur, and (iii) calculating one or more summary measures for the variation in occurrence of health problems between the groups.[48]

Each of these steps will be introduced briefly in this section. Readers who are already familiar with these measurement issues can go immediately to section 2.2 'Generalized but uneven', but should be aware that the arithmetic of health inequalities can be tricky.

Measuring socioeconomic position

Class, status, position

'Social class', 'socioeconomic status' and 'socioeconomic position' are terms commonly encountered in the literature on health inequalities, and although they are often used interchangeably it may be useful to briefly outline the different traditions from which they originate. All three derive from the idea that societies are 'stratified', in the sense that different social roles or positions in society give different levels of control over resources, such as money, power, or prestige, which then generates 'social inequality'.[49]

The concept of *social class* is mainly used in the Marxist tradition. German philosopher and founder of communism Karl Marx (1818–83) defined positions in society in terms of their relationship to the 'means of production', because in his view this was the main determinant of an individual's control over material resources. Nowadays this perspective implies an emphasis on occupational class as a measure of socioeconomic position, and making distinctions between employers and employees with varying levels of autonomy.[50,51]

The concept of *socioeconomic status* originates with German sociologist Max Weber (1864–1920), who recognized that societies may be stratified along several dimensions (e.g. education, occupation, and income), and that the 'status' or 'prestige' attributed to people in different social roles may be equally important for their 'life chances' as their access to material resources.[50,51] In this book we will use the term *socioeconomic position* as a neutral alternative to social class and socioeconomic status, while retaining the idea that it indicates people's position within a stratified society.

It is important to note that however we label these positions in society, these are inherently relational concepts which cannot be completely reduced to the characteristics of individuals. When we determine a person's socioeconomic position on the basis of his or her individual level of education, occupational class, or income, we may interpret these as different routes that the individual has to gain access to material and non-material resources.[52] However, when doing so we should not forget that the uneven distribution of resources over different social positions is something that happens between individuals, not within them. The unequal distribution of money, power, and prestige is the result of a game or struggle in which there are winners and losers.[50,51,i]

The hotel metaphor

Austrian economist Joseph Schumpeter (1883–1950) has compared the occupational structure of society with a hotel—a hotel that is always occupied, but always by different persons. Schumpeter asks us to imagine a hotel with several floors, of which the lower ones contain small rooms with few amenities, and the higher ones contain much nicer rooms. Even if the guests are allowed to change their rooms every night, at any given moment there will be guests in uncomfortable as well as guests in more comfortable rooms.[53]

There are three similarities between this imaginary hotel and the structure of society, and each of these indicates a key element of social stratification:[49] the floors represent the different positions in society; the different levels of luxury of the rooms represent the resources that different positions in society can access; and the placement of guests on floors represents the recruitment of individuals into different social positions—at first when they are born and then during their lives when they acquire educational credentials, enter the labour market, move up or down the occupational ladder during their careers, retire with a larger or smaller pension allowance, and gradually build up or lose wealth.

However, there is also a large difference between a hotel and society: a hotel is a physical structure, built of durable stone and glass, whereas society does not have such an equally tangible reality, but exists only in the actions and interactions of its members. The 'invisibility' of society may even lead one to think that 'you know, there's no such thing as society. There are individual men and women and there are families', according to British Prime Minister Margaret Thatcher (1925–2013) in an interview in 1987. But as sociological research shows, despite the non-physical nature of society all three elements of social inequality mentioned above do exist, and are to some extent durable over time.

What persists over time, however, is something more subtle than the precise placement rules, or the precise outfit of the rooms, or the exact number of floors and number of rooms per floor in the imaginary hotel, because all of these change gradually over time. What does persist is that there *are* different social positions, that these *do* give access to different levels of resources, and that individuals are *not* distributed at random over social positions, but according to implicit or explicit rules that create inequality of opportunity for achieving the higher social positions.[49]

The defining characteristics of lower and higher social positions which determine smaller or greater access to resources has clearly changed over time. For example, in the industrialized societies of the later nineteenth and early twentieth centuries occupational class became the most important predictor of a person's access to material and immaterial resources, whereas in post-industrial societies with a large service sector a person's level of education has become relatively more important, due to the greater importance of knowledge in the economy.[54]

There is also evidence for the recent emergence of a new wealth 'elite' as well as a new 'precariat', with less easily distinguishable groups in the middle, which are not a simple continuation of the social classes of the past. Although these changes illustrate that the 'floors' in the metaphorical 'hotel' may have been rebuilt, the structure of society is still layered to some extent, as is evident from the systematic differences between these groups in access to a variety of resources.[55]

Level of education

In health inequalities research the most commonly used measures of socioeconomic position are level of education (e.g. classified by highest obtained diploma), occupational class (e.g. classified according to one of the available occupational class schemes) and level of income (e.g. classified by quintile of net household income adjusted for household size). Indicators of wealth are also sometimes used, as are area-level indicators (e.g. prevalence of deprivation in the neighbourhood where people live).[51]

All these measures of socioeconomic position are potentially relevant, but preferences for one or the other differ between countries, and as a result whether data are available for one or the other also differs between countries. Schematically, level of education is the preferred measure on the European continent, and occupational class is the preferred measure in the United Kingdom, with level of income coming second or third (but being relatively more popular in the United States).[46,56]

In many analyses presented in this book, socioeconomic position will be indicated by highest level of completed education. Although this has partly pragmatic reasons, there are also good theoretical reasons to use education. The most important is that, as mentioned above, in post-industrial societies education becomes increasingly important as a 'social stratifier'. When the economy becomes dominated by the service sector, as has happened in most European countries, educational credentials partly replace social origins as the 'entrance ticket' to well-paid jobs and many other social benefits.[54,57] As we will see later in this chapter, nowadays in most European countries inequalities in health by education are also larger than inequalities in health by occupational class.

Formal education more specifically indicates investment in human capital, because it develops skills and abilities of general value, such as communication, problem solving, and complex thinking, and fosters a sense of personal control which encourages and enables a healthy lifestyle.[58] Furthermore, education is the most stable measure of socioeconomic position because it is normally completed early in adulthood, which avoids most problems of 'reverse causation' (i.e. health outcomes at older ages cannot change a person's level of education).[46,56]

When we use level of education in this book, this will be in the form of a three-fold classification: 'low' (no primary or lower secondary education), 'mid' (higher secondary education) and 'high' (tertiary education).[ii] Diplomas as obtained within each national educational system were reclassified into the International Standard Classification of Education, from which this three-fold classification was then easily derived. Analyses will be restricted to ages 35–79 years because higher levels of education become increasingly uncommon in older age-groups.

Occupational class

A second indicator that we will use, whenever it is available, is occupational class. As indicated above, there are good theoretical reasons to use occupational class, and in contrast to education it will also more directly reflect the influence of work-related factors such as work stress, control and autonomy at work, and occupational hazards. While education is attained at younger ages and remains more or less fixed in adult life, occupational class can change throughout the life course, which may be seen as a disadvantage as well as an advantage for the analysis of health inequalities.[46,56]

Although there are good theoretical reasons for using occupational class, data on morbidity and mortality by occupational class are only available for a limited number of European countries. Also, international comparability of measures of occupational class is more difficult to achieve than that of measures of educational achievement. One important problem is that a complete classification by occupational class of all those without current paid work is often not available in national data sources. Think of pensioners, for whom one would have to retrieve their last or main occupation before retirement, and think of women with no or part-time jobs, for whom one may have to use the occupation of their husbands.

When we use occupational class in this book, this will be in the form of a five-fold classification: upper non-manual workers (professionals, managers), lower non-manual workers (clerical, service, sales workers), manual workers, farmers, and self-employed. Depending on data availability some of these groups will sometimes be combined. Detailed occupations are usually registered according to the International Standard Classification of Occupations, which we collapsed into this five-fold classification using the Erikson-Goldthorpe-Portocarero scheme.[59]

Level of income

A third indicator that we will sometimes use is level of income. Income is often available as a measure of socioeconomic position in health interview and level of living surveys, and there are therefore abundant European data on self-reported morbidity by income level. However, inequalities in mortality (or other objective health outcomes) by income are available for a few countries only, such as the Nordic countries[60–62] and the Netherlands, as could be seen in Figure 1.1.

Apart from limitations in terms of data availability, the measurement of income also presents more technical difficulties than the measurement of educational level or occupational class. We may be interested in gross income (e.g. because we are interested in a person's control over economic resources in general) or in net income (because we are interested in the availability of financial means to live a healthy life). In the latter case taxes and transfers have to be taken into account, and we may then also want to measure household instead of individual income.[46,56] All these aspects represent measurement challenges, particularly in an international-comparative context.

'Intersectionality'

Differences in access to resources within society are not only determined by people's socioeconomic position (as indicated by their level of education, occupational class, income, and other strictly 'socioeconomic' measures), but also by other social factors, such as age, gender, sexual orientation, migrant status, ethnicity, race, urban vs. rural residence, etc. Some scholars have therefore challenged the idea that there is only one social hierarchy, and have argued that people's access to resources is determined by how they are located within 'intersecting systems of power', that is, by how different social factors combine.[63] 'Intersectionality' has been proposed as a promising alternative to one-dimensional approaches to social inequality.[64]

Although this approach needs further development before it can be applied on a larger scale, it is important to be aware of the interactions between socioeconomic position and other social factors. We illustrate this for migrant status in Box 2.1.

Measuring health in different socioeconomic groups

Leaving aside the important question of how health should be measured, we will take the simplistic but common view that health can be equated with the absence of health problems in the form of disease, disability, or an untimely death. We restrict ourselves here to describing the health measures that are available for the international-comparative work to be presented in this book. Although many more health measures have been used in studies within single countries, we have used two types of measures for which comparable data are available in many countries: mortality and self-reported health problems.

Mortality

Data on inequalities in mortality come from data sources with a population-wide coverage in which mortality could be related to indicators of socioeconomic position as reported in a census.

Box 2.1 Migrants and socioeconomic inequalities in health

Due to immigration European countries are increasingly diverse in their composition by country of origin. For example, in 2010 Switzerland (23%), Ireland (20%), Austria (16%), and Spain (14%) had a relatively high percentage of international migrants in their national populations. Because first generation migrants usually have a low level of education and work in less well-paid jobs, and because they were born in countries with worse average health, it is often thought that immigration from low income countries aggravates health inequalities in the countries of destination. However, this is a mistake.[65]

The effect of immigration on the health inequalities that we observe, for example in the data in this book, first of all depends on whether or not migrants are included in the data. For mortality, in most countries migrants are included, but they are not fully included in Switzerland where non-nationals are excluded from the data. This implies that in most countries it is a relevant question whether or not the presence of large numbers of migrants affects the magnitude of health inequalities. (For Switzerland there may be an issue of non-representativeness of the mortality data for the whole Swiss population.) In the surveys used in this book, migrants are formally included, but may be under-represented due to non-response.

What the effect of migrants and their health is on the magnitude of health inequalities, depends on how migrants are distributed over socioeconomic groups, and what their relative health (dis)advantage is as compared to natives in the same socioeconomic group. Many European studies have shown that migrants often have different average morbidity and mortality rates as compared to natives in their country of destination, also after controlling for socioeconomic position. However, migrants from some low income countries have higher morbidity or mortality rates, and migrants from other low income countries have lower rates than natives in their country of destination.[66–68]

Some recent 'double comparative' work, that is, studies which have simultaneously examined immigrants from multiple countries of origin in multiple countries of destination, have shown that the situation is actually even more complex: migrants from the same country of origin often have worse health than the native population in one European country, and better health than the native population in another European country. For example, women from North Africa had higher mortality than the native population in Spain, and England and Wales, similar mortality in Denmark, and lower mortality in the Netherlands and France. It is unknown what the background is to these differences.[69,70]

More relevant than migrants' average morbidity and mortality rates is how their health relates to natives in the same socioeconomic groups in their country of destination, which is a function of both the average morbidity and mortality rates and the magnitude of socioeconomic inequalities in health among migrants. If health inequalities among migrants are larger than those among the native population, the presence of large numbers of migrants will tend to aggravate health inequalities in the population as a whole. However, some European studies have found smaller socioeconomic inequalities in morbidity or mortality among migrants,[71,72] whereas some other studies have found inequalities of a similar magnitude as in the native population.[73]

These perplexing patterns—which may in part be due to various unsolved data problems—imply that it is impossible to make general statements about the effect of migrants and their health on the magnitude of health inequalities.

For the analyses reported in this book, we selected all European countries for which population-wide data on socioeconomic inequalities in mortality were available for the period ca. 1980 to ca. 2010.

While mortality—and its derivate, life expectancy—is an obviously important health indicator, it captures only part of the health spectrum. As we will see in section 2.2 'Generalized but uneven', by studying specific causes of death we catch a glimpse of whether and how socioeconomic position is associated with a large number of specific diseases, but non-fatal diseases such as mental disorders and musculo-skeletal diseases will remain hidden from view. It is also important to keep in mind that inequalities in mortality may arise from either inequalities in incidence of disease, or inequalities in case fatality, or both.

Measuring health inequalities requires that we have socioeconomic and health information for the same individuals. In surveys (see below) this is straightforward, because one and the same respondent reports on his or her socioeconomic position and health status. For mortality data this is somewhat less straightforward. Most data that we use stem from a longitudinal mortality follow-up after a census, in which socioeconomic information of the population-at-risk and of the deceased has been recorded in the census. However, some Central-Eastern and Eastern European countries only have so-called cross-sectional data in which socioeconomic information on the deceased comes from the death certificate, and that for the population-at-risk from the census.[iii]

Self-reported morbidity

The other main source of information is health and level of living surveys.[iv] Many of these surveys contain questions on disability (e.g. in the form of the Global Activity Limitations Indicator: 'For at least the past six months, to what extent have you been limited in activities people usually do?', 'Yes, a lot', 'Yes, a little', 'No') and self-assessed health (a simple question like 'How is your health in general', with answers ranging from 'Bad' to 'Very good').

The Global Activity Limitations Indicator focuses on a specific consequence of health problems, which should reduce the scope for subjectivity. In evaluation studies against other health measures it has been shown to correlate well with other measures of disability, such as activities of daily living, instrumental activities of daily living, and functional limitations. However, because the strength of these associations differs between countries it is likely that there are cross-country differences in the perception of functioning and limitations, or in the understanding of the question in the survey.[75]

The abundant availability, and convenience of use, of data on self-assessed health, in combination with individual-level measures of socioeconomic position in the same data source, makes them attractive for measuring and comparing health inequalities. However, it is likely that both between-country and within-country inequalities in self-assessed health are distorted by differences in reporting styles. This has been documented fairly extensively, both on the basis of comparisons between self-reports and objective measurements,[76,77] and in studies using 'anchoring vignettes', that is, standard descriptions of fixed health states that respondents are asked to rate.[78-80]

The general picture is that within Europe, some countries have a tendency to report more optimistically about their health than others, and *vice versa*. Equally importantly, highly educated respondents tend to respond more negatively than lower educated respondents, and as a consequence inequalities in self-assessed health are likely to underestimate true differences in health status.[78] One therefore has to be very careful in using these data for more than a general impression.

Of course, before we can even start to look at the magnitude of health inequalities we have to take away the effect of age: because of educational expansion and the growth of the professional class over time, younger generations tend to be more highly educated and to have a higher occupational class than older generations. Because younger people also have lower morbidity and mortality, morbidity and mortality rates have to be age-standardized.[v]

Measuring variation in health between socioeconomic groups

The 'magnitude' of socioeconomic inequalities in health can be measured in different ways, ranging from simple measures like Rate Ratios and Rate Differences to more complex measures like the Relative Index of Inequality and the Slope Index of Inequality.[48,82–87] We list some of the commonly used measures in Table 2.1 and explain their main differences in Box 2.2, which classifies health inequality measures along four dimensions: 'relative' versus 'absolute', 'effect' versus 'impact', 'based on hierarchical ordering' versus 'not based on hierarchical ordering', and 'gap' versus 'gradient'.[vi]

Table 2.1 Measures of the magnitude of health inequalities

Measure	Relative or absolute?	'Effect' or 'impact'?	Hierarchical ordering required?	'Gap' or 'gradient'?
Rate Ratio	Relative inequalities	Effect of being in a lower position	Yes, compare low to high	Gap between low and high
Rate Difference	Absolute inequalities	Effect of being in a lower position	Yes, compare low to high	Gap between low and high
Population-attributable risk (%)	Relative inequalities	Impact on population health	Yes, non-exposed (=high) needs to be identified	All groups with reference to non-exposed (=high)
Population-attributable risk (abs)	Absolute inequalities	Impact on population health	Yes, non-exposed (=high) needs to be identified	All groups with reference to non-exposed (=high)
Average Inter-group Difference (%)	Relative inequalities	Impact on population health	No	All groups with reference to each other
Average Inter-group Difference (abs)	Absolute inequalities	Impact on population health	No	All groups with reference to each other
Relative Index of Inequality	Relative inequalities	Effect of being in a lower position	Yes, stepwise from low to high	Linear gradient throughout population
Slope Index of Inequality	Absolute inequalities	Effect of being in a lower position	Yes, stepwise from low to high	Linear gradient throughout population
Concentration Index (rel)	Relative inequalities	Effect of being in a lower position	Yes, stepwise from low to high	All groups with reference to best off
Concentration Index (abs)	Absolute inequalities	Effect of being in a lower position	Yes, stepwise from low to high	All groups with reference to best off

Box 2.2 Explanation of measures of the magnitude of health inequalities

As shown in Table 2.1, there is a bewildering array of measures of the magnitude of health inequalities, which differ conceptually as well as technically. The four differences highlighted in the table are:

1. 'Relative' versus 'absolute'.

The most basic, and probably most important, distinction is that between relative and absolute measures of health inequalities. One can express differences in the frequency of health problems between socioeconomic groups in relative terms, for example, as the ratio of the morbidity or mortality rates of the lowest as compared to the highest group (Rate Ratio (RR)). One can also express these differences in absolute terms, for example, as the difference between the morbidity or mortality rates of the highest and lowest group (Rate Difference (RD)). For example, suppose that the mortality rate among the low educated is 1000 deaths per 100,000, and that among the high educated is 500 deaths per 100,000. In this case, the Rate Ratio would be 1000/500 = 2.0, indicating that the mortality rate among the low educated is twice as high as that among the high educated, whereas the Rate Difference would be 1000 – 500 = 500, indicating that the mortality rate among the low educated is 500 per 100,000 higher than that among the high educated. Relative differences are usually more readily understood, but suppose that the mortality rates have declined to 100 per 100,000 and 50 per 100,000 among the low and high educated, respectively. In the new situation the Rate Ratio would still be 2.0, but the Rate Difference would be 50 per 100,000, indicating that absolute inequalities have become much smaller and implying that health inequalities have become a less important problem. The scientific literature is undecided about whether one should give preference to relative or to absolute measures, and includes both mathematical[xi] and more policy-oriented arguments in favour of one or the other.[90,91] In this book we will therefore systematically use both. Fortunately, all measures mentioned in Table 2.1 have a relative and an absolute version.

2. 'Effect' versus 'impact'

The main difference between measures of 'effect' and measures of 'population impact' is that the latter take into account not only the health effect of being in a lower socioeconomic position, but also the magnitude of the groups with a lower socioeconomic position. The larger the groups with a disadvantaged socioeconomic position, the higher a measure of total impact will be. One such measure, commonly used in epidemiology, is the Population-Attributable Risk (PAR). Its interpretation is intuitive and useful: the relative version of the PAR gives us the proportion of all health problems in the population which is attributable to the presence of people with a lower-than-high socioeconomic position in the population. Measures of 'effect' and measures of 'impact' answer different questions. Explanatory studies most often use measures of 'effect', but as what ultimately matters for population health is how many people are affected by health inequalities, policy reports may decide for a more comprehensive measure of 'impact'.[48,84]

Box 2.2 **Explanation of measures of the magnitude of health inequalities** (*continued*)

3. 'Based on hierarchical ordering' versus 'not based on hierarchical ordering'

Most of the measures mentioned in the table require socioeconomic groups to be hierarchically ordered from low to high. This may be problematic, especially when we use occupational class as the indicator of socioeconomic position, because some occupational classes (e.g. the self-employed) cannot unambiguously be placed above or below other groups.[92] The Average Inter-group Difference (AIG) is an alternative for other summary measures when no hierarchical ordering is possible.[xii] Regression-based measures also have to make assumptions about the form of the relationship between socioeconomic position and health outcomes—usually, the assumption is one of linearity, which is not always unrealistic.

4. 'Gap' versus 'gradient'

Some measures of health inequalities simply look at the difference between two extreme groups (and thus measure the 'gap') while others take into account all socioeconomic groups (and thus measure the whole 'gradient', if there is an association between socioeconomic groups all along the distribution). The latter are of course more informative, and whereas 'gap' measures will more easily suggest remedial policies targeted at the worst off, 'gradient' measures will naturally suggest remedial policies with a more universal character.[93] Nevertheless, because 'gradient' measures are technically more complex, and usually also are based on more demanding assumptions, the simpler 'gap' measures are still often encountered, and because of their ease of understanding will also be used frequently in this book.

A special case among the 'gradient' measures are the Relative Index of Inequality (RII) and the Slope Index of Inequality (SII). These measures have become quite popular in social epidemiology, partly because they use a clever way of creating an interval scale for socioeconomic position which can then be used to perform regression analyses.[12,48] These measures take into account the fact that the size of socioeconomic groups may change over time, or differ between countries, in ways that suggest that the relative social position of groups has also changed. The idea is that a smaller size of the lower or higher socioeconomic groups implies a more 'extreme' social position, which could in itself lead to a wider gap in mortality.[48] The RII and SII can be interpreted as the rate ratio and rate difference respectively, comparing those with the very lowest to those with the very highest socioeconomic position in the population.[xiii]

The Concentration Index (CI) is a measure for the magnitude of health inequalities that is often used by health economists. It takes into account all socioeconomic groups, which need to be ordered hierarchically and whose relative position in society is derived from their size—just as in the calculation of the RII and SII. Its values can range between −1 and + 1, with negative values indicating 'pro-rich inequality', that is, better health among those with a higher socioeconomic position.[xiv] Whereas the standard version of the CI has a relative interpretation, it is also possible to construct a version with an absolute interpretation.[82,84] It has been shown that the RII and SII are conceptually similar to, although numerically different from, the Concentration Index.[84]

An explanation of the calculation methods for each of these measures can be found in several papers and reports.[48,84,87]

The gradient

Several of these measures are illustrated in Figure 2.1. We will often come back to the intriguing patterns that can be seen in this figure, because they were one of the reasons for writing this book. Let's start with the top panel, which shows recent mortality rates by education among men and women in a range of European countries, from Finland and other Nordic countries on the left hand side, to Eastern European countries on the right, with Western, continental, Southern, and Central-Eastern countries in between. In order to facilitate a quick recognition of variations between geographical regions we will use the same ordering of countries throughout this book.

We show two results each for both Spain and Italy, one for an urban region (Barcelona and Turin, respectively) and one for the whole country. The reason for this is that national data have become available only recently, and that data for Barcelona and Turin have already been collected for several decades, so that the latter have to be used for analyses of time trends and determinants of inequalities in mortality. Fortunately, Figure 2.1 shows that inequalities in mortality in Barcelona and Turin are similar to those in Spain and Italy as a whole.[97,98]

Panels a and e of Figure 2.1 show that in all countries mortality is greater among the low than among the mid, and also greater among the mid than among the high educated. In other words, there is a socioeconomic 'gradient' of mortality in all countries. This gradient is not only seen in a three-group comparison as in Figure 2.1, but also and even more clearly when more fine-grained distinctions are made. The gradient even exists within the group of university educated, among whom those with a PhD degree have lower mortality rates than those without.[99]

The existence of this graded relationship has often been used to argue that social inequality affects the health of nearly everybody, not only the worst-off. This has been seen to imply that explanations should be sought in factors operating across society and not only among the worst-off,[100,101] and that policies to reduce health inequalities should do more than close the gap between the worst- and best-off.[93] Although this is true, the specific 'factors operating across society' that could explain a gradient are many, and range from genetics and cognitive ability[102] to income and the 'psychological pain of low[er] social status'.[103]

Patterns of relative and absolute inequalities in mortality by education

Whatever the explanation, the size of the gap in mortality between lower and higher educational groups varies importantly. In absolute terms the gap between low and high is widest in Central-Eastern and Eastern Europe, and smallest in Southern Europe. Northern Europe does not stand out as having a smaller gap than most other countries, although the gap is somewhat smaller in Sweden than elsewhere.

These impressions are confirmed by panels B and F of Figure 2.1 which show two summary measures for *absolute* inequalities in mortality: the simple Rate Difference and the somewhat more complex Slope Index of Inequality. Both represent the difference in mortality rates between low and high, but they differ importantly in how this difference is calculated (see Box 2.2). The Slope Index of Inequality has higher values than the Rate Difference, because it quantifies the difference between the lowest and highest individual in society—not the difference between the lowest and the highest group.

Although the geographical patterns are similar between the two measures, the difference between the Rate Difference and the Slope Index of Inequality is larger in countries like Hungary and Poland, because the low educated groups in these countries combine a large size (and thus a less extreme social position, and a steeper regression line) with a high mortality rate.

Panels C and G of Figure 2.1 show two summary measures for *relative* inequalities in mortality: the simple Rate Ratio and the more complex Relative Index of Inequality. Both represent the ratio of the mortality rates between low and high. Among men, the Rate Ratio hovers around 2, indicating twice as high mortality among the low than among the high educated. The Relative Index of Inequality is higher than the Rate Ratio for the same reason as why the Slope Index of Inequality is higher than the Rate Difference. Although Central-Eastern and Eastern Europe again have larger inequalities than most other European countries on these measures, the contrast is somewhat less than for measures of absolute inequalities, because the latter are also influenced by the higher average mortality rates in these countries.

Absolute and relative inequalities are both important. Focusing on relative inequalities makes sense from a strictly egalitarian position, in which what matters is equality in itself, independent of other considerations such as the absolute rates of disease or death for each group. Focusing on absolute inequalities, on the other hand, makes sense if we take the view that absolute rates of disease or death matter most for people in lower socioeconomic groups, and that a smaller absolute excess of disease or death is to be preferred even if it goes together with a larger relative excess. For example, although relative inequalities in mortality (as indicated by the RII) among men in England and Wales are larger than in many other European countries, smaller absolute inequalities (as indicated by the SII) suggest a less alarming situation.

Finally, panels D and H of Figure 2.1 show two simple measures of *population impact*, the absolute and relative versions of the Population Attributable Risk. These represent the part of mortality in the whole population that can be attributed to the higher mortality among those with less-than-high education, or, in other words, the part of mortality in the whole population that would be eliminated if the low and mid educated had the same mortality rate as the high educated. This ranges between 10% among Italian women and more than 50% among Polish men. Again, according to this measure inequalities in mortality are largest in Central-Eastern and Eastern Europe, and smallest in Southern Europe, with other countries in between.

Patterns of inequalities in mortality by occupational class

Comparable data on mortality by occupational class are available for a smaller number of European countries, and for men only (Panel A of Figure 2.2). In all countries, there is a clear gradient of rising mortality from the upper non-manual class, through the lower non-manual class, to the manual class.

Panel B of Figure 2.2 presents two summary measures for inequalities in mortality by occupational class: the Rate Ratio (comparing manual with upper non-manual men) and the Population-Attributable Risk (relative version, using upper non-manual men as reference category). Both indicate that the magnitude of these inequalities is substantial, with Rate Ratios hovering around 2.0 and Population Attributable Fractions hovering around 35%.

The Rate Ratios and Population-Attributable Risks seem to be of a similar magnitude as those seen for education in Figure 2.1, but cannot directly be compared because educational inequalities were calculated for the age-range 35–79 years, whereas occupational class inequalities apply to the age-range 35–64 years only. When we restrict the calculation for education to the same, younger age-range, it becomes clear that educational inequalities in mortality are somewhat larger than occupational class inequalities in mortality, particularly in continental Europe. For example, in England and Wales the Population Attributable Risks for education and occupational class among 35–64 years olds are 33% and 31%, respectively, whereas in Switzerland they are 36% and 26%.[vii]

2.2 **Generalized, but uneven**

One of the most striking aspects of health inequalities is that they occur in a highly generalized way: in all age-groups and both genders, and across a wide range of diseases and other health

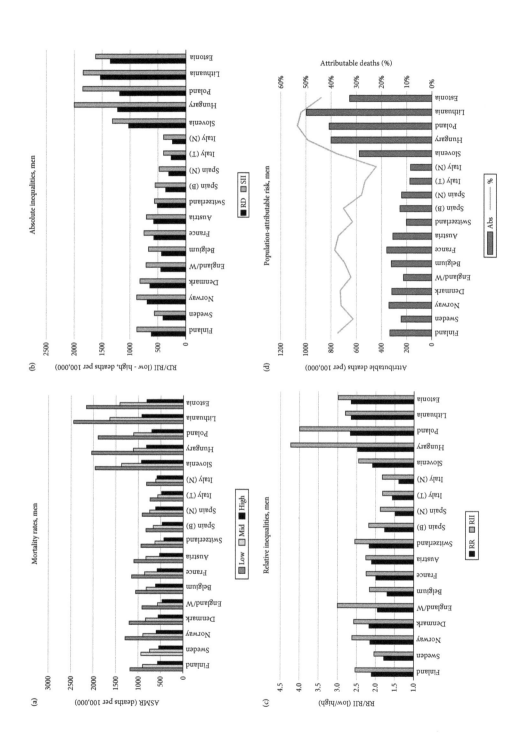

(a) Mortality rates, men

ASMR (deaths per 100,000)

Legend: Low, Mid, High

Countries (top to bottom): Estonia, Lithuania, Poland, Hungary, Slovenia, Italy (N), Italy (T), Spain (N), Spain (B), Switzerland, Austria, France, Belgium, England/W, Denmark, Norway, Sweden, Finland

(b) Absolute inequalities, men

RD/RII (low - high, deaths per 100,000)

Legend: RD, SII

(c) Relative inequalities, men

RR/RII (low/high)

Legend: RR, RII

(d) Population-attributable risk, men

Attributable deaths (%)

Attributable deaths (per 100,000)

Legend: Abs, %

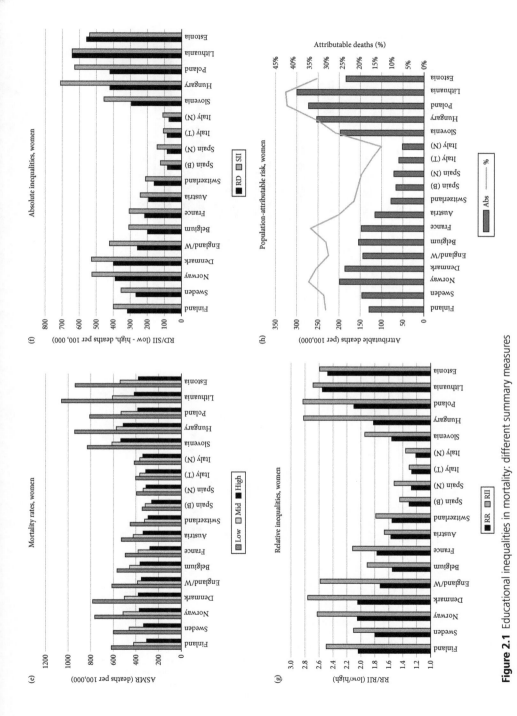

Figure 2.1 Educational inequalities in mortality: different summary measures

Notes: ASMR = Age-Standardized Mortality Rate. RR = Rate Ratio, RII = Relative Index of Inequality, RD = Rate Difference, SII = Slope Index of Inequality. Spain (B) = Barcelona, Spain (N) = Spain as a whole, Italy (T) = Turin, Italy (N) = Italy as a whole. Most recent period available for each country (central year = ca. 2010). For explanation of inequality measures, see Box 2.2.

Source: dataset constructed in DEMETRIQ/LIFEPATH projects, with harmonized data from national/regional mortality registers.

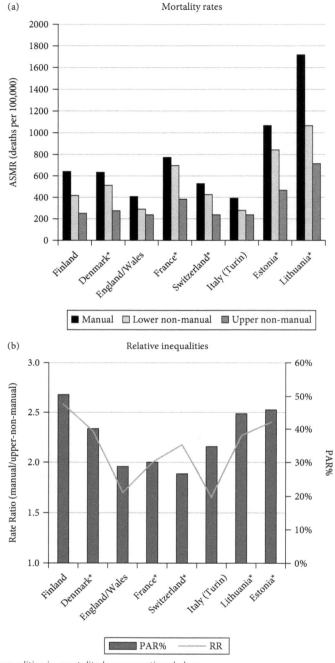

Figure 2.2 Inequalities in mortality by occupational class

Notes: ASMR = Age-Standardized Mortality Rate. PAR = Population-Attributable Risk. RR = Rate Ratio. Men aged 35–64 years. Most recent period available for each country (central year = ca. 2010). Data on mortality among farmers not available for England and Wales, and data on self-employed not available for Estonia. Inactive men classified by last occupational class, except in countries marked by * where occupational class of inactive men was unknown, and data have been adjusted for proportion of inactive by occupational class.[104,105]

Source: dataset constructed in DEMETRIQ/LIFEPATH projects, with harmonized data from national/regional mortality registers.

problems. However, the magnitude of health inequalities does vary by age and gender, and be-tween different diseases and health problems, and these variations sometimes hold important clues to explanation.

Variations by age and gender

Children

Health inequalities are found in all age-groups, from the very young to the very old. Actually, health inequalities even start before birth as is evident from inequalities in rates of still-birth, low birth weight and perinatal mortality by socioeconomic position of the mother—even in the Nordic countries and other advanced welfare states.[106]

After birth, children with parents who are low educated, have a low occupational class or live on a low income, have higher rates of health problems and developmental disorders, as is clear from several reviews of European studies of inequalities in child health and development.[107,108] These inequalities do not only express themselves in higher rates of various illnesses, but also in higher rates of infant and child mortality—again, even in advanced welfare states.[109–111]

For adolescents the picture is more mixed. Some studies have suggested that in adolescence, the period between childhood and adulthood, there is a narrowing of health inequalities, per-haps as a result of the transition between socioeconomic position of family of origin and own socioeconomic position. However, family affluence does correlate strongly with a range of health outcomes and health behaviours among adolescents throughout Europe.[112,113]

Height is often used as a summary measure of the effect of children's living conditions on their overall health and development. Although height partly depends on children's genetically de-termined growth potential, it also depends on the restrictions imposed by the environment, for example, in terms of nutrition, the occurrence of disease, psychosocial stress, and housing condi-tions. Inequalities in height, with people in higher socioeconomic groups being taller than people in lower socioeconomic groups, are not only found among current adults and elderly people who grew up in the sometimes distant past,[114,115] but also among children growing up now.[116,117]

Adults and elderly

Beyond adolescence, inequalities in health continue or—if they have temporarily faded out—re-emerge. Despite the secular decline in mortality and the concomitant rise in life expectancy, data on inequalities in mortality remain one of the most striking illustrations of health inequalities. Mortality rates increase exponentially with age—with various demographic 'laws of mortality' predicting that adults' risk of dying roughly doubles with every eight years that they age.[118]

However, this rise of mortality with advancing age differs between socioeconomic groups, and as a result the magnitude of inequalities in mortality changes with age as well (Figure 2.3). Relative inequalities in mortality are largest among young adults and strongly decline with age, to reach their lowest values among the elderly, whereas absolute inequalities in mortality follow a reverse pattern, and are smallest among young adults and rise with age. These age-patterns extend into even higher ages than shown in Figure 2.3, with average Rate Ratios going down to around 1.10 among nonagenarians.[119]

What lies behind these striking age-patterns? In mathematical terms, the paradox of increasing absolute and declining relative inequalities is not difficult to resolve: due to the fact that average mortality rates rise strongly with age, smaller relative inequalities at higher ages can easily go together with wider absolute inequalities. But why do absolute inequalities in mortality increase with age? This has been interpreted as evidence that people in lower socioeconomic classes age more rapidly than do those in higher classes, due to the unhealthy environments to which they

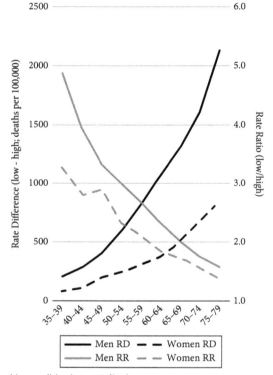

Figure 2.3 Educational inequalities in mortality by age

Notes: RD = Rate Difference. RR = Rate Ratio. Pooled data of 16 European countries. Most recent period available for each country (central year = ca. 2010).

Source: dataset constructed in DEMETRIQ/LIFEPATH projects, with harmonized data from national/regional mortality registers.

are exposed.[120,121] Low educated men have a mortality rate at the age of 55–59 years that is equal to that of high educated men at the age of 65–69 years, which in this reasoning would imply a ten-year difference in 'biological age'.[viii]

Increasing absolute inequalities in mortality suggest that with advancing age people in lower socioeconomic groups accumulate more insults to their bodies, and/or experience more decline of their bodies' capacity for repair, than people in higher socioeconomic groups. Further ideas about the biological mechanisms involved will be discussed in Chapter 3.

Figure 2.3 also shows that there is more 'premature mortality', that is, mortality below the age of 65, among the low than among the high educated.[122] Analyses of the distribution of deaths by age have shown that lower socioeconomic groups do not only have higher mortality in all age-groups, but also have larger variation in their age at death (or 'lifespan variation') than higher socioeconomic groups.[ix]

Men and women

Health inequalities differ between men and women. *Relative* inequalities in all-cause mortality are somewhat smaller among women than among men, but because average mortality rates are also lower among women than among men, *absolute* inequalities in mortality are much smaller among women than among men (Figure 2.3).

This is true in nearly all countries, but the differences between men and women in the magnitude of relative inequalities are very small in Northern Europe, as a result of a stronger increase of inequalities in mortality among women over the past decades in Northern Europe than in other parts of the subcontinent (see section 2.3, 'Persistent, but dynamic'). Surprisingly, women in Northern European countries (with the exception of Sweden) now have larger inequalities in mortality than women in most other European regions (Figure 2.1).

When we look behind these smaller inequalities in mortality among women to see where they come from in terms of specific diseases, we find that they are due to two distinct phenomena: women have smaller inequalities in mortality than men from most causes of death, and causes of death for which inequalities are small among both men and women happen to be more important among women.[123] Relative inequalities in mortality are smaller among women for most causes of death, and mortality from cancer, for which inequalities are smaller than for other causes of death among both men and women, makes up a larger share of total mortality among women than among men.

These differences between men and women must reflect differences between men and women in the social patterning of risk factors for mortality, but at a more general level they signal the greater vulnerability of men to the mortality risks associated with social disadvantage. Larger inequalities in mortality among men have also been found for other social determinants, for example marital status: excess mortality among divorced and widowed men is much higher than excess mortality among divorced and widowed women.[124]

Possible explanations are that the health behaviour of married men is to some extent controlled by their wives, more so than women's health behaviour being controlled by their husbands, and that men, more than women, respond to social problems with mortality-increasing behaviours such as excessive alcohol consumption.[125] It should not surprise us, then, that socioeconomic inequalities in mortality are larger among divorced than among married men.[126]

However, this greater vulnerability of men to various forms of social disadvantage does not universally apply to all health problems. It is widely known that 'women get sicker but men die quicker', that is, that although women outlive men by several years, their rates of ill-health are higher for many non-fatal conditions.[127,128] Socioeconomic inequalities in these non-fatal conditions are *not* larger among men than among women. Taking all European countries together, relative inequalities in self-assessed health and activity limitations are about equal in magnitude for men and women, but because average rates of less-than-good health and activity limitations are somewhat higher for women than for men, absolute inequalities tend to be somewhat larger among women.

Variations between health problems

Diseases and causes of death

Socioeconomic inequalities can also be found for many specific diseases. In the large majority of studies, incidence or prevalence of specific diseases has been found to be higher in lower than in higher socioeconomic groups.[129] Possible exceptions, for which 'reverse' gradients have been found with higher socioeconomic groups having a higher incidence or prevalence, include hay fever[130] (where the reverse gradient may be due to less or later exposure to infection of children from higher socioeconomic status parents[131]), anorexia nervosa[132] (where the reverse gradient may be a negative side-effect of the higher frequency of dieting among women in higher socioeconomic groups[133,134]), as well as several cancers.

Cross-country comparability of data on the incidence or prevalence of specific diseases, for example, as collected in health interview or even health examination surveys, is usually not so good, but it is likely to be better for cause-specific mortality. Data on cause-specific mortality therefore allow us to create a comprehensive and Europe-wide picture of inequalities in a wide range of diseases, although at the expense of combining the effect of inequalities in incidence with that of inequalities in case fatality.

Because case fatality is usually higher among people with a lower socioeconomic position, mortality data will tend to overestimate inequalities in the incidence of diseases. Ischemic heart disease patients with a lower socioeconomic position have a greater likelihood of dying than ischemic heart disease patients with a higher socioeconomic position,[135-137] and the same is true for cancer.[138-140] However, incidence remains the main driver of trends and patterns of mortality.

Figure 2.4 shows that, although cause-specific mortality is usually higher among lower educated people, the magnitude of these inequalities is strongly variable between diseases. Diseases have been ordered on the basis of the average Rate Ratio (comparing the low to the high educated) in all countries with available data, from Chronic Obstructive Pulmonary Disease (RR = 4.0, indicating a fourfold excess mortality among low educated men) to melanoma (RR = 0.8, indicating a 20% excess mortality among high educated men).

Some general observations

Several important observations can be made. First, in Europe as a whole 'reverse' inequalities are rare: these are seen only for melanoma among men and for Hodgkin's disease among women. When we look behind these averages to the Rate Ratios by country, we also find higher mortality among the high educated in some European countries for lung cancer (women only) and breast cancer.

These reverse gradients have been attributed to patterns of diffusion of some of the relevant risk behaviours. For melanoma the reverse gradient is probably due to more recreational sunlight exposure in higher socioeconomic groups.[141] For lung cancer among women the reverse gradient that we see in some Southern European countries is due to an earlier uptake of smoking among high educated women.[142] For breast cancer the reverse gradient is due to more delayed childbearing among high educated women.[143] Both for lung and breast cancer there is clear evidence from trend studies that these reverse gradients are a temporary phenomenon, and—in those countries where they can still be found—will turn into 'normal' gradients in the years to come, thereby contributing to a further widening of inequalities in mortality among women.[142,143]

A second observation that we can make on Figure 2.4 is that some of the largest inequalities are seen for causes of death that are eminently avoidable, either by addressing the underlying behavioural risk factors or by applying widely available medical interventions. Among men, the top five consists of COPD (closely linked to smoking[144]), homicide (interpersonal violence[145]), alcohol-related conditions (excessive alcohol consumption[146]), tuberculosis (medical treatment[147]) and suicide (depression and mental health care[148]). Among women, the largest inequalities are found for diabetes, which is linked to another avoidable risk factor, obesity.[149,150]

On the other hand, apart from tuberculosis Figure 2.4 contains many more causes of death that are amenable to medical intervention, but which nevertheless are in the bottom half of the figure, and thus have inequalities that are smaller than those we see for all-cause mortality: leukaemia, Hodgkin's disease, rheumatic heart disease, appendicitis. Although inequalities in mortality from amenable conditions do suggest deficiencies in the delivery or uptake of medical care,[151] these findings also suggest that medical care may have a dampening effect on inequalities in mortality. We will more systematically look at whether greater 'actionability' is indeed associated with larger health inequalities in Chapter 4.

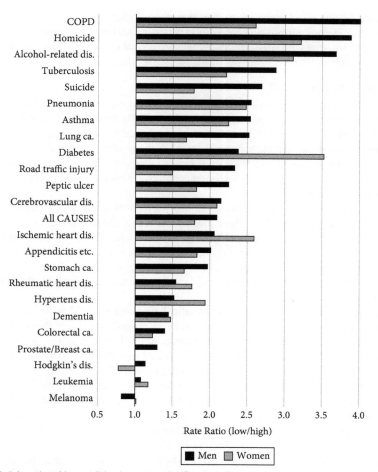

Figure 2.4 Educational inequalities in cause-specific mortality

Notes: COPD = Chronic Obstructive Pulmonary Disease. Ca. = cancer. Most recent period available for each country (central year = ca. 2010). Pooled dataset of 16 European countries.

Source: dataset constructed in DEMETRIQ/LIFEPATH projects, with harmonized data from national/regional mortality registers.

And then a third observation: the striking range of health problems for which inequalities in mortality are found. These range from tuberculosis to dementia, and from ischemic heart disease to injuries—conditions which at first sight seem to have completely different aetiologies.

Inequalities in ischemic heart disease (IHD) mortality have been studied extensively, because of their important role in generating inequalities in all-cause mortality. Since the start of the decline of IHD mortality in the 1970s and 1980s, it has been observed that the timing and magnitude of the decline have been different between socioeconomic groups, with higher socioeconomic groups experiencing an earlier and/or a faster decline than lower socioeconomic groups.[152]

This has been attributed to socioeconomic differences in uptake of heart-healthy behaviours (e.g. stop smoking, physical exercise, less saturated fats) or of health care interventions (e.g.

hypertension detection and treatment, statins, thrombolytic therapy), or both. As a result, people with a lower socioeconomic position currently experience a higher IHD mortality in most industrialized countries—but with large differences between countries, partly depending on the timing of the IHD epidemic. [153-155]

Injuries and mental health

It is not immediately obvious what the common underlying factor is between inequalities in ischemic heart disease mortality and inequalities in mortality from injuries (road traffic injury, suicide, homicide). The latter are among the health conditions for which inequalities in mortality tend to be substantial—at least among men (Figure 2.4). Inequalities in mortality from road traffic injuries are smaller among women than among men, because the higher risks of injury and case fatality among women from lower socioeconomic groups are compensated by their lower participation in motorized traffic.[156]

Rates of suicide are systematically higher among people with a lower socioeconomic position in most European countries.[148,157] These inequalities reflect inequalities in underlying mental health problems, such as depression and anxiety disorders, which have also been found in many studies.[158, 159] The higher prevalence of mental illness in lower socioeconomic groups is likely to have a complex explanation, involving 'social drift' (a greater likelihood of downward social mobility for people with mental health problems) as well as effects of unfavourable living conditions on mental health.

Inequalities in mental health problems are also found among children of parents in lower socioeconomic groups who cannot yet be affected by downward mobility.[160] Exposure to stressful living conditions (in the form of financial insecurity, unemployment, family violence, ...) plays a role, which may lead to chronic arousal of the body's stress response systems and then result in depression, anxiety disorders or other mental health problems.[161]

Because mental health problems are a risk factor for somatic health problems, and increase the risk of mortality from many other causes than suicide,[162] inequalities in mental health may play an independent role in generating the other health inequalities that we discuss in this book.

Perhaps the most remarkable cause of death in this group is homicide for which large inequalities in mortality are found throughout Europe, both among men and women.[145] People in lower socioeconomic groups are not only more likely to be victims of homicide, but also more likely to be perpetrators.[163] Many factors are likely to be involved: more impulsivity, lower problem solving skills, occurrence of alcohol-fuelled disputes, availability of lethal weapons, exposure to organized crime, etc.[145]

The fact that violent crime is more frequent in lower socioeconomic groups should not be taken as evidence that people in lower socioeconomic groups are more prone to unethical behaviour—studies of driving behaviour and laboratory experiments actually suggest the reverse: people in higher socioeconomic groups are more likely to break the law while driving, and to lie and cheat.[164] Larger income inequalities at the national level are associated with higher average homicide rates, suggesting that the erosion of social cohesion in more unequal societies increases the likelihood of violent crime.[165]

(Healthy) life expectancy

As a result of differences in mortality rates, people from lower socioeconomic groups live considerably shorter lives than those with more advantaged social positions. A recent study by the Organization of Economic Cooperation and Development (OECD) found that, across the 23 member countries analysed, life expectancy from age 25 years was 49 years for men with low education, and 57 years for men with high education. The corresponding values for women were 55 and 60 years, suggesting a gap of eight years, on average, among men and of five years among women.[166]

The fact that morbidity rates in the lower socioeconomic groups are higher too, implies that inequalities in 'healthy life expectancy' (the number of years which people can expect to live in good health) are even larger than inequalities in (total) life expectancy.[167,168] This could already be seen for the Netherlands in Figure 1.1.

Inequalities in total and disability-free life expectancy are particularly relevant around the age of retirement. In most European countries, the statutory age of retirement is still about 65 years (sometimes a little lower, sometimes a little higher).[169] In order to reach this retirement age in good health, people should have a disability-free life expectancy of at least 65 years, but there is no European country where this is the case for low educated men. In some Eastern European countries, many low educated men cannot even expect to be alive at the age of 65 years. For high educated people, it is much easier to continue working until pension age, and they can also expect to live longer after retirement, so that they draw greater benefits from their pension premiums than low educated people.[167]

2.3 **Persistent, but dynamic**

Mortality

Health inequalities are at the same time remarkably persistent, and remarkably dynamic. Although health inequalities seem to be a constant nuisance for public health, below the surface the changes are more remarkable than is often appreciated.

All-cause mortality

Studies of trends in inequalities in mortality stretching over three or more decades are rare.[60,170–174]. Long-term trends in mortality by education in a wide range of European countries are shown in Figure 2.5. In these graphs we introduce a way of denoting countries that we will often use in this book: the Nordic countries are denoted by black dotted lines, England and Wales, and Ireland by grey dotted lines, continental European countries by grey continuous lines, Southern European countries by grey dashed lines, Central-Eastern countries by black dashed lines, and Eastern European countries by black continuous lines.

In most European countries, mortality has steadily declined among both the low and the high educated. Whether the decline was faster among the low than the high educated or *vice versa*, often depends on whether we calculate relative declines (i.e. declines in mortality expressed as a proportion or percentage of the starting level) or absolute declines (i.e. declines in mortality expressed as a difference between the mortality rates at the beginning and end of the study period). Relative declines were usually faster among the high educated, so that relative inequalities as measured by the Rate Ratio or Relative Index of Inequality have generally increased considerably. However, absolute declines were sometimes larger among the low educated, so that absolute inequalities as measured by the Rate Difference or Slope Index of Inequality have often decreased, particularly among men.

However, trends in all-cause mortality in Central-Eastern and Eastern Europe were different. After a dramatic increase of mortality among the low educated in the 1980s and 1990s, and a concomitant increase in mortality inequalities, particularly in Hungary, Lithuania, and Estonia, a trend reversal has occurred. Mortality has started to decline among the low educated, and as a result absolute inequalities in mortality have also started to drop.

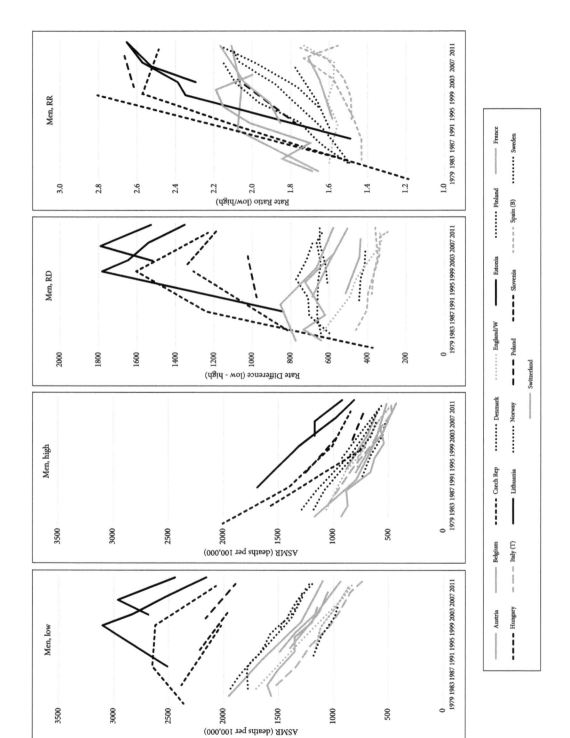

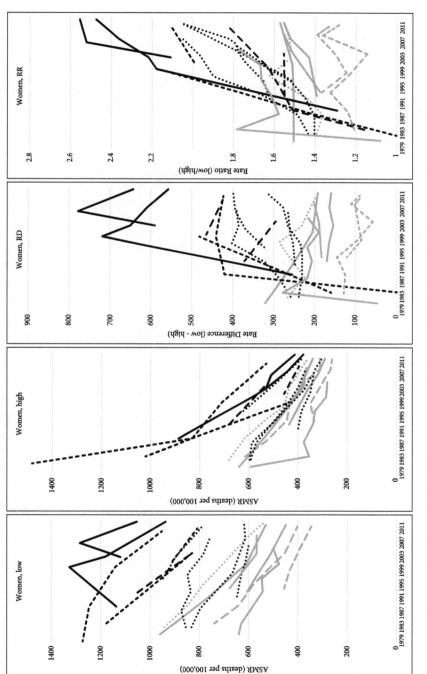

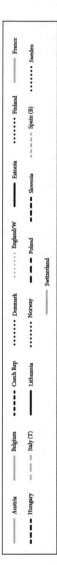

Figure 2.5 Trends in mortality by level of education

A. Men

B. Women

Notes: ASMR = age-standardized mortality rate, RR = Rate Ratio. RD = Rate Difference. Italy (T) = Turin. Spain (B) = Barcelona. Trends in RII/SII largely similar to those in RR/RD.

Source: dataset constructed in DEMETRIQ/LIFEPATH projects, with harmonized data from national/regional mortality registers.

We note in passing that the Great Recession following the 2008 financial crisis has left no visible traces in the mortality trends as illustrated in Figure 2.5—which may well be a testimony to the buffering effects of European welfare states.[175] Trends in mortality by occupational class were similar to those by level of education.[174]

Causes of death

Trends in all-cause mortality and their inequalities are, of course, driven by what happens to mortality from specific causes of death. In Western Europe, mortality has declined for most specific causes of death, and like we saw for all-cause mortality decline has usually been faster in relative terms among the high than among the low educated (Figure 2.6).

Causes of death for which mortality has increased among the high educated are few, and include alcohol-related causes, other heart disease, and dementia among men (Figure 2.6), and other infectious diseases, lung cancer, alcohol-related causes, and dementia among women (not shown in Figure 2.6). In most of these cases trends have been even less favourable among the low educated.

Trends in all-cause mortality and their inequalities are, to an important extent, driven by what happens to mortality from cardiovascular diseases. The role of cardiovascular diseases in generating inequalities in all-cause mortality has changed considerably over time, particularly in the North and West of Europe. For example, among Finnish women the contribution of cardiovascular diseases to inequality in all-cause mortality decreased from 72% in the early 1970s to 36% in the late 2000s. As a result, cancer has now replaced cardiovascular disease as the main contributor to inequalities in mortality in several countries.[174]

Life expectancy

As a result of declines in mortality, life expectancy has increased almost continuously for several decades in Western Europe, and has been increasing since the mid-1990s or early 2000s in Central-Eastern and Eastern Europe as well.[176]. Figure 2.7 shows how the gap in life expectancy between low and high educated has developed in selected European countries. During the 1980s and 1990s a huge gap in life expectancy between low and high educated opened up in Central-Eastern Europe (represented by Hungary) and Eastern Europe (represented by Estonia), particularly among men. It is only recently that this gap has started to narrow again.

In other European countries the gap in life expectancy has been both smaller and more stable, although when we look more carefully we do see some changes. Among men, the gap has widened in Norway[177] (as it has in Finland[178] and Denmark[179]), to reach values about twice the size of the gap in England and Wales and Italy where the gap has either been stable or has narrowed. Among women, the gap is considerably smaller than among men, but the trends are similar.[x]

Other health outcomes

The trends that we see for mortality cannot be generalized to other domains of health. One other health outcome for which trend data on inequalities is available is self-assessed health (SAH). A study covering 10 European countries between the 1980s and 1990s already showed that it is difficult to discern trends in these inequalities,[180] and that is still the case.

Figure 2.8 shows trends in the prevalence of less-than-good self-assessed health by occupational class in selected European countries. Over the past three decades, the prevalence went up in some countries, and down in others, but where it went down, like in Central-Eastern and Eastern Europe, the declines were stronger in higher socioeconomic groups, which led to an increase in relative inequalities. Whereas reductions of absolute inequalities were common for mortality, they are uncommon for less-than-good self-assessed health.[181]

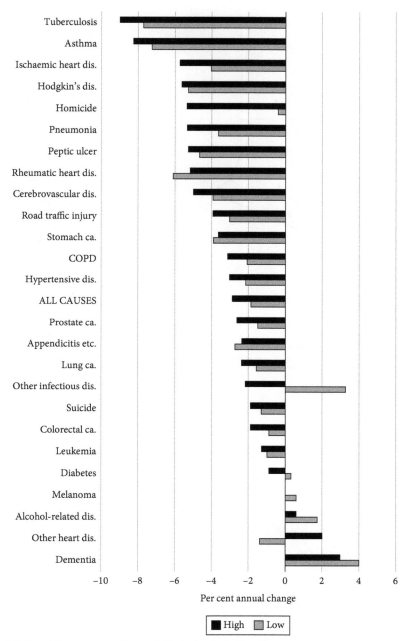

Figure 2.6 Trends in cause-specific mortality by level of education

Notes: COPD = Chronic Obstructive Pulmonary Disease. Ca. = cancer. Pooled dataset of 12 Western European countries, ca. 1980–ca. 2014.

Source: dataset constructed in DEMETRIQ/LIFEPATH projects, with harmonized data from national/regional mortality registers.

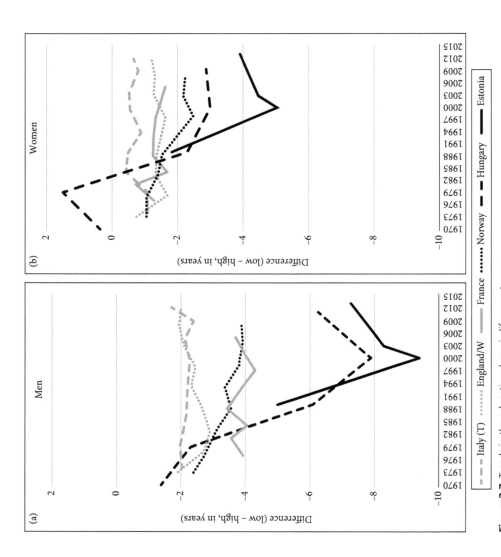

Figure 2.7 Trends in the educational gap in life expectancy

Notes: Graph shows absolute difference between low and high educated in partial life expectancies between ages 35 and 80 years.

Source: dataset constructed in DEMETRIQ/LIFEPATH projects, with harmonized data from national/regional mortality registers.

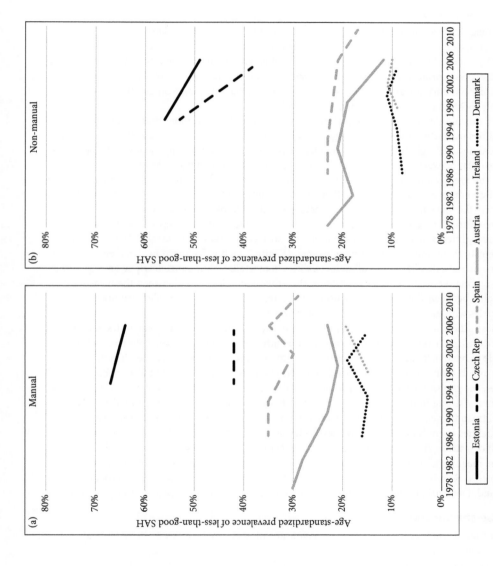

Figure 2.8 Trends in self-assessed health by occupational class

Notes: SAH = Self-Assessed Health. Men 35–64 years.

Source: dataset constructed in DEMETRIQ/LIFEPATH projects, with harmonized data from National Health Interview Surveys.

2.4 **Ubiquitous, but variable**

Mortality

Although health inequalities are present in all countries that collect the data, a closer look at their magnitude reveals that countries are actually quite different in their patterns of health inequalities.

All-cause mortality

The magnitude of inequalities in all-cause mortality varies substantially between European countries, as Figure 2.1 has already shown. Relative inequalities in mortality, as indicated by the Relative Index of Inequality, vary more than threefold among men, from less than 2.0 (indicating 100% excess mortality among the low educated) in Spain and Italy to more than 4.0 (indicating 300% excess mortality among the low educated) in Hungary. Among women, they vary from 1.3 in Italy to 2.8 in Denmark, Hungary, and Poland.

The magnitude of absolute inequalities in mortality varies even more than that of relative inequalities in mortality, because average mortality rates tend to be high in countries where relative inequalities are large. This is not a coincidence: whereas mortality among the high educated is rather similar between countries, mortality among the low educated varies substantially, and drives both the average mortality rate and the magnitude of relative inequalities in mortality. It is as if the high educated manage to keep their mortality levels low, regardless of national conditions, whereas the low educated are more vulnerable to unfavourable national conditions.

These variations manifest themselves in clear geographical patterns. Regardless of what measure for inequalities is used, inequalities in mortality are clearly largest in Central-Eastern and Eastern Europe, both among men and among women (Figure 2.1). It is Southern Europe, represented by Spain and Italy, that has the smallest inequalities in mortality—but more clearly so among women than among men. The relative position of the other countries varies between the measure used and also between the sexes. As mentioned before, inequalities in mortality are not smaller in countries with more advanced welfare arrangements.

These differences are the result of differences between countries in how inequalities in mortality have developed over time. As could be seen in Figure 2.5, variation between countries in the magnitude of relative inequalities in mortality was small in the 1980s, but since then inequalities have risen much more in some countries than in others. In Spain and Italy, but also in England and Wales, the rise of relative inequalities in mortality has been modest or even absent, while it has been very strong in most countries in Central-Eastern and Eastern Europe, and also in Norway and Finland (men only). In other words, the between-country variations in the magnitude of inequalities in mortality that we witness today are a relatively recent phenomenon, which is the result of a strong divergence between countries starting in the 1980s.[174]

The magnitude of occupational class differences in mortality also varies substantially between countries. Relative and absolute inequalities in all-cause mortality are more pronounced in Finland, Denmark, Lithuania, and Estonia than in other countries, as we have seen in Figure 2.2.

Cause-specific mortality

Countries do not only differ in the magnitude of their inequalities in total mortality, but also in the causes of death contributing to higher mortality in lower socioeconomic groups (Figure 2.9). For example, among men in Finland, Estonia, and Lithuania cardiovascular diseases make a more important contribution than cancer to occupational class inequalities in mortality among men, but in Denmark, France, Switzerland, and Italy cancer is more important.

In Central-Eastern and Eastern Europe inequalities in mortality are larger than elsewhere for most causes of death, particularly among men, whereas in Southern Europe inequalities in

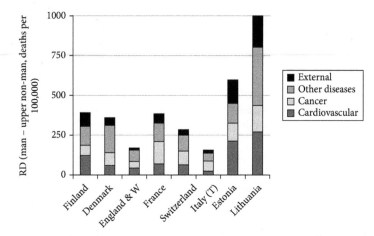

Figure 2.9 Contribution of causes of death to occupational class inequalities in mortality

Notes: RD = Rate Difference. Man = manual occupation. Upper non-man = upper non-manual occupation. Most recent period available for each country (central year: 2010).

Source: dataset constructed in DEMETRIQ/LIFEPATH projects, with harmonized data from national/regional mortality registers.

cause-specific mortality are smaller than elsewhere. Inequalities in cardiovascular mortality are even practically non-existent among women in Italy, and inequalities in cancer mortality are practically non-existent among women in Spain.

There is a clear North-South gradient for ischemic heart disease mortality, with relative and absolute inequalities being larger in Northern Europe and the United Kingdom than in Southern Europe. This international pattern for ischemic heart disease results from differences between countries in how the 'epidemic' of ischemic heart disease has developed over time.[153,154,182]

In many countries, particularly in the North of Europe, mortality from ischemic heart disease increased substantially after the World War II, probably as a result of changes in health-related behaviours, such as smoking, increased intake of saturated fats, and less physical exercise. During the 1970s, however, a decline set in, and is still continuing. During this epidemiological development, important changes occurred in the association between socioeconomic position and ischemic heart disease mortality. In the North of Europe, during the 1950s and 1960s ischemic heart disease mortality was higher in the higher socioeconomic groups, leading to the notion of ischemic heart disease being a 'manager's disease'.[153,154,182]

It was only during the 1970s, coinciding with the start of the decline of ischemic heart disease mortality in the population as a whole, that a reversal occurred, and the current association emerged. This is due to differences between socioeconomic groups in both the timing and the speed of decline of ischemic heart disease mortality. In the South of Europe, however, a similar 'epidemic' of ischemic heart disease mortality has not occurred, and similar inequalities in ischemic heart disease mortality have not arisen, partly as a result of the protection of traditional Mediterranean living habits against ischemic heart disease.[153,154,182]

Self-reported morbidity

Activity limitations and disabilities are also more prevalent among lower socioeconomic groups. This higher frequency applies to many aspects of functioning (e.g. mobility, vision, hearing, grip strength, walking speed) and translates into more problems with activities of daily living (ADL) such as dressing and bathing, and with instrumental activities of daily living (IADL) such as preparing hot meals and making telephone calls.[183] As shown by studies using objective measures of grip strength and walking speed, inequalities in self-reported disability are not only a matter of reporting bias.[184,185]

Figure 2.10 shows inequalities in disability on the basis of the Global Activity Limitation Indicator (GALI). While the prevalence of activity limitations is higher among the low than the high educated in all countries, we do not see a clear geographical pattern in the magnitude of these differences.

For self-assessed health our data cover a very large number of European countries, including countries for which other comparative data are very scarce, such as Serbia and other countries in the Western Balkans, and Belarus, Ukraine, Moldova, and Russia (Figure 2.11). Again, the prevalence of less-than-good self-assessed health is higher among the low than the high educated in (almost) all European countries.

The prevalence of less-than-good self-assessed health is high among both the low and the high educated in many countries in Central-Eastern and Eastern Europe, and as a result prevalence rate ratios are often surprisingly low in these countries. In Belarus, Moldova, and Russia the rate ratios are even lower, sometimes even below 1.00 when the prevalence of less-than-good self-assessed health is actually higher among the high than the low educated.

The prevalence of less-than-good self-assessed health is usually lower in countries in the Northern, Western, Continental, and Southern European regions, and prevalence rate ratios are often as high or higher than those in more Eastern parts of the European subcontinent. Clearly, we find a different geographical pattern for inequalities in less-than-good self-assessed health than for mortality.

There is a strong correlation between the prevalence of less-than-good self-assessed health and measures of overall well-being, particularly the prevalence of low life satisfaction: both are high in Central-Eastern and Eastern Europe among the low and the high educated. It is therefore likely that the high levels of less-than-good self-assessed health in Central-Eastern and Eastern Europe partly reflect the unfavourable psychological conditions in these countries, and are less reliable as indicators of the health conditions prevailing in these countries, although both are of course linked.

2.5 **Health inequalities outside Europe**

The United States and Canada

This book exploits European data to investigate why health inequalities persist despite the welfare state—for good reasons, because the welfare state is a European invention, and European countries have implemented it in different forms. Nevertheless, it is important to put the European data in perspective by comparing them to data from other high-income countries.

In terms of welfare arrangements, most existing classifications include the United States and Canada, as well as Australia and New Zealand, with the 'liberal' type (see section 1.2, 'The great paradox of public health').[18] It is as if there is an 'Anglo-Saxon' preference for low social expenditure levels and targeted social benefits, perhaps because these countries have majoritarian two-party systems, in which there is less opportunity for the middle classes to form political coalitions with the lower classes to create a more generous welfare state.[13]

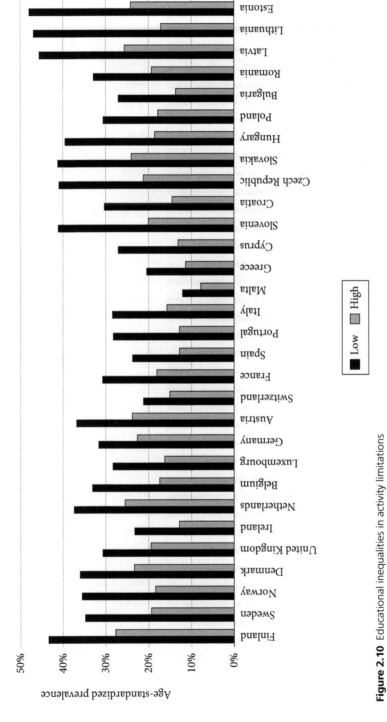

Figure 2.10 Educational inequalities in activity limitations

Note: 'Yes, limited' on GALI (Global Activity Limitations Indicator). Women; patterns similar for men. Average of all waves of 3 surveys, held between 2002 and 2014, adjusted for average of each survey.

Source: dataset constructed in DEMETRIQ/LIFEPATH projects, with harmonized data from European Social Survey, EU Statistics on Income and Living Conditions, and European Health Interview Survey.

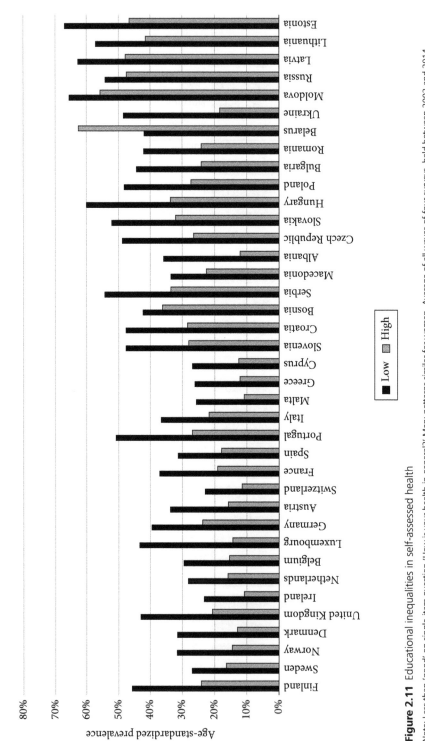

Figure 2.11 Educational inequalities in self-assessed health

Note: Less than 'good' on single-item question 'How is your health in general?' Men; patterns similar for women. Average of all waves of four surveys, held between 2002 and 2014, adjusted for average of each survey.

Source: dataset constructed in DEMETRIQ/LIFEPATH projects, with harmonized data from European Social Survey, EU Statistics on Income and Living Conditions, and European Health Interview Survey.

Although these countries all have restrictive welfare arrangements, they differ importantly in the way health care is financed, and in the existence of financial barriers to health care use. Whereas in the US a large fraction of the population has no health insurance at all—even after the introduction of President Obama's Affordable Care Act—Canada has a system of universal health insurance, and inequalities in access to health care are much less in Canada than in the US.[186]

'Health disparities' research in the US has traditionally focused more on race than on socioeconomic position, but socioeconomic inequalities in morbidity and mortality are also well documented—much better than in Canada for which most nationally representative data derive from aggregate level studies. Based on area-level data, inequalities in mortality in Canada appear to be smaller than those in the US,[187] but due to a lack of internationally comparable data it is difficult to accurately determine Canada's position in a broader international context.

Patterns of health inequalities in the US are roughly similar to those described above for European countries, with a clear gradient of lower mortality, higher life expectancy, and lower morbidity in higher socioeconomic groups—but with variations in the magnitude of health inequalities between different geographic regions, as would be expected in a country of this size.[188]

That the US is much more diverse than any European country is also clear from the enormous disparities in health and life expectancy that are seen when small areas are compared.[189] This has led to the distinction of 'Eight Americas', with a life expectancy gap of 20 years between the worst-off (high-risk urban black males) and the best off subgroup (Asian females).[190]

There is some evidence that health inequalities as measured between small areas are narrowing,[191,192] but otherwise trends are roughly similar to what we have seen for Western European countries, in the sense that falling average death rates in the US have been accompanied by rising relative inequalities in mortality.[170,193]

However, there is one important exception to these similarities. Recently, unfavourable trends in mortality among the lower educated have been reported from the United States.[194] Since the early 2000s total mortality and self-reported morbidity rates have risen among middle-aged white Americans, as a result of rising rates of suicide and poisonings, partly due to an epidemic of misuse of opioid painkiller drugs.[195] These deaths have been labelled 'deaths of despair', because the increases in mortality were concentrated among the low educated who have experienced increasing economic and social disadvantage.[196] Similar setbacks have not been observed in Western European countries,[175] although alcohol-related mortality has been increasing among the low educated.[197]

A few studies have tried to harmonize data across the Atlantic to compare the magnitude of health inequalities in the US with those in one or more European countries. Comparisons on the basis of self-reported morbidity suggest that both lower and higher socioeconomic groups have worse health in the US, but that the magnitude of health inequalities is larger in the US than in Western Europe.[198,199]

A study comparing the US with a wide range of European countries found educational inequalities in mortality in the US to be larger than in most European countries. The US has larger educational disparities in mortality than Western European countries—but smaller inequalities than Central-Eastern and Eastern European countries. The US also has lower life expectancy at birth than most Western European countries. High educated Americans have life expectancies roughly similar to those of their European counterparts, whereas low educated Americans have lower life expectancies—which largely explains the lower average life expectancy in the US.[200]

Australia and New Zealand

Socioeconomic inequalities in morbidity and mortality in Australia and New Zealand are not unlike those in European countries. Reviews of the situation in Australia show that socioeconomically disadvantaged groups have higher morbidity and mortality, and also have higher health risks in terms of poorer health-related behaviours, less favourable psychosocial factors, and lower use of preventive health care services.[201–203]

The situation is similar in New Zealand,[204] but in this country inequalities in mortality are better documented than in Australia due to the development of an anonymous linkage procedure between the census and mortality follow-up.[205] Inequalities in cause-specific mortality resemble those seen in Western Europe,[206,207] and relative inequalities in mortality have widened over time as they have in Western Europe.[208]

Interestingly, because smoking is recorded in the census in New Zealand, researchers are in a very good position to study the role of smoking, and have shown that it is the greatest single contributing factor to inequalities in mortality in this country, as it is in many Western European countries.[209,210]

Although data collection systems for the measurement of mortality inequalities are somewhat different between New Zealand and European countries, comparative studies have plausibly shown that the magnitude of inequalities in mortality among New Zealand men is somewhere in the middle of the range observed in Western Europe.[211,212] However, among women New Zealand is closer to Norway with its huge and rapidly rising inequalities, which may well be due to large inequalities in smoking.[211,213]

Japan and South Korea

Following the World War II, East Asian countries such as South Korea, Taiwan, Singapore, and Japan have achieved high levels of average income and life expectancy, comparable to or even exceeding those of many Western European countries. They have also built up welfare states, and studies of these countries' welfare arrangements have suggested the existence of a specific 'Confucian' welfare state regime. This is characterized by low levels of government intervention and expenditure, and a strong reliance on family and the voluntary sector in providing social safety nets, in accordance with the Confucian ideals of a strong work ethic and obligation to care for immediate family members.[18,214]

For both South Korea and Japan a reasonable number of research studies is available to assess the magnitude and pattern of health inequalities. This is particularly true for South Korea where research and policy attention to health inequalities have risen substantially in the last 15 years.[215] Studies based on mortality linkage to the National Health and Nutrition Examination Survey have shown independent effects of education, occupation, and income on mortality, with lower socioeconomic status generally being associated with higher mortality rates.[216] Cross-sectional unlinked mortality studies from South Korea have shown educational inequalities in mortality from many causes of death,[217] which may be explained by inequalities in material, psychosocial, and behavioural factors.[218]

However, below a surface of similarity there is one important deviation of the patterns of health inequalities in South Korea as compared to the patterns seen in Western Europe: recently, that is, after the 2008 financial crisis, mortality among men in non-manual occupational classes has risen, and because mortality among manual classes has continued to decline, the pattern of occupational class inequalities in mortality has reversed.[219]

This mirrors a similar but earlier development in Japan. At first sight, health inequalities in Japan resemble those seen in Western Europe, but they are not as clearly expressed, with gradients being less monotonous and the magnitude of health inequalities often being somewhat smaller.[220] Occupational class inequalities in mortality in Japan used to be regular but small in the 1990s, but have reversed more recently due to a rise of mortality among men in higher non-manual occupations. This may be due to the economic crisis of the early 1990s, which because of the associated work-related stress may have had a stronger effect on mortality among higher non-manual occupations. The rise in mortality was seen for a range of causes of death, but most strongly for suicide.[219,221,222]

The explanation for these deviant patterns in Japan and South Korea still eludes us. A study set up to explain the differences in health inequalities between Japan and Western European countries compared health inequalities among civil servants in London (Whitehall study), Helsinki (Helsinki Health study), and Japan (Japanese Civil Servants Study). It confirmed smaller inequalities in health in Japan, measured as inequalities in self-reported physical functioning and perceived health,[223] but could not clearly identify the factors contributing to smaller inequalities in Japan, with one exception: differences in smoking by occupational class are large in Britain and Finland, but small in Japan.[224,225]

Here again, as on the smaller scale of Europe, international comparisons suggest that health inequalities are more variable than is often assumed, and the findings from Japan and South Korea even challenge the often assumed universality of socioeconomic inequalities in health.

Key points

♦ There is not one single measure of the magnitude of health inequalities that we can rely on for all purposes, and it is often necessary to look at the underlying data by socioeconomic group before summary measures of health inequalities can be properly interpreted.

♦ Health inequalities are one of the most replicated findings in public health, but at the same time their magnitude is highly variable between different diseases and health problems, in patterns suggesting that health inequalities are larger when health problems are more 'actionable'.

♦ Health inequalities are persistent, but some are also highly dynamic. Relative inequalities in mortality have generally widened over time, due to faster mortality declines in higher socioeconomic groups, whereas absolute inequalities in mortality have sometimes narrowed.

♦ Health inequalities are ubiquitous, but their magnitude varies enormously between countries, suggesting that there is great scope for their reduction. Inequalities in mortality are unexpectedly large in Northern Europe, surprisingly small in Southern Europe, and massive in Central-Eastern and Eastern Europe.

♦ Health inequalities as found in European countries have also been documented in other high-income countries, in largely similar patterns suggesting that the European experience has worldwide relevance. The main exception is Japan and South Korea where occupational class inequalities in mortality do not follow the usual pattern.

Chapter 3

Explanatory perspectives

3.1 Methodological issues

Two big questions

*What explains health inequalities? The answer to this question is important for an obvious reason: it determines what can be done to reduce health inequalities. But it may also influence our normative judgement of whether health inequalities are unfair or not: dying younger because of living in poverty will generally be considered unfair, but this is less clear for dying younger because of binge drinking.

There are two big questions with regard to the explanation of health inequalities: (1) do differences in socioeconomic position cause differences in health, or does the 'causal arrow' point from health to socioeconomic position? and (2) what are the specific factors and mechanisms linking socioeconomic position to health (or vice versa)? Finding a scientifically valid answer to these questions poses great methodological challenges, to which we provide an introduction in this paragraph. Readers who wish to skip this technical introduction are of course free to do so, but should be aware of the fact that these methodological difficulties imply that much of our current understanding of the explanation of health inequalities is somewhat provisional.

Causation

Causation versus selection

Starting with the publication of the Black report,[20] which brought health inequalities back into the focus of public health research, the question whether 'causation' (i.e. socioeconomic position determining health) or 'selection' (i.e. health determining socioeconomic position, by influencing the selection of people into and out of socioeconomic groups) was the more important mechanism involved in generating health inequalities, has been central to debates about the explanation of socioeconomic inequalities in health.[226] And although some progress has been made, this is true to the present day.

There are several reasons why this issue occupies such a central place. The first is that if socioeconomic position causally determines health, the most effective countermeasures against health inequalities will be providing more years of education to those at the bottom of the social hierarchy, or reducing income inequalities, or other 'egalitarian' social and economic policies. By contrast, if there is no causal relationship between socioeconomic position and health, such policies are unlikely to be effective, at least as far as reducing health inequalities is concerned, although they may still help in achieving other social goals.

A second reason why this issue has been so hotly debated is that selection mechanisms are often considered to be less of a problem for public policy than causation mechanisms. Health inequalities due to causation mechanisms are often perceived to be more unfair, particularly by those who feel that the underlying social inequalities are already unfair in themselves.[227] Scientific disagreements on this issue are therefore to some extent fuelled by ideological differences, with causation explanations being more popular among those leaning towards the political left, and selection explanations being more popular among those with a more conservative or economically liberal outlook.[47 (p. 109)] However, health-related selection is an equally legitimate object of public policy as causation, as is clear from the fact that many countries have policies in place that reduce the effects of health problems on labour participation and income, and the polarization of this debate has not always been conducive to reaching nuanced conclusions.

Selection explanations stipulate that a person's health determines his or her socioeconomic position, and as this is not less of a causal claim than that of causation explanations, health-related selection can better be called 'reverse causation'.[i] Like health, socioeconomic position is not a fixed characteristic but changes during a person's lifetime.[228] Because of this 'social mobility' there is, in theory, ample scope for health-related selection processes. For example, health problems may form barriers to achieving a high educational level or to moving up the occupational ladder, and may lead to downward mobility when they experience temporary or permanent loss of paid work. However, whether this mechanism plays an important role in generating health inequalities cannot be determined on theoretical grounds, but needs to be demonstrated empirically.

Confounding

Causation and health-related selection are not the only possible explanations for health inequalities. There is a third possibility, in the form of 'confounding' by 'third factors'.

There are many other factors involved in generating health inequalities than socioeconomic position and health alone, but not all of these should be seen as confounders.[229 (pp. 129–134)] Confounders are third factors which are related to both socioeconomic position and health, but are not on the causal pathway linking socioeconomic position to health.[ii]

Confounders should be distinguished from 'mediators'.[231] These are third factors that represent an intermediate step in the causal pathway between socioeconomic position and health.[iii] Just as in the case of confounders, mediators are involved in the relationship between socioeconomic position and outcome, but in contrast to confounders which *may not* lie on the causal pathway, mediators *must* lie on this causal pathway.[229 (p. 186)] For example, to the extent that inequalities in smoking or bad working conditions are actually determined by people's socioeconomic position, they have to be considered possible 'mediators', not 'confounders'.[iv]

Nevertheless, there are third factors that can legitimately be considered confounders, because they partly determine people's socioeconomic position, instead of vice versa. For example, the higher prevalence of obesity in lower socioeconomic groups is not only due to an effect of socioeconomic disadvantage on the risk of becoming obese, but also to the fact that obese people are discriminated against during recruitment for jobs or promotion.[132,232] Also, alcohol-related health problems may stand in the way of upward occupational mobility, and may even lead to loss of income.[233] To the extent that the 'causal arrow' points from obesity and alcohol-related health problems to socioeconomic position, their contribution to health inequalities should be considered a form of confounding, not mediation.

Potentially more important as confounders are personal characteristics such as cognitive ability, coping styles, control beliefs, personality, and bodily and mental fitness. These influence educational and occupational achievement, and at the same time partly determine later health, either directly or indirectly through health-related behaviours such as consumption and exercise patterns and use of health services.[234,235,236] To the extent that the 'causal arrow' points from these personal characteristics to socioeconomic position, their contribution to health inequalities should be considered a form of confounding, not mediation.

Social epidemiologists, in recognition of the mechanism through which these personal characteristics are sorted across socioeconomic groups, sometimes use the term 'indirect selection' to denote this mechanism, which should be distinguished from the 'direct selection' involved when health or health problems affect social mobility.[230]

Genetic factors that predispose to ill-health and of which the prevalence varies between socioeconomic groups should also be seen as potential confounders, because a person's genotype temporally precedes his or her socioeconomic position. Again, an association between socioeconomic status and a certain genotype is most likely to arise when that genotype affects social mobility, through an effect on the likelihood of getting a disease that affects social mobility (e.g. mental health problems that stand in the way of educational achievement or upward occupational mobility), through an effect on health-related behaviour that affects social mobility (e.g. predisposition to alcohol addiction), or through an effect on personal characteristics that affect social mobility (e.g. cognitive ability or personality traits).[237]

Such selection effects may occur in each new generation, but may also lead to intergenerational transmission of disadvantage. Genetic factors predisposing to ill-health that have contributed to the low socioeconomic position of parents may be transmitted to their children, and will make it even more difficult for these children to reach a higher socioeconomic position than their parents. This illustrates that we should not be misled by the somewhat depreciating term 'confounding': like 'health-related selection', 'confounding' can be as policy-relevant as 'causation'.

Observation versus experimentation

Because associations between low socioeconomic position and ill-health may be due to health-related selection or confounding by third variables, demonstrating that low socioeconomic position causes ill-health requires more than showing that morbidity or mortality rates are higher in lower socioeconomic groups.[238] At the very least, our study design must enable us to establish that low socioeconomic position precedes ill-health instead of vice versa, and that confounding by other factors can be excluded, either by careful study design (e.g. by randomization, or by limiting the study to people who are identical in terms of other factors) or by controlling for these other factors in the analysis.

In the empirical sciences, the most reliable evidence of causation can be obtained by conducting experiments, but this is mostly unfeasible in the area of socioeconomic inequalities in health. This area therefore relies almost completely on clever observation, in which one tries to approach as closely as possible the 'clean' contrast of a controlled experiment. Such a clean contrast is, however, made difficult by the multiple links between socioeconomic position, health and third variables over a person's lifetime.

Consider the example of two groups of 35-year old and perfectly healthy persons of whom the first has a primary level of education, a routine manual job and an income in the lowest quintile, and the second a tertiary level of education, a professional occupation and an income in the highest quintile. When we follow these two groups over time, we will most likely find a higher incidence of ill-health and premature deaths in the first than in the second group. We have ruled out the possibility of health-related selection because both groups were perfectly healthy at the start of follow-up. But how do we rule out the possibility of confounding by third factors?

One option is to restrict the comparison to 35-year old and perfectly healthy people who are identical in terms of all the personal characteristics that predispose to good or bad health, and that were formed before the individuals had attained their adult socioeconomic position. Candidate factors would include cognitive ability, personality traits, some health-related behaviours already formed in adolescence, bodily and mental fitness, and genetics, as mentioned above. Another option is to accept a certain degree of heterogeneity of the two groups, and to statistically control for all these potential confounders in the analysis.

However, in the unlikely case that it were practically feasible to select on, or control for, all the confounders, how would we avoid over-adjustment? Over the life-course socioeconomic position and health are linked in a mutually reinforcing way. In our example, removing the effect of third variables that preceded the attainment of their current socioeconomic position of 35-year olds, will also remove some of the effect of socioeconomic conditions in preceding life stages. For example, a person's cognitive ability is not only dependent on his or her genotype, but also on the socioeconomic conditions in which he or she has grown up. In other words, the paradox is that the closer we get to identifying a true causal effect, the farther we may get from a good understanding of how socioeconomic position affects health.

A fundamental divergence of opinion

It is often thought that quasi-experimental studies, which try to mimic randomized experiments by cleverly exploiting 'natural experiments', hold a lot of promise for isolating the causal effects of socioeconomic position on health.[239,240] Some of these 'quasi-experimental' methods, which have only recently come to be applied in the study of health inequalities, are explained in Box 3.1. While these methods may indeed avoid confounding by both observed and unobserved third variables,[241] they do not escape the paradox just mentioned.

This paradox actually relates to a fundamental divergence of opinion among scientists on how to approach issues of causality, particularly when it comes to relatively vague concepts such as socioeconomic position. These quasi-experimental studies are often inspired by the 'counterfactual' approach to causal inference that is increasingly popular in many empirical disciplines, including epidemiology and economics. This uses the 'potential outcomes' framework for assessing causality, which requires that putative causes can be manipulated in experiments, at least in theory.[245]

In the case of smoking, it is not difficult to imagine the counterfactual of an otherwise identical person who has never smoked, but in the case of social exposures like low socioeconomic position (or gender, or race), this is much more difficult. Adherents of the counterfactual approach have therefore argued that assigning causal status to non-manipulable attributes like socioeconomic position (or gender, or race) is problematic, and that only more specifically defined and manipulable exposures qualify as possible causes of health problems.[246]

For the study of health inequalities, this point of view implies that it is not useful to ask 'does low socioeconomic position cause ill-health?' For adherents of the counterfactual approach this is an unanswerable question that should be replaced by more specific questions, such as 'does an extra year of education cause better health?' or 'does raising the social assistance benefit level cause better health?' It is the latter type of questions that—in their view—can be answered scientifically, in quasi-experimental (or even truly experimental) studies, and that is also more directly policy relevant.[247]

However, other epistemological positions have been defended as well. A more pluralistic approach to causality recognizes the evident existence of causes of ill-health that cannot be manipulated, such as earthquakes, non-white race, or low socioeconomic position. Although the effects of these exposures cannot be studied according to the rigorous framework prescribed by the counterfactual approach, their role as possible causes of ill-health is considered too important to be ignored.[248,249] In this alternative view it is precisely because low socioeconomic position often implies life-long exposures which are inextricably linked to social processes—and thus cannot be construed as a counterfactual cause—that it has such pervasive and persistent health effects.

British sociologist John Goldthorpe has argued that the counterfactual approach to causal inference has limited applicability to the central concerns of sociology as a population science. In

Box 3.1 Assessing causality between socioeconomic position and health

Schematically, the following design options could be considered to assess whether there is a causal relationship between socioeconomic position and health:[238,241]

Purely observational studies (i.e. the investigators exploit naturally occurring variations in exposure):

- cross-sectional and case control studies, for example, in which current health is related to current or previous socioeconomic position, with regression adjustment for observed confounders
- longitudinal studies, for example, cohort or panel studies relating socioeconomic position to health at a later point in time, with regression adjustment for observed confounders, or fixed effects adjustment for unobserved confounders
- twin studies, relating socioeconomic position to health of twins who are discordant on socioeconomic position, thereby controlling for genetic factors

Quasi-experimental studies (i.e. investigators exploit 'natural experiments' that have created quasi-random variations in exposure):

- cross-sectional or longitudinal studies with statistical creation of quasi-randomness in the allocation of socioeconomic resources, for example, by propensity score matching, differences-in-differences, instrumental variables, regression discontinuity, ...
- cross-sectional or longitudinal studies exploiting naturally occurring randomness in the allocation of socioeconomic resources, for example, lotteries, random roll-out of intervention programs, ...

Purely observational studies potentially suffer from many of the problems mentioned in the main text, although (partial) solutions have been proposed. For example, fixed effects adjustment (e.g. analyses which link changes in socioeconomic position to changes in health within the same individual) can be used to remove bias by both observed and unobserved confounders. Also, studying twins who have ended up in different socioeconomic positions guarantees extensive control for genetic factors.

Quasi-experimental studies are potentially more powerful in avoiding these problems. For example, in a regression discontinuity analysis one can exploit income thresholds in the allocation of financial benefits to compare health outcomes among people falling just below or above the threshold and therefore getting or just not getting the benefit. Because people just below and just above the threshold are likely to be otherwise similar, this may produce an unbiased estimate of the effect of the financial benefit.[242] However, getting close to a clean contrast carries a price: the external validity of the results of regression discontinuity studies for the wider problem of income-related inequalities in health is dependent on whether the health effect of the small difference in financial benefits around the threshold correctly represents the health effects of income along the whole income ladder.

Sometimes, socioeconomic resources are allocated at random in real life. The prime example is lotteries which at first sight offer an excellent opportunity to evaluate the causal effects of money on health—but whether the health impact of an incidental amount of money

> **Box 3.1 Assessing causality between socioeconomic position and health** (*continued*)
>
> obtained in a lottery adequately represents the health effects of years of living on a higher income is unclear.[243] Another example is the roll-out of certain intervention programmes which sometimes occurs more or less at random, as in the roll-out of a higher age of compulsory education across Swedish municipalities in the 1930s.[244]
>
> Box 3.1 has been reproduced from J.P. Mackenbach and J.P. de Jong, 'Health inequalities; an interdisciplinary exploration of socioeconomic position, health and causality.' Copyright © 2018 Federation of European Academies of Medicine (FEAM), All European Academies (ALLEA), and the Royal Netherlands Academy of Arts and Sciences (KNAW). Published under creative commons licence [Attribution 3.0 Netherlands]: https://creativecommons.org/licenses/by/3.0/nl/

his view, sociology primarily aims to explain observed regularities at the population level (such as in our case, health inequalities), and the counterfactual approach addresses different and much more restricted questions. Also, the counterfactual approach does not provide any insight into the underlying mechanisms, and cannot take into account the voluntary nature of human activity, and the fact that human beings are not passive recipients of manipulated exposures. In Goldthorpe's view, a more fruitful approach is elucidating the mechanisms underlying observed regularities at the population level.[250]

In this book we will try to follow a middle road between the two positions, by acknowledging both the strengths and limitations of the counterfactual approach to assessing a causal effect of socioeconomic position (or its more specific components) on health.

Mediation

Mediators

A scientific approach to the explanation of health inequalities cannot stop at the demonstration of an effect of socioeconomic position on health, but also requires an understanding of the factors and mechanisms involved in generating this effect. We need to be able to identify plausible causal pathways before we can reasonably conclude that socioeconomic position has an effect on health.[251]

This is, of course, also important from a policy perspective. Broadly speaking, one can distinguish two strategies for reducing health inequalities.[252] The first and most radical option is equalizing the distribution of socioeconomic factors, for example by reducing inequalities in educational attainment, employment, or income. To the extent that there is a causal effect of socioeconomic factors on health, this can be expected to also reduce health inequalities.

A second, more pragmatic strategy for reducing health inequalities is to equalize (by 'levelling up') the distribution of specific health determinants across socioeconomic groups.[253] For example, to the extent that socioeconomic inequalities in mortality are determined by differences in working conditions or access to health care, reducing these differences by improving working conditions and access to health care for lower socioeconomic groups can be expected to also reduce health inequalities.[v]

The most commonly used analytical technique for identifying the specific health determinants involved in generating health inequalities is 'mediation analysis'. This technique allows one to quantify the contribution of one or more 'mediators' to the effect of an independent variable (in this case: socioeconomic position) and a dependent variable (in this case: a health outcome).

Mediation analysis is based on the notion that health inequalities can be explained by differences in exposure to health determinants between people in lower and higher socioeconomic groups. This is the type of explanation we know most about, and will therefore be the focus of this chapter. However, third variables can not only act as mediators, but also as 'moderators' of the relationship between socioeconomic position and health.[231,254] A moderator is defined as a variable that affects the strength of the relationship between an independent variable and a health outcome.[vi]

This may give rise to 'differential susceptibility' or 'differential vulnerability', that is, health inequalities may partly be explained by the fact that people in lower socioeconomic groups are more 'susceptible' or 'vulnerable' to the negative health effects of various determinants, due to a range of other biological, psychological, and social factors.[255,256] Although empirical evidence on such moderation effects is still scarce, there is evidence that it may play a more important role than previously recognized.

For example, it has been shown that excessive alcohol consumption leads to more alcohol-related hospitalizations and deaths in lower socioeconomic groups, perhaps because drinkers from higher socioeconomic groups are protected by better dietary habits, a safer drinking environment, or more support from work and family to address emerging alcohol problems.[257,258]

Similarly, some studies have found that lower educated smokers have a greater likelihood of developing lung cancer than smokers with a higher level of education. This may be due to subtle differences in smoking behaviour (e.g. deeper inhalation of tobacco smoke or more carcinogenic types of tobacco smoked), but also to differences in biological susceptibility. In either case the contribution of smoking to inequalities in lung cancer will be larger than estimated on the basis of a simple mediation analysis.[259]

How can mediation be demonstrated?

One approach to assessing mediation is to take the prevalence rates of the health determinant of interest in each socioeconomic group, extract the relative risk of the determinant on morbidity or mortality from the literature, and then estimate the contribution of the determinant to morbidity or mortality inequalities using the method of population-attributable fractions.[260]

Because data requirements for this approach are modest, it can be applied in many settings, and has produced estimates of the contribution of various risk factors to inequalities in mortality for many European countries.[261-264] For example, it suggests that the contribution of smoking to inequalities in mortality ranges between 4% and 26% among men, and between 1% and 20% among women.[262]

This is, however, a rather crude approach, and a more accurate assessment of the contribution of health determinants to health inequalities requires a multivariate analysis of the three-way relationships between socioeconomic position, health determinant and health outcome. This is what 'mediation analysis' does.

The practice of mediation analysis in social epidemiology (and in other disciplines, such as psychology and sociology) has long been based on the so-called Baron and Kenny approach which was developed in the 1980s.[231,265] Current insights into the contribution of health determinants to health inequalities therefore largely derive from this approach, in which one studies whether the statistical relationship between socioeconomic position and health disappears, either completely or partly, upon controlling for the mediator(s).

This usually takes the form of the so-called 'difference method', in which one estimates the difference between the 'effect' of socioeconomic position on a health outcome before and after controlling for the mediator(s).[231,265] This reduction in the size of the 'effect' of the independent variable on the health outcome is called 'attenuation'.[vii]

For example, in a cohort study in the Netherlands it was found that the Rate Ratio of mortality among low as compared to high educated men decreased from 1.84 to 1.66 upon controlling for the higher prevalence of smoking among the low educated, suggesting that the contribution of smoking to educational inequalities in mortality is 21% in this setting (calculated as 100*(1.84–1.66)/(1.84–1.00)).[268]

Recently, the 'difference method' has been criticized for a number of methodological short-comings.[254,265,269] More specifically, it has been shown that it often gives biased results.[viii] New methods of mediation analysis have therefore been designed that remove some of these sources of bias.[254,265] Social epidemiologists have started to apply the new techniques, and found that these may lead to substantially different conclusions as compared to the conventional 'difference' method.[270–272]

Apart from technical difficulties, a more fundamental shortcoming of mediation analysis is that the results can only be interpreted as evidence for mediation *sensu stricto*, if we assume two causal relationships: socioeconomic position causes exposure to the health determinant, and exposure to the health determinant causes ill-health. Unfortunately, most datasets to which mediation analysis is applied, do not allow us to test that assumption.

In the example of the cohort study on the role of smoking in generating health inequalities in the Netherlands, despite its longitudinal design and adjustment for a range of confounders, due to the possibility of unobserved confounders there is no guarantee that the higher prevalence of smoking among the low educated is caused entirely by their lower socioeconomic position, nor is there a guarantee that the higher mortality among smokers found in the dataset is caused entirely by smoking.[268]

In order to acknowledge all these uncertainties we will therefore refrain from using the term 'mediator' and use the term 'contributing factor' instead, and we will also largely refrain from presenting quantitative estimates of the role of differences in exposure to health determinants, and instead present our conclusions on the role of contributing factors in more qualitative terms.

3.2 Education, occupation, income, and health

Education and health

From a sociological point of view, socioeconomic position is a multi-faceted phenomenon, which cannot be completely captured by measures of education, occupational class, and income. Nevertheless, the best evidence that we have on the causal effects of low socioeconomic position on health comes from quasi-experimental studies in which socioeconomic position has been dis-aggregated in its component parts. In this paragraph we review the scientific evidence on the health effects of education, occupational class and income.

Causation, reverse causation, confounding

Many longitudinal studies have shown that adults with a lower level of education have a higher likelihood of falling ill or dying prematurely: indeed, these inequalities have been found in all countries which take the trouble to collect the information.[273] Because most of these health problems arise long after the age at which people complete their education, health-related selection is unlikely to be involved,[51] although some health-related selection may have occurred in a previous life-stage, as children with chronic diseases are somewhat less likely to achieve a higher level of education.[274]

The main question is whether and, if so to what extent, the association between education and health is confounded by third variables. The short answer is 'yes, it is likely to be confounded, but we do not know by how much, and confounding is certainly not the only explanation, because there is good evidence from quasi-experimental studies that there is also a causal effect of education on health'.

Although variations in educational achievement are partly dependent on parental socioeconomic position, educational achievement is also strongly dependent on a person's own cognitive ability during childhood and adolescence.[275] And although children's cognitive ability is partly dependent on the environment in which they grow up, variations in cognitive ability among children are also strongly genetically determined.[276] We explain some of the concepts and methods of population genetics in Box 3.2.

It is therefore very likely that the association between education and health is partly confounded by genetic factors. Empirical evidence comes from molecular studies which have recently identified many genetic variants related to education, with 'polygenic scores' now explaining up to 10% of all inter-individual differences in educational achievement.[284–287] These associations do not necessarily arise from a causal effect of children's genotype on their own educational achievement, but could theoretically also arise from an effect of their parents' genotype (which is, of course, partly similar to that of their children) on how they are raised. However, there is evidence that 'polygenic scores' predicting education also predict upward educational (and occupational class) mobility of children as compared to their parents, suggesting a truly causal effect.[288]

The pathways linking genotype to education are likely to include, first of all, cognitive ability. We will more extensively review the evidence on the genetic determinants of cognitive ability in section 3.3, 'Six groups of contributing factors'. The pathways are also likely to include genetically determined aspects of personality such as the Big Five personality traits ('openness to experience', 'conscientiousness', 'extraversion', 'agreeableness', and 'neuroticism'), or the personality traits studied in behavioural economics ('self-control', 'risk aversion', and 'time preferences').[285,289] Because cognitive ability and other (partly) genetically determined personal characteristics are independent predictors of health in later life, one can reasonably infer that genetic factors must to some (as yet unknown) extent confound the relationship between education and health.

Furthermore, the relative contribution of genetic factors to differences in educational achievement has increased over time, due to a decreasing influence of environmental barriers. This is shown, for example, by the fact that the heritability of educational achievement is larger among twins born more recently, after the introduction of educational policies which decreased the influence of family background.[290,291] Although the evidence on trends is not entirely consistent,[277,292] between-country comparisons show that the heritability of educational achievement is higher in countries where the environment puts less constraints on educational achievement, such as the Nordic countries.[293]

Quasi-experimental evidence

In the presence of these and other risks of confounding, which are difficult to control in observational studies, experimental and quasi-experimental studies may provide more reliable evidence for a causal effect of education on health. Truly experimental evidence is limited to a few studies from the US that have assessed the long-term health effects of early childhood (or pre-school) education. These showed that children receiving preschool education were healthier and less likely to be smoking or obese as adults were.[294]

The effect of school education on health in later life has repeatedly been assessed in a quasi-experimental set-up. The most common approach has been the evaluation of the impact of compulsory schooling laws.[238,294–296] During the twentieth century, many countries have introduced such laws, and thereby increased the minimum school leaving age. Because the resulting changes in years of schooling can be regarded as 'exogenous' (i.e. independent of personal attributes of the children involved), any improvements in health occurring in cohorts that left school after the change can reasonably be attributed to the extra years of schooling.

Box 3.2 Genetic analysis: selected concepts and methods

Heritability

Heritability is defined as the proportion of all variation in a 'phenotypic trait' (i.e. observed characteristic, such as cognitive ability or health) between individuals in a population that is due to genetic variation between individuals in that population. The total variation in a 'phenotypic trait' is thought to consist of three components: genetically induced variation, environmentally induced variation, and random error. This implies that the measured degree of heritability of a 'phenotypic trait' depends on the degree of both genetic and environmental variation in a population. In a population in which the environment is more homogeneous, heritability will be higher, and vice versa.[277]

Twin studies

The classical approach to estimating heritability in human populations is by comparing resemblances between dizygotic and monozygotic twins. Other but conceptually similar approaches involve comparisons between adoptive and biological siblings and between parents and their adoptive and biological offspring. Dizygotic twins on average share half their genes, whereas monozygotic twins share all their genes and therefore are twice as genetically similar as dizygotic twins. The heritability of a particular 'phenotypic trait' can thus—under certain assumptions, such as the environmental similarity between the two types of twins being the same—be estimated as approximately twice the difference in correlation between monozygotic and dizygotic twins.[277]

The heritability gap

Estimates of the heritability of cognitive ability calculated from twin and similar studies range between 30% and 80%, and increases from a value of about 30% in early childhood to much higher values in adulthood and old age.[278] Genome-Wide Association Studies (GWAS) have identified many specific genetic variants that are associated with cognitive ability,[278,279] but there still is a big 'heritability gap', that is, the combined effects of all genetic variants that have until now been identified cannot fully account for the heritability estimated from twin studies. This may either be due to violations of the assumptions underlying estimates from twin studies, or be a matter of slow advances in filling the gap as the findings of more and more molecular studies accumulate.[277,280]

Genome-wide complex trait analysis

Recently a new technique, genome-wide complex trait analysis (GCTA), has been proposed which does not require the often tenuous assumptions of twin studies and other studies based on known family relationships. In this technique, the degree of genetic similarity between unrelated individuals in the population is determined directly on the basis of an analysis of their DNA, using the presence of common single-nucleotide polymorphisms.[281] Applications of this method have grown explosively, and have produced new estimates for the heritability of many 'phenotypic traits' including level of education, socioeconomic position, cognitive ability, personality traits, smoking, alcohol consumption, many chronic diseases, etc. The estimates are often somewhat lower than those from twin studies, but almost always substantial.

> **Box 3.2 Genetic analysis: selected concepts and methods** (*continued*)
>
> Although promising, it is still a new technique and there is no consensus yet about its relative merits.[282]
>
> ## Mendelian randomization
>
> This approach uses the genetic determinants of a particular 'phenotype' (e.g. a high serum cholesterol, or a low level of education) to study the causal effects of that phenotype on health. The idea behind this analytical strategy is that whether people have certain genes or not is the outcome of a natural experiment occurring at conception, when each child inherits half of each of their parents' genomes. Because whether a child inherits a particular gene from its father or mother is the outcome of a random process, the association between that part of the variation in phenotype (high serum cholesterol, low education) induced by the gene and a health outcome is considered to be less subject to confounding than the association between most other variations in the phenotype and a health outcome.[56] Application of this idea is, however, challenging, for example, because children's genotypes are only randomly assigned conditional on their parents' genotype, and the latter therefore needs to be controlled.[283]

Most of these studies found that longer schooling led to a reduction in mortality in mid-life and beyond, with large variations in effect size.[294] Education also reduces the risk of taking up smoking,[294,295] and better-educated parents have healthier children.[295] Although studies exploiting compulsory schooling laws have important limitations (e.g. it is unclear whether the effect of one year of extra schooling at the age of, say, 16 can be generalized to the whole range of variation in length of education currently seen), these findings clearly suggest that there is a causal effect of education on mortality, and that the association between the two seen in observational studies is not only due to confounding by genetic or other usually unobserved factors.

This conclusion is strengthened by the results of recent studies using Mendelian randomization, a technique exploiting the natural experiment occurring at conception when genes from the mother and father are allocated at random to the child. Using genetic determinants of education as an 'instrumental variable' to mimic randomly occurring variation in educational achievement, these studies found clear evidence for a protective effect of more years of education on dementia,[57] ischemic heart disease,[58] and mortality.[60]

Occupational class and health

As in the case of education, many studies have shown that a lower occupational class is associated with higher rates of morbidity and mortality.[104,105,297] The main issue is whether this is due to a causal effect of occupational class on health, or due to 'reverse causation' or confounding. Perhaps because of the difficulties involved, no studies with rigorous identification strategies to isolate a causal effect of occupational class on health have been conducted (although there is reasonably strong evidence of the effect of specific working conditions on ill-health).[298]

Because educational achievement usually precedes entry to the labour market, and because a higher level of education is a requirement for entry into higher occupations, education should be considered a potential confounder of the association between occupational class and ill-health. Studies from the US have sometimes found that the association between occupational class and health disappears after controlling for level of education,[299,300] but studies from several European countries often show independent (although attenuated) effects.[51,301,302]

A big difference between education and occupational class is that whereas one's level of education remains constant after the age of, say, 25, one's employment status and occupational class can still change after entering one's first job. This implies that the scope for reverse causation by health-related conditions is much larger in the case of occupational class than in the case of education. A rigorous analysis of the labour market effects of health-related conditions in a range of high-income countries has indeed shown that having a chronic disease, and being a smoker or obese, have negative effects on employment, wages, sick leave, and early retirement [303].

That health-related selection in and out of employment, and during occupational careers does occur is thus undisputed, but there is no consensus on whether these selection effects widen or narrow health inequalities. Several studies have found that the health of people who move downward is worse than that of those who remain in their class of origin, and better than that of those in their class of destination, whereas the health of those who move upward is better than that of others in their class of origin, and worse than that of others in their class of destination. On the basis of this it has been claimed that health-related occupational mobility will tend to 'constrain' or 'dilute' health inequalities.[304, 305]

While this may seem straightforward, others have demonstrated that this is not necessarily true. Even if the health of the socially mobile is in-between that of their classes of origin and destination, the net effect of health-related selection may be to widen health inequalities. This is because the effect of health-related selection does not depend on the difference in health between the socially mobile and *all those in the class they join*, but on the difference in health between the socially mobile and those *whom they replace* in the class they join.[306,307]

If the health of those who move upward into a higher class is better than that of those who move out of this class, or if the health of those who move downward into a lower class is worse than that of those who move out of this class, health inequalities will widen, not narrow. Detailed studies of the relative numbers and health status of incomers and out-goers to each occupational class have confirmed that health-related selection during intragenerational mobility may indeed widen health inequalities in the population as a whole.[306,307]

However, whatever the direction of the effect is, the contribution of health-related selection to the explanation of occupational class inequalities in health at adult and higher ages is likely to be limited, because most health problems occur in late middle or old age, after people have reached their final occupational class. This reasoning is confirmed by the fact that longitudinal studies in which occupational class has been measured before health problems are present, and in which the incidence of health problems has been measured during long-term follow-up, also show clearly higher risks of health problems in the lower occupational classes.[297,308,309]

Income and health

Many studies have also found a positive association between income and health: people with a higher income tend to have better health and live longer.[238,295,310] The relationship is non-linear: at the lower end of the income distribution, the relationship is steeper than at the upper end, suggesting that whatever mechanisms explain these inequalities, their effects are stronger among those living on a very low income.[62,311] Studies that have assessed whether the association between income and health still holds after controlling for education and/or occupational class have often (but not always) found that this is indeed the case[51,301,312,313]

Causation, reverse causation, confounding

As in the case of education and occupational class, an important question is whether this association is due to a higher income leading to better health (causation), to better health leading to a higher income (reverse causation), or to confounding by third variables. The common view among public health scientists is that causation accounts for a substantial part of this relationship, whereas the dominant view in the economics literature is that reverse causation is far more important.[314]

Both directions of causality are certainly plausible. A higher level of income may produce better health through several mechanisms. For example, it increases access to healthy foods and good housing conditions, it reduces the stress of financial insecurity and boosts self-confidence, and it removes financial barriers to health care. But better health may also produce a higher income, for example by increasing capacity to work, labour productivity, and wages.[315] As compared to health inequalities by education and occupational class, health inequalities by income probably have the largest scope for health-related selection.

In addition to these two directions of causality, there is also the possibility of third variables (such as cognitive ability or personality traits) influencing both. Some studies have indeed shown that differences in cognitive ability and other personal attributes—whose formation plausibly predates the attainment of various income levels in adult life—explain part of the income-related inequalities in health. There is also emerging evidence of genetic determinants of income and material deprivation, again probably acting through cognitive ability and other personal attributes.[316]

Quasi-experimental evidence

For an assessment of a causal effect of income on health it is therefore best to rely on experimental and quasi-experimental studies, but it is important to recognize from the outset that most of these studies have a number of important limitations. They often study the effect of rather small variations in income, sometimes in settings (such as lotteries or stock market gains) that may not represent the experience of a lower or higher regular income over longer periods of life. It is also more difficult to demonstrate causation (i.e. the effects of a change in income on health, which may take a long time to materialize) than to demonstrate reverse causation (i.e. the effects of a 'health shock' on income, which can be seen within a couple of years).

Nevertheless, experimental and quasi-experimental studies potentially provide the strongest evidence for a causal effect of income on health. Recently, a number of reviews on these types of studies have been carried out. Overall, the main conclusion is that in high-income countries there is clear evidence for a causal effect of major changes in health on income, but there is no consistent evidence for a causal effect of modest and short-term changes in income on physical health in adulthood. However, all reviews emphasize that the available evidence does not rule out the possibility that there is a causal effect of larger variations in lifetime income on physical health in adulthood. Also, they agree that the evidence for a causal effect of parental income on the health of children is more consistent[238,295,314,317,318]

The evidence for reverse causation is generally considered convincing. In a range of studies exploiting 'exogenous' changes in health (i.e. health events that are abrupt and unforeseen), ill-health in adulthood had a modest negative effect on wages among those who work, and a stronger effect on income through decreasing the employment rate and reducing the hours worked among the employed.[314]

In addition, ill-health in early life and childhood had substantial effects on lifetime earnings, through decreasing the build-up of cognitive and non-cognitive abilities, constraining the acquisition of education, and by continuing into ill-health in adulthood which then interferes with labour productivity in adulthood. Ill-health can thus have a very long reach from childhood to constrained economic opportunities in adulthood.[314]

On the other hand, studies trying to find evidence for a causal effect of income on physical health in adulthood in high income countries using a quasi-experimental set-up have had inconsistent results. One review summarizing the results of 16 studies found eight studies with no effect, two studies with a negative effect (i.e. more money, worse health), and six studies with a positive effect (i.e. more money, better health). Based on a further evaluation of the methodological quality of these studies, the authors conclude that the evidence that income does have a causal impact on health in adulthood is 'weak'.[314] For low- and middle-income countries the evidence for a causal effect of income on health—which partly comes from true experiments—was considered to be more convincing.[314]

A second recent review summarizing the results of nine studies of income effects on health in adulthood (six of whom were also included in the first review) found four studies with no effect, two studies with a negative effect, and three studies with a positive effect. When looking at other outcomes, the review did find strong evidence that additional financial resources during adulthood make people happier and reduce mental health problems, but also that more money can lead to less healthy behaviours such as more drinking and smoking. The authors conclude that for physical health in adulthood the evidence is 'mixed'.[318]

Some of the reviewed studies focused on so-called windfall gains in income, for example, lottery winnings, which closely approximate a true experimental setting. Some European studies found that the recipients of lottery prizes experience positive changes in self-reported health. These positive effects are particularly seen for mental health and less so for physical health, perhaps because winning a lottery also tends to increase smoking and drinking.[314]

The weakness of this research strategy is, of course, that this variation in 'income' does not necessarily correspond to that of normal monthly or yearly income. This limitation has to some extent been circumvented in a recent study of a Swedish lottery, not included in the reviews quoted above, that distributed sizable prizes and paid them out over longer periods of time, but this study also found largely null effects on physical health in adulthood.[319]

The reviews also agree that the evidence for a causal effect of parental income on children's health is considerably stronger than that for adults' income on their own health. As the likelihood of reverse causation is less, because children's health will not directly affect their parents' income, observational evidence does not have to be discarded altogether, provided there is sufficient control for confounding by third variables. Although evidence from experimental and quasi-experimental studies is again somewhat mixed, reviews conclude that a causal effect of parental income on children's health is likely to exist.[295,314,317]

This conclusion is further supported by the fact that parental income has positive effects on intermediate outcomes, such as the quality of parenting, the physical home environment, maternal depression, smoking during pregnancy, and children's cognitive ability, school achievement, and behaviour.[317] Long-term increases in incomes of lower socioeconomic groups may thus have health benefits that accumulate over generations.[238]

Nevertheless, the lack of convincing evidence for an effect of income on adult physical health in high-income countries makes one wonder whether this does not partly resolve the paradox of the persistence of health inequalities in modern welfare states. Has the welfare state perhaps reduced the importance of one mechanism—low income causing ill-health—so that we are now mainly left with other mechanisms—ill-health leading to low income, and confounding by cognitive ability and other personal characteristics?

Provisional conclusions

Surprisingly, after decades of research, there is still uncertainty about whether there is a causal effect of socioeconomic position on health, and if so about how much of the observed association between socioeconomic position and health is due to such a causal effect.

Social epidemiologists have generally tended to interpret the association between socioeconomic position and health as being largely due to a causal effect of socioeconomic position on health. However, recent research in other disciplines, such as genetics and economics, has cast doubt on this interpretation. The new evidence reviewed above suggests that both health-related selection (in the case of the association between income and health) and confounding by unobserved personal attributes (in the case of the association between education, occupational class, and income) play a more important role than previously recognized.

At the same time, the importance of the new (quasi-)experimental evidence should not be overrated. As mentioned above, the paradox here is that the closer we get to identifying a true causal effect, the farther away we may get from a good understanding of how socioeconomic position affects health. We have to sail between the Scylla of being strict on causality (but not capturing the full effects of living in socioeconomic disadvantage) and the Charybdis of more fully capturing the effects of living in socioeconomic disadvantage (but being too lenient on causality). In other words, the new evidence may well underestimate the full causal effects of a life spent in socioeconomic disadvantage.

Nevertheless, at this stage of advancing knowledge we cannot claim to know that all or even most of the associations between socioeconomic position and health are due to a causal effect of socioeconomic position on health. The most we can say is that there is a causal effect of education on health, and that the observed association between education and health is therefore partly due to such a causal effect. It is also likely that there is a causal effect of parental income on children's health, and while there is no clear evidence for an effect of modest changes in income on adult health, it is plausible that larger changes in income, particularly at the low end of the income distribution and particularly in countries with lower average incomes, do have an effect on adult health.

3.3 **Six groups of contributing factors**

Life-course models

Six groups of specific factors are likely to play a role in the explanation of health inequalities—although not necessarily in a strictly 'mediating' role (see section 3.1 'Methodical issues'). These are: genetics, childhood environment, material living conditions, social and psychological factors, health-related behaviours, and health care.

Before we discuss each of these in turn, we introduce the life-course perspective that will be used to structure the presentation—and after presenting the contributing factors we end by briefly discussing the biological pathways linking socioeconomic position to health. This has resulted in this section being very long, reflecting the enormous productivity of research in this area in the past three decades.

What transpires from all this research is a rather complex picture of how individuals in lower socioeconomic groups are exposed over their lifetime to a wide variety of unfavourable living conditions, and how these exposures and the behavioural responses to them lead to ill-health—but also of how health influences socioeconomic position and how both are influenced by personal characteristics, like cognitive ability and personality traits, which partly reflect childhood environment and are also partly genetically determined. All these bits and pieces can be brought together in a 'life-course' perspective.

At conception, all individuals are endowed with a particular set of genes, and after birth move from a situation that is still largely determined by their parents' socioeconomic position to one that is determined by their own socioeconomic position. They enter the labour market with certain educational credentials, and during their adult life move through various occupations and varying levels of income, reaching retirement with or without some wealth. During each of these life stages health problems may be a consequence of their previous and current socioeconomic position, and a determinant of their current and future socioeconomic position. Moreover, both health and socioeconomic position may be determined by personal characteristics that are themselves the consequences of socioeconomic conditions in previous stages of life.

A life-course approach then sees the higher rates of illness and premature death among adults and older persons in lower socioeconomic groups as the cumulative result of socially patterned exposures acting at different stages of the life-course, and at the same time as possible determinants of future changes in socioeconomic position.[320] This has proven to be a very useful way of integrating different strands of evidence.

The simplest conceptual model for life-course influences is that of 'accumulation of risk'. Different forms of material and immaterial disadvantage tend to cluster in the same persons, with one disadvantage increasing the likelihood of another at a later point in time, and with health disadvantage arising as a result of cumulative social disadvantage.[321,322] Such accumulation models can incorporate both 'selection' and 'causation' mechanisms, because a low socioeconomic position in one stage of the life-course may translate into a health disadvantage in the next, which may then lead to a still lower socioeconomic position some years later, and so on.[323]

Life-course models may also incorporate 'critical periods': time windows of exposure that are particularly important for health at later ages. One possible example of a 'critical period' is intra-uterine life, as elaborated in the 'foetal origins of adult disease' hypothesis which holds that foetal growth and other factors during pregnancy are linked to the risk of developing cardiovascular and other diseases in adulthood.[324] Another is childhood: the child's physical, cognitive, and emotional development is strongly influenced by socioeconomic circumstances, which in its turn influences both adult socioeconomic position and adult health in many ways ('the long arm of childhood').[325]

Circumstances in early life also set up a pattern of social learning, which may generate a sense of powerlessness reinforced by others in the social network who have been similarly disadvantaged and socially excluded, sometimes over generations.[326] Such intergenerational transmission of social and health disadvantage may therefore be one of the mechanisms contributing to the persistence of health inequalities over time.

Genetics

A life-course approach to health inequalities starts by clarifying the role of genetics.[ix] Investigating the role of genetics in generating social and health inequalities is not only scientifically challenging—Box 3.2 listed some of the complexities—but also surrounded by intense dispute, fuelled by fears that research findings may be (mis)used to justify existing inequalities.[327] However, as we will see in Chapter 5, inequalities originating in genetic differences are not necessarily less inequitable than inequalities based on differences in living conditions, and even if they were we cannot close our eyes to the results of genetic studies.

These results clearly show that genetic factors are likely to play a role in generating health inequalities, by partly determining cognitive ability and other personal characteristics, which in their turn also partly determine both a person's socioeconomic position and his or her health. Technically speaking, genetically determined variations in these personal characteristics are confounders of the relationship between socioeconomic position and health, strengthening a relationship that would otherwise have been present in a weaker form.

The important role of genetic determinants for children's cognitive ability has first been convincingly shown in twin studies, which found substantial heritability in the order of at least 50%.[278,328] Molecular studies have more recently identified many specific genetic variants that are associated with cognitive ability,[278, 279] and although there is still a big gap between the combined effects of all genetic variants that have until now been identified, and the heritability estimated from twin studies, this 'heritability gap' is being slowly filled as the findings of more molecular studies accumulate.[277,280]

The transmission of genetic material from parent to child should not be seen as a completely pre-determined process. Cognitive ability and personality are complex traits that are determined by many genes, and a complete set of genes associated with a particular level of intelligence or personality profile cannot be transmitted intact from parent to child, because the relevant genes are located on different chromosomes and will become re-assorted during cell division and meiosis.[329] Nevertheless, as a result of both intergenerational transmission and random re-assortment children do differ in their genetic predisposition towards low or high cognitive ability and towards various personality profiles.

The role of genetics in the explanation of health inequalities is not limited to 'gene-environment correlation' (i.e. genetic factors occurring more frequently in lower than in higher socioeconomic groups or vice versa), but may also include 'gene-environment interaction' (i.e. genetic factors determining the effects of the socioeconomic environment).[330,331] Some genotypes may increase or decrease the susceptibility to a disadvantaged environment,[332], and in twin studies the heritability of cognitive ability has been found to be larger in higher than in lower socioeconomic groups, probably because the effect of the environment overwhelms the effect of genetic determinants in lower socioeconomic groups.[333]

The role of genetics in explaining health inequalities may also involve 'epigenetics', that is, heritable changes in gene function that do not involve changes in the DNA sequence, for example, due to methylation of DNA. Such changes may be the result of various exposures, such as smoking, nutrition, psychosocial stress, and environmental toxicants, and may play a role in the generation of health inequalities and their intergenerational transmission.[334,335] However, epigenetic mechanisms would be an instance of mediation, not of confounding.

Childhood environment

Moving on through the life-course, what happens after conception is pregnancy and childhood. Whether or not pregnancy and childhood conditions can mediate the effect of socioeconomic position on health, depends on whether we look at health inequalities in childhood or in adulthood. In the latter case—which is what we are focusing on in this chapter—they logically cannot, because pregnancy and childhood conditions temporally precede adulthood. But if we take into account the fact that a person's socioeconomic position often has a high degree of continuity over the life-course, it does certainly make sense to consider the role of pregnancy and childhood conditions as contributing factors.

This continuity is illustrated in Figure 3.1—which, however, also shows that the degree of continuity of socioeconomic position over the life-course should not be exaggerated. On the one hand, many more low than high educated people come from lower occupational class families. On average in Europe as a whole, 58% of low educated men had a father with a manual occupation, against 35% of high educated men. This continuity indicates that inequalities in exposure to socioeconomic disadvantage during childhood may indeed play a role in explaining health inequalities in adulthood.

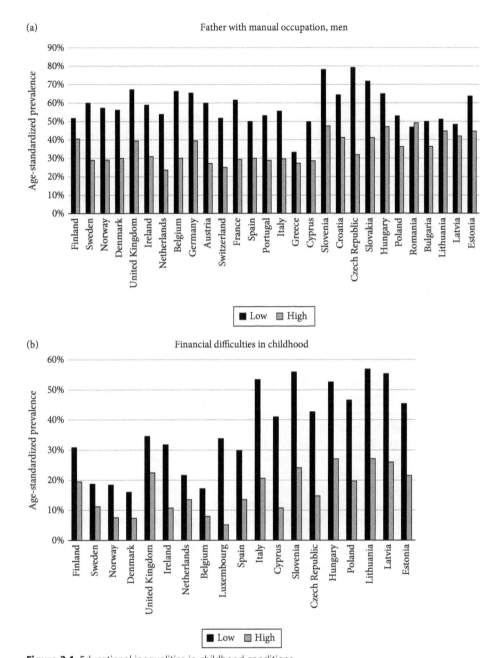

Figure 3.1 Educational inequalities in childhood conditions

Notes for panel a: Men aged 35–79 years (women similar). Data for ca. 2010.

Source: dataset constructed in DEMETRIQ/LIFEPATH projects, with harmonized data from European Social Survey.

Notes for panel b: Financial hardship = self-reported financial difficulties (most of the time/often) when growing up. Women aged 35–79 years (men similar). Data for 2005.

Source: dataset constructed in DEMETRIQ/LIFEPATH projects, with harmonized data from EU Statistics on Income and Living Conditions.

On the other hand, not all low educated men had a father with a manual occupation, and only 31% of high educated men had a father with an upper non-manual occupation—which really counts as growing up in advantage. Thus, although there is a certain degree of continuity in socioeconomic position, this is diluted by social mobility.

Adverse childhood conditions

Socioeconomic conditions already have an impact on children's health and development before they are born. Low socioeconomic position of the mother is associated with impaired foetal growth, low birth weight, and premature birth,[336,337] which may all contribute to a higher frequency of health and developmental problems after birth—and perhaps even into adulthood.[324] Mechanisms linking socioeconomic disadvantage of the parents to impaired foetal growth include impaired maternal health (e.g. gestational hypertension and diabetes), more psychosocial stress (e.g. due to financial and relational problems), and parental health behaviours (e.g. smoking during pregnancy).[338]

After birth, there are also substantial inequalities in exposure to a range of unfavourable childhood conditions. Retrospectively, having experienced serious conflict or hardship in childhood is much more common among adults with a lower than with a higher socioeconomic position. This is illustrated in panel B of Figure 3.1, which also shows that financial hardship in childhood is reported much more frequently in Southern, Central-Eastern and Eastern Europe, probably reflecting lower levels of prosperity in the past.

Systematic reviews show that growing up in disadvantaged socioeconomic circumstances is associated with many negative health and development outcomes in childhood, ranging from impaired growth to general ill-health and from impaired neurocognitive functioning, structural brain development, and mental health to higher rates of asthma and dental caries.[107,283,339–341]

This is commonly thought to reflect a causal effect of socioeconomic disadvantage on health, because there is less potential for reverse causality in the case of children's health and development than in the case of adult health outcomes.[47] However, it is also possible that there are common underlying factors in the association between parents' socioeconomic disadvantage and children's health and development, such as genetic factors shared by parents and their children.[285]

Systematic reviews also show that growing up in disadvantaged socioeconomic circumstances is associated with many negative health outcomes in adult life, independent from the socioeconomic position children achieve for themselves, including higher increased all-cause mortality, mortality from various specific causes, cardiovascular risk factors, impaired cognitive and physical functioning, and less good self-rated health.[342,343]

Several mechanisms are likely to be involved in these delayed effects.[107] Health inequalities initiated in childhood may continue into health inequalities later in life when ill-health in childhood continues into ill-health in adulthood, and even more so when it also negatively affects adult education or income.[340]

Adverse childhood conditions may also contribute to health inequalities at older ages through other, more indirect mechanisms.[344,345] Growing up in unfavourable socioeconomic conditions impairs the neurocognitive development of children, particularly their language ability and executive functioning (i.e. the cognitive processes necessary for the control of behaviour, such as attentional control and working memory).[341,346] Neuroimaging studies have even found a biological substrate for some of these effects, such as reduced grey matter volumes of certain parts of the brain.[347]

These effects of socioeconomic disadvantage on neurocognitive development are probably due to a combination of prenatal exposures (such as higher levels of maternal stress hormones), parental care (such as harsh discipline), and lack of cognitive stimulation.[348] Stimulation of learning by parents raises children's intelligence, and the comparatively harsh living conditions of families with a lower socioeconomic position increase family stress and hamper family investments in children, which harm the development of their cognitive ability and personality.[349]

The socioeconomic environment in which children grow up may also have an impact on their epigenome with effects on health and development throughout the life-course.[350] For example, some studies have found an association between childhood socioeconomic status and DNA methylation of genes regulating stress reactivity and inflammation, suggesting a specific biological pathway linking childhood disadvantage to adult ill-health.[351,352]

Simpler mechanisms may, however, also play a role. For example, the higher prevalence of smoking in lower socioeconomic groups can partly be explained by the fact that children from low educated or poor parents copy the behaviour of their parents, or do not acquire the skills or motivation to resist the temptations of smoking.[353]

Cognitive ability and personality

At this juncture, after having presented some evidence on the roles of both genetics and childhood environment, we can also more fully discuss the role of personal characteristics such as cognitive ability and personality. As a result of both genetics and childhood environment, adults in lower and higher socioeconomic groups differ in a number of personal characteristics that promote good or bad health, and that contribute to health inequalities. This has been convincingly documented for both cognitive ability and personality traits.

'Cognitive ability' or 'intelligence' has been defined as 'a very general mental capability that involves the ability to reason, plan, solve problems, think abstractly, comprehend complex ideas, learn quickly, and learn from experience'.[354] Although cognitive ability has many dimensions, as illustrated by this definition, these are usually strongly inter-correlated, which has given rise to the idea that the underlying general ability (often called 'g') can be measured along a single scale of intelligence.

On average, people in lower socioeconomic groups have substantially lower scores on intelligence tests. This is not only true when we group people by their level of education, but also when we group them by their occupational class or level of income.[355] For example, in Britain the average scores on a general intelligence test were found to be almost twice as high for men in professional occupations than for men in unskilled manual occupations,[356] and in Sweden one third of men in unskilled manual occupations was found to have a very low intelligence test score against only one tenth of men in the whole population.[357]

As explained above, differences in cognitive ability reflect a mixture of the effects of genetics and childhood environment, but regardless of the ultimate causes children with low cognitive abilities are less upwardly mobile,[358,359] and thus are over-represented in lower socioeconomic groups as adults.

Lower cognitive ability is also very strongly and independently associated with a range of unfavourable health outcomes, from health-related behaviours and specific diseases and injuries to all-cause mortality.[360 361, 362] A recent meta-analysis estimated that one standard deviation higher cognitive test score in childhood or youth was associated with 24% lower mortality during several decades of follow-up.[363]

As was to be expected in view of these strong interrelations, differences in cognitive ability have been found to account for a sizable part of socioeconomic inequalities in health.[357,362,364] For example, a long-term follow-up study of schoolchildren in the Netherlands who had undergone intelligence testing in the 1940s, found that about half of the observed inequalities in mortality by level of attained education could be explained by differences in cognitive ability as measured in the last grade of primary school.[365] In the British Whitehall study about one third of inequalities in various health outcomes by 'employment grade' (a measure of occupational class among civil servants) could statistically be explained by differences in cognitive ability.[362]

People in lower and higher socioeconomic groups also differ in their personality profiles as measured with the so-called Big Five personality traits. People in lower socioeconomic groups have been found to have higher levels of 'neuroticism' and 'agreeableness', and lower levels of 'extraversion', 'openness', and 'conscientiousness'. Because some of these factors are also predictors of mortality, differences in personality statistically explain part of inequalities in mortality.[366,367]

Material living conditions

Poverty

Although differences in income level across the whole income distribution may not play an important role in generating health inequalities in high income countries (as discussed in section 3.2 'Education, occupation, income, and health'), poverty does plausibly play a role, but to a different extent in different European countries, depending on its depth and impact on access to other resources important for health.

Poverty can be measured in different ways, for example, as a net household income level below 60% of the median, or below a threshold deemed to represent the minimum income necessary for a decent life.[368] It can also be measured more directly as material deprivation, in the form of lack of access to a number of items deemed necessary for a decent life (e.g. having a telephone, having a refrigerator, being able to receive friends, having at least one week of holiday per year, etc.).

Figure 3.2 shows that the prevalence of material deprivation is very unevenly distributed between people with lower and higher socioeconomic positions. Although there is some material deprivation among the high educated, its prevalence is much higher among the low educated. The gap in material deprivation between low and high educated differs substantially between countries: countries with more generous welfare policies, as indicated by higher social expenditure (see Figure 1.2) tend to have lower levels and smaller inequalities in material deprivation.

Many studies show that poverty is associated with a range of adverse health outcomes,[369,370] and a few mediation analyses which link indicators of socioeconomic position to health outcomes via poverty suggest that differences between socioeconomic groups in the prevalence of poverty do indeed contribute to the explanation of health inequalities.[371–373]

The plausibility of a causal effect of poverty on health is supported by the existence of a range of well-documented pathways through which poverty may affect health. It reduces financial access to activities and products that are important for the maintenance and promotion of health (such as a healthy diet, sports, social contacts). This includes reduced access to health care services, particularly when out-of-pocket payments are required. And it often leads to psychosocial stress, which has negative biological and mental effects and increases the likelihood of risk-taking behaviours (such as smoking and excessive alcohol consumption).[368,374,375]

Work and working conditions

A second group of living conditions contributing to health inequalities are working conditions. Poor working conditions are more prevalent among employed people with lower levels of occupation: many studies have shown physical, chemical, and psychosocial exposures to be more common in lower occupational groups.[376,377] Figure 3.3 illustrates this for one harmful physical working condition (carrying heavy loads) and one unfavourable psychosocial working condition (not being able to choose or change the order of one's tasks). Both are much more frequent in the lower occupational classes in all European countries.

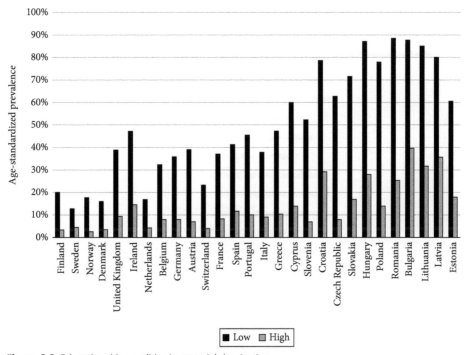

Figure 3.2 Educational inequalities in material deprivation

Notes: Material deprivation = at least 3 out of 9 necessities missing. Men only; women similar. Data for 2010.

Source: dataset constructed in DEMETRIQ/LIFEPATH projects, with harmonized data from EU Statistics on Income and Living Conditions.

There is also moderate to good evidence that these exposures lead to various forms of ill-health, and a recent systematic review of mediation analyses using the 'difference method' confirms a role in generating health inequalities for both the physical/chemical work environment (higher exposure to physical demands, biomechanical strains, and chemical substances in certain lower occupations) and the psychosocial work environment (higher prevalence of demand-control and effort-reward imbalance in certain lower occupations).[378] An imbalance between effort and reward at work has also been found to have a mediating role in the higher prevalence of depressive symptoms in lower occupational classes.[378]

Under the broad heading of working conditions we also need to consider unemployment and precarious employment. These conditions are more common in lower socioeconomic groups.[379] The health effects of unemployment have been a long-standing issue for scientific debate, partly because there is strong selection of unhealthy persons out of employment. Such selection is, however, less pronounced during mass unemployment, and several studies have used this insight to look at health consequences during and after episodes of mass unemployment. It appears that deep recessions do cause excess mortality among those who experience unemployment, for instance from suicide, alcohol-related conditions, and cardiovascular diseases, in particular if the unemployed have a low education.[380–382] Moreover, precarious employment, high job insecurity, and wages that are low or perceived to be unfairly paid are associated with elevated risks of stress-related disorders.[379]

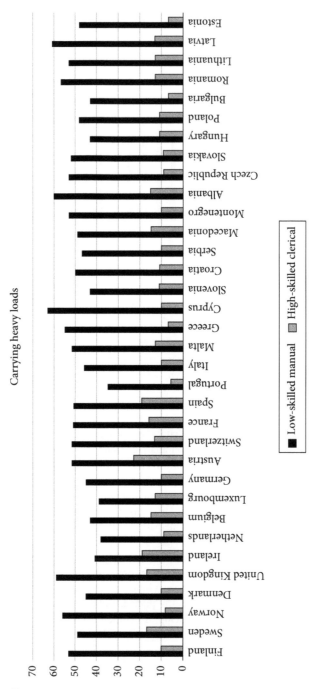

Carrying heavy loads

(a)

■ Low-skilled manual   ■ High-skilled clerical

(b)

Not able to change order of tasks

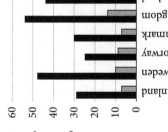

Figure 3.3 Occupational class inequalities in working conditions

Notes: Carrying heavy loads = Q: 'Does your work involve carrying or moving heavy loads?' A: 'Yes, at least ¼ of the time.' Not able to change order of tasks = Q: 'Are you able to choose or change your order of tasks?' A: 'No.' Only two occupational classes shown. Men and women combined.

Source: data from European Working Conditions Survey (https://www.eurofound.europa.eu/data/european-working-conditions-survey, accessed July 2018).

Housing, neighbourhood, wider environment

A third group of factors are the conditions under which people live, both in the immediate sense of quality of housing (e.g. crowding, dampness, and accident risks),[383] and in the more indirect sense of their neighbourhood conditions (access to amenities such as sports facilities and groceries with fresh fruit and vegetables, presence of psychosocial stressors, levels of social capital),[384–386] all of which tend to be less favourable for lower socioeconomic groups. People with a low socioeconomic position also tend to be more exposed to general environmental health risks such as air pollution and toxic waste dumps.[387,388]

Social and psychological factors

Another group of specific determinants which likely contribute to the explanation of health inequalities are non-material factors such as social and psychological factors.

Psychosocial stress

People with a low socioeconomic position on average are exposed to more psychosocial stressors than people with a high socioeconomic position, in the form of more negative life events (e.g. loss of beloved ones or loss of paid work), more 'daily hassles' (e.g. in the form of financial difficulties), and a combination of high demands and low control in life as a whole.[389] At the same time, they also tend to have smaller social networks, lower levels of social support, and less 'social capital' generally,[390] as well as less effective coping styles (e.g. a more external 'locus of control').[391] People with a higher socioeconomic position have a stronger sense of control over their own lives, including their work, and this is associated with healthier behaviour, and lower rates of morbidity and mortality.[392,393]

This combination of a higher exposure to psychosocial stressors and less capacity to remove or buffer these exposures may explain part of the higher frequency of health problems in the lower socioeconomic groups. At least two pathways may be involved. The first is a behavioural pathway: psychosocial stress and other unfavourable psychosocial factors increase the likelihood of unhealthy behaviours, such as smoking, excessive alcohol consumption and lack of physical exercise.[394–397]

The second is a more direct biological pathway. The experience of stress affects the neural, endocrine, and immune systems of the body, and chronic stress may lead to maladaptive responses in the form of, for example, high blood pressure, a prolonged high level of cortisol, higher blood viscosity, or a suppression of the immune response, which may in turn increase the susceptibility to a range of diseases.[398–400] We will further discuss the biological pathways linking low socioeconomic position to ill-health at the end of this paragraph.

Although the evidence suggests that higher exposure to psychosocial stressors, in combination with less capacity to remove or buffer these exposures, has negative health effects, consensus has not yet emerged.[401] If there is an independent health effect of psychosocial factors—which seems plausible—then this may explain part of the higher frequency of health problems in lower socioeconomic groups. This has been best documented for psychosocial factors related to work organization, such as job strain, which have been shown to contribute to socioeconomic inequalities in cardiovascular health, including in mediation analyses.[378] Mediation analyses focusing on the role of psychosocial stressors outside the work environment are less common, but have also suggested a role for psychosocial factors in generating health inequalities.[371,402]

Other non-material factors

The role of non-material factors is not limited to psychosocial stressors and their moderators. Socioeconomic groups differ profoundly in their exposure to a wide range of social, cultural, and psychological factors, use of media like television and the internet, living with a partner, having someone to confide in, loneliness, trust, being religious, feeling depressed, life satisfaction, happiness, etc.[403]

Figure 3.4 shows this for a few examples. The low educated are almost always worse off, but the magnitude of these inequalities differs importantly between European regions. Northern Europe almost always has a lower average prevalence of unfavourable conditions, but relative and/or absolute inequalities are not always smaller than in other European regions, suggesting that the welfare state has probably reduced material inequalities more than non-material inequalities.

Health-related behaviours

The role of health-related behaviours, such as smoking, excessive alcohol consumption, inadequate diet, lack of physical exercise and obesity, in generating health inequalities has been relatively well documented. These are established causal determinants of morbidity and mortality, and are often more prevalent in the lower socioeconomic groups in many high-income countries.[132,404–407] This is also the group of factors for which most formal mediation analyses have been carried out, which generally show that health-related behaviours make substantial contributions to the explanation of health inequalities.[408] Despite the fact that almost all mediation analyses followed the conventional 'difference method', so that we cannot attach too much importance to their quantitative results, a non-trivial role of health-related behaviours in generating health inequalities is highly plausible.

Smoking

By far the most widely available data on a specific determinant of health inequalities relate to smoking. In many European countries cigarette smoking is the leading determinant of health problems. Systematic reviews have shown the prevalence of smoking to differ strongly between socioeconomic groups in many high-income countries,[404,409] particularly among men, and mediation analyses have found that smoking alone accounts for a substantial part of socioeconomic inequalities in mortality.[408,410,411]

There are, however, major differences between European countries in the magnitude of inequalities in smoking, and consequently in the contribution of smoking to inequalities in mortality and other health outcomes.[262,412] As has been shown in a number of comparative studies, inequalities in smoking follow a North-South gradient within Europe, with larger inequalities in the North and smaller (sometimes even 'reverse') gradients in the South.[413,414]

This is particularly clear in the case of women: high educated women smoke considerably less than low educated women in the North of Europe, but the reverse is true in several Southern European countries, such as Portugal, Italy, and Cyprus (Figure 3.5).

Among men, the gap between low and high educated is large in the North and West of Europe, not so much because the prevalence of smoking among the low educated is so high, but primarily because the prevalence among the high educated is so low. The gap is smaller in Spain, Portugal, and Italy, mainly because the prevalence among the high educated is so high. Among women, the gap is small in Southern Europe too, partly because smoking prevalence is low among the low educated, and partly because it is high among the high educated (Figure 3.5).

This all fits with the idea that Southern European countries are in an earlier phase of the 'smoking epidemic', in which smoking among high educated men and women has not yet declined strongly, and in which smoking among low educated women has not yet risen strongly.[409] The concept of the smoking epidemic will be further discussed in section 3.4 'Theories about the explanation of health inequalities'.

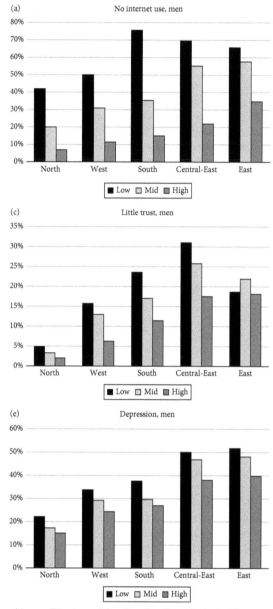

Figure 3.4 Educational inequalities in social, cultural and psychological factors

Notes: The survey questions are given below:

No internet use = Q: 'Personal use of internet/e-mail/www'; A: 'No access' or 'never use'. Not living with partner = Q: 'Lives with husband/wife/partner in same household'; A: No. Little trust = Q: 'Most people can be trusted or you can't be too careful'. A: 0,1,2 on scale of 11. Security values = Positive score on scale consisting of two items: 'It is important to him to live in secure surroundings. He avoids anything that might endanger his safety' and 'It is very important to him that his country be safe from threats from within and without. He is concerned that social order be protected.'. Depression = Q: 'Felt depressed, how often last week'; A: 'Some of the time', 'Most of the time' and 'All or almost all of the time'. "Little life satisfaction = Q: 'How satisfied with life as a whole'; A: 0–4 on a scale from 0–10.

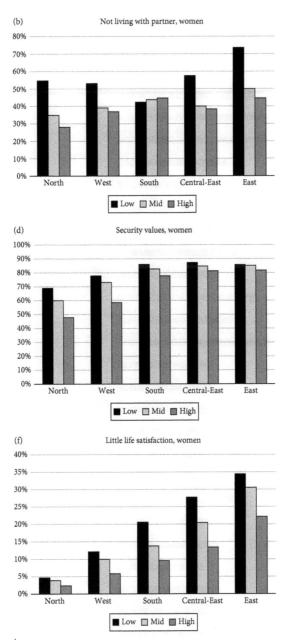

Figure 3.4 Continued

Men and women show similar findings for all variables. Pooled dataset of 25 countries. North = Finland, Sweden, Norway, Iceland, Denmark. West = Austria, Belgium, France, Germany, Ireland, Netherlands, Switzerland, United Kingdom. South = Portugal, Spain, Italy, Greece, Cyprus. Central-East = Croatia, Czech Republic, Hungary, Poland, Slovakia, Slovenia. East = Estonia, Lithuania, Russia, Ukraine.

Source: data from European Social Survey cumulative data file 2002–14 (https://www.europeansocialsurvey.org/data/, accessed 2 April 2017)

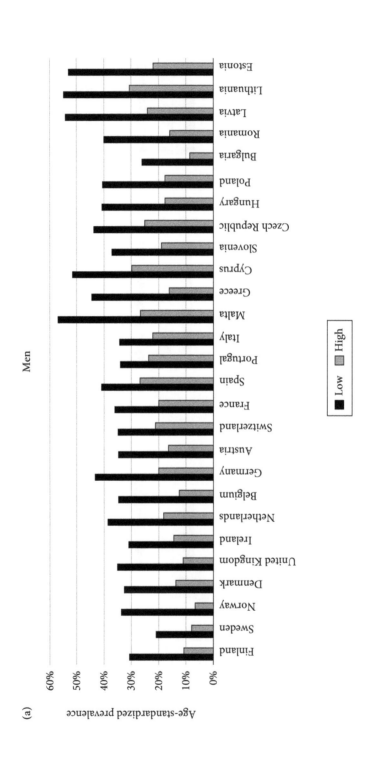

(a)

Men

Age-standardized prevalence

Legend: ■ Low ▨ High

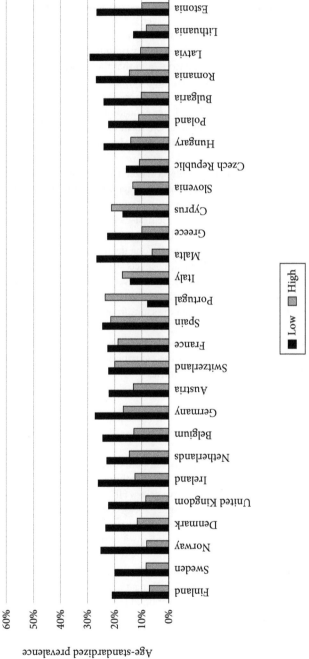

Figure 3.5 Educational inequalities in smoking

Notes: Smoking = current smoking. Data for ca. 2010. Average of 3 surveys, adjusted for average per survey.

Source: dataset constructed in DEMETRIQ/LIFEPATH projects, with harmonized data from European Health Interview Survey, European Social Survey, and National Health Interview Surveys.

Diet, physical activity, and obesity

Men and women in lower socioeconomic groups tend to eat less fresh vegetables and fruits, particularly in the North of Europe. Differences in fresh vegetable and fruit consumption are smaller in the South of Europe, probably because of the larger availability and affordability of vegetables and fruits in Mediterranean countries.[406] Literature reviews have shown that it is likely that many other aspects of diet, such as consumption of meat, dairy products, and various fats and oils, also are socially patterned in many European countries, and that these social patterns differ between countries, reflecting long-standing differences in food culture.[415,416]

Little or no leisure time physical activity tends to be more common in the lower socioeconomic groups. Survey data show that people with a higher education on average have a lot more physical exercise in their leisure time, for example in the form of sports activities. Although people with a lower education used to be more physically active during work, this is no longer the case today.[417,418]

As a result of differences in food intake and physical exercise, overweight and obesity are usually more common in lower socioeconomic groups, but the magnitude (and sometimes even the direction) of these inequalities again differs strongly between countries.[132,419] For example, among men absolute inequalities are small in Scotland and in Central-Eastern and Eastern Europe because of a very high prevalence among the higher educated, whereas among women inequalities are large in Southern Europe because of a very low prevalence among the higher educated (Figure 3.6).

Interestingly, this is one of the very few health aspects where socioeconomic inequalities are larger for women than for men. Women with a higher level of education are far less often overweight or obese than men with the same educational level, probably because they are more worried about their weight than boys and men from the same groups, and more actively try to manage their weight.[132]

Mediation analyses show that inequalities in physical activity and obesity play a role in generating health inequalities,[410,411,420,421] but the contribution of inequalities in obesity to inequalities in health differs strongly between countries.[263]

Excessive alcohol consumption

Excessive alcohol consumption is bad for health too, raising the risk of a wide range of health problems including various cancers, cardiovascular disease, liver cirrhosis, psychiatric disorders, and unintentional and intentional injuries.[422]

As in the case of smoking and obesity, the social patterning of harmful drinking differs between countries and between men and women. Whereas the association between socioeconomic position and *drinking status* is uniformly positive across all countries and genders (i.e. whether one drinks alcohol at all is more common in higher socioeconomic groups), the association between socioeconomic position and *harmful drinking* (either in the form of regular consumption of hazardous amounts exceeding recommended limits, or in the form of heavy episodic or 'binge' drinking) is very heterogeneous.[423,424]

Among men drinking regular hazardous amounts is more frequent in lower socioeconomic groups in some countries (Switzerland, Spain, Hungary, …), but more frequent in higher socioeconomic groups in other countries (Finland, England, Germany, …).[424] Similarly, although heavy episodic drinking is more frequent among men in lower socioeconomic groups in most countries, in some countries (England, France, Czech Republic) the reverse seems to be the case.[423,424] Among women, drinking regular hazardous amounts is uniformly more frequent in higher socioeconomic groups, but heavy episodic drinking is more frequent in higher socioeconomic groups in some countries, and in lower socioeconomic groups in other countries.[423,424]

At the same time, studies consistently show that alcohol-related problems, such as alcohol dependence, social and financial difficulties, and alcohol-related diseases and injuries, are more common in lower socioeconomic groups, even after taking alcohol consumption patterns into account. This may be due to the fact that the risks of harmful drinking can be buffered by a favourable social environment, for example, friends and relatives helping to prevent problems.[257,425] Mediation analyses confirm that excessive alcohol consumption does contribute to the explanation of health inequalities in some countries, but less so in others.[410,411,421]

Determinants of health-related behaviour

The systematic nature of these differences in health-related behaviour clearly demonstrates that these are not only a matter of free choice, but at least partly determined by constraints imposed by conditions beyond the control of the individual. If smoking, eating fruits and vegetables, physical exercise, and excessive drinking were a matter of free choice, one would expect random patterns, not the systematic differences between socioeconomic groups that we have seen in the previous pages.[374]

A lot of research, from various angles, has been done to try to understand why people in lower socioeconomic groups tend to have less healthy behaviour patterns. A recent review identified nine different causal mechanisms that have found empirical support.[426]

Four of these mechanisms are about incentives or motivations for healthy behaviour. The general idea is that people in lower socioeconomic groups have less reason to forego the short-term pleasures of unhealthy behaviour (smoking, sedentary living, over-eating, excessive drinking) in exchange for a long-term gain in longevity because: (i) they face more psychosocial stress that encourages coping through engaging in unhealthy behaviour; (ii) they gain less longevity benefits from healthy behaviour, because they have lower life expectancy anyway; (iii) they have less need to gain prestige by setting themselves apart with healthy behaviour; and (iv) they have less 'health literacy', and thus knowledge of health risks.[426]

Some other mechanisms are about the means to reach health goals. The general idea here is that, even if lower and higher socioeconomic groups would have a similar motivation for healthy behaviour, lower socioeconomic groups would still have more difficulty in realizing their goals, because: (v) they have less self-efficacy, problem-solving skills, ability to process information, and general sense of control needed to overcome obstacles for healthy behaviour; (vi) they have less financial resources for healthy behaviour, as in the case of costly healthy diets and sports; (vii) they have less opportunities in their neighbourhood for healthy behaviour, such as grocery stores with fresh fruits and vegetables and green spaces for leisure-time physical activity; and (viii) they receive less social support and less positive peer influence to promote healthy behaviours.[426]

A ninth mechanism affects both motivations and means: lower socioeconomic groups have (ix) latent traits, such as lower cognitive ability and certain personality characteristics, that are not conducive to healthy behaviour.[426] To this we might add a tenth mechanism: (x) some of these inequalities in health behaviour may be due to reverse causation: as mentioned in section 3.1 'Methodological issues', obesity and excessive alcohol consumption may affect social mobility.

Health care

A final group of contributing factors is health care: if people with a lower socioeconomic position receive less, or lower quality, health care than people with a higher socioeconomic position, this exacerbates the inequalities in health generated by all the other contributing factors. Less use of effective preventive services by lower socioeconomic groups may contribute to a higher incidence or higher case fatality rate of diseases, and less use of effective treatment services may contribute

Men

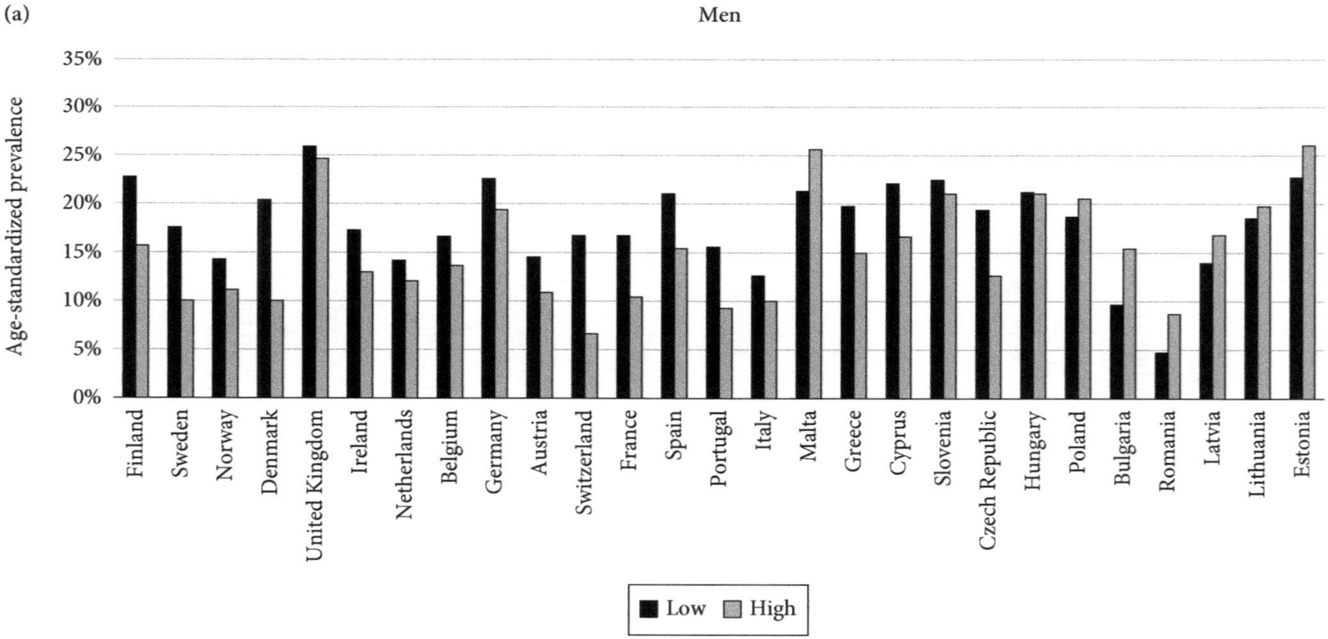

(a)

Age-standardized prevalence

Low ■ High ▨

Finland
Sweden
Norway
Denmark
United Kingdom
Ireland
Netherlands
Belgium
Germany
Austria
Switzerland
France
Spain
Portugal
Italy
Malta
Greece
Cyprus
Slovenia
Czech Republic
Hungary
Poland
Bulgaria
Romania
Latvia
Lithuania
Estonia

0% 5% 10% 15% 20% 25% 30% 35%

(b)

Women

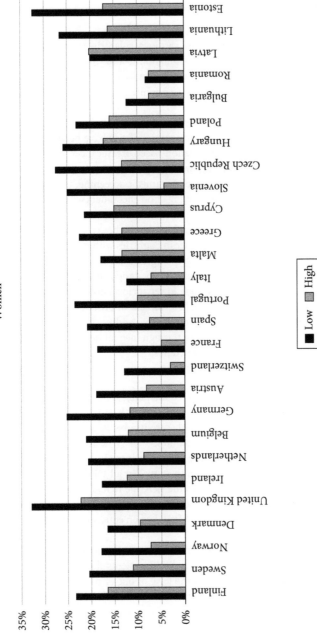

Figure 3.6 Educational inequalities in obesity

Notes: Obesity = Body mass index > 30 kg/m2, calculated from self-reported weight and height. Data for ca. 2010. Average of 3 surveys, adjusted for average per survey.

Source: dataset constructed in DEMETRIQ/LIFEPATH projects, with harmonized data European Health Interview Survey, European Social Survey, and National Health Interview Surveys.

to a lower recovery rate or higher case fatality rate of diseases. There are good reasons to suspect that this plays a role, depending on the degree to which countries have, or have not, eliminated inequalities in access and quality of health care.

Preventive health care

Prevention programmes, such as vaccinations, cardiovascular risk management, and cancer screening, can be very effective in improving population health. In order to avoid inequalities in health outcomes, it is important to implement them in such a way that lower socioeconomic groups participate at the same rate as higher socioeconomic groups, and receive the same quality of care. However, this is not always the case.

Many countries have cancer screening policies, particularly for cervical cancer, breast cancer and colorectal cancer. Of these breast cancer screening policies have been studied most extensively. More and more countries now have population-based breast cancer screening programmes, in which all members of the target group (e.g. women aged 50–75 years) are individually identified and invited to attend screening. However, opportunistic screening, in which invitations depend on the individual's decision to ask for screening or on encounters with health-care providers, has been more common in the past.[427]

Women from higher socioeconomic groups tend to have higher rates of participation in breast cancer screening, but these inequalities are smaller in countries with population-based screening than in countries with opportunistic screening or regional screening programmes.[428] Within population-based screening programmes, variations in design also affect participation rates. Some designs enhance access to screening among lower socioeconomic groups, such as low cost (free tests and reducing geographical barriers), involvement of primary-care physicians, and individually tailored pro-active communication policies that address barriers to screening.[429] It is therefore likely that some screening programmes, through inequalities in participation rates, contribute to a widening of inequalities in health outcomes.

Curative health care

Although most high-income countries have created financing systems that have substantially reduced financial barriers to health care use, these and other barriers have not been completely eliminated and still generate differences in health care use between socioeconomic groups, as shown by an important series of comparative studies.[430–432] The most recent of these studies found 'horizontal inequities' in health care use (i.e. differences in health care use between income groups after adjustment for 'need', or health status) in all OECD countries. Whereas the poor are as likely to see a general practitioner as the rich, the rich are much more likely so see a specialist and a dentist, and to participate in cancer screening.[433] Similar differences in doctor visits and use of a range of preventive services are found when education is used as an indicator of socioeconomic position.[428,434,435]

Although these inequalities are found nearly everywhere, countries differ substantially in their magnitude. Some of these differences are related to health systems characteristics, particularly the extent of public health insurance coverage and the level of out-of-pocket payments for different services. Countries with less public, and more private insurance coverage have larger inequalities in doctor visits, and so do countries with higher out-of-pocket payments.[433]

That financial barriers may play an important role in generating inequalities in health care use, but to a differing extent in different countries, can be seen in Figure 3.7. This shows differences between low and high educated in 'unmet needs for medical care' for financial reasons. In many European countries, the proportion of people reporting such unmet needs is very low, even among people in the lowest income quintile. However, proportions exceeding 5% among those with a low

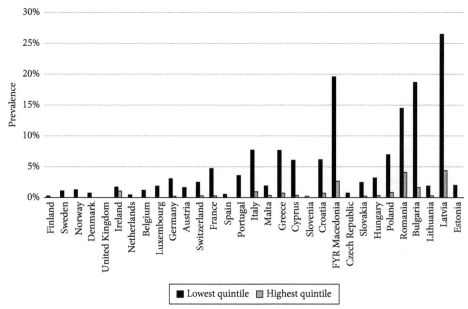

Figure 3.7 Inequalities by income in unmet need for medical care

Notes: Unmet need = self-reported assessment of whether respondent needed medical examination or treatment (dental care excluded), but did not have or seek it, because 'too expensive'. Income in quintiles of equivalized net household income. Data for 2010.

Source: data from EU Statistics on Income and Living Conditions via Eurostat (http://ec.europa.eu/eurostat/data/database; accessed 28 February 2018).

income and large inequalities between income groups are found in several Southern European countries (Italy, Greece, Cyprus) as well as in many Central-Eastern and Eastern European countries.[436] Similar results are found for low versus high education.

Whether these inequalities in health care use generate inequalities in health outcomes depends on the effectiveness of the specific interventions that the services deliver, and are forgone by those who do not use the service. Two separate pieces of evidence suggest that this is indeed the case. First, for many specific interventions inequalities in use favouring people with a higher socioeconomic position have been found in many European countries. These include interventions of proven effectiveness: cardiac revascularization (by coronary bypass grafting or percutaneous coronary intervention),[437] common surgical procedures,[438] statins,[439] various treatments for lung and colorectal cancer,[139,440] diagnosis and control of diabetes mellitus,[441] and many others.

Despite low levels and small inequalities in unmet need (Figure 3.7), these inequalities have also been found in Finland, where they can be studied in detail thanks to the availability of linked administrative databases. The Finnish experience suggests that it is reasonable to expect other Western European countries to have similar inequalities in use of specific therapeutic interventions, and to expect many Southern, Central-Eastern and Eastern European countries to have even larger inequalities in use of specific therapeutic interventions.

Inequalities in health care outcomes

A second type of evidence suggesting that inequalities in health care use generate inequalities in health outcomes is that inequalities in case fatality rates have been found for many diseases, and that these are likely due, at least partly, to inequalities in treatment. European studies of socioeconomic inequalities in survival after myocardial infarction have often found short- and long-term case fatality after the event to be higher among patients with lower socioeconomic position.[135-137] Also, studies of inequalities in cancer survival have almost universally shown case fatality to be higher among patients with lower socioeconomic status[138-140]—a finding that can only partly be explained by inequalities in diagnosis stage or other patient or tumour characteristics, suggesting that inequalities in treatment must also play a role.[442]

Whereas these two pieces of evidence clearly indicate that inequalities in health care play a role in exacerbating inequalities in health, particularly in countries where inequalities in health care access and utilization are large, it is unknown what their quantitative contribution is. Formal mediation analyses are rare and fraught with methodological problems (such as incomplete measurement of non-health care determinants of survival and confounding by indication[443]). The most suggestive (but still indirect) evidence comes from studies of inequalities in mortality from conditions amenable to medical intervention, such as cerebrovascular disease, tuberculosis, appendicitis and perinatal mortality (see Chapter 4).

Biological mechanisms

Health inequalities can thus be thought of as resulting from differences between socioeconomic groups in a wide range of contributing factors, playing out over the life-course: genetics, childhood environment, material living conditions, social and psychological factors, health-related behaviours, and health care. But before these factors can cause disease, they have to 'get under the skin', to use a popular expression among social epidemiologists.

Embodiment

American social epidemiologist Nancy Krieger has introduced the concept of 'embodiment'— the notion that 'we [human beings] literally embody, biologically, our lived experience', that 'our living bodies tell stories about our lives, whether or not these are ever consciously expressed', and that differences in health status between population groups are the biological expression of social relations.[444 (p. 350)] This is a powerful idea that can potentially capture a wide variety of pathways linking the social to the biological, including the effects of exposure to toxic substances in the work environment, tobacco smoking, major life events, and many other 'social-biological transitions'.[445]

Attention to these biological pathways has increased importantly with the rise of interest in biomarkers, that is, indicators of some biological state or condition that measure exposure to determinants of disease or early harmful effects of such exposures on the body. The rise of interest in biomarkers has been propelled by technological developments in areas such as molecular biology and imaging, which have greatly expanded the scope for measuring the physiological state of the human body.

There must be many different biological pathways linking lower socioeconomic position to ill-health and premature death, but it may well be that some of these pathways have a more generic effect, in the sense that they link several different health outcomes to lower socioeconomic position. The 'embodiment' of psychosocial stress is an important candidate for such a more generic mechanism.

The biological response to psychosocial stress

As mentioned above, the experience of stress affects the neural, endocrine, and immune systems of the body, and chronic stress may lead to maladaptive responses in the form of, for example, high blood pressure, a prolonged high level of cortisol, higher blood viscosity, or a suppression of the immune response, which may in their turn increase the susceptibility to a range of diseases.[398–400]

The neuroendocrine response to psychosocial stressors comes in the form of a fast response mediated by the sympathoadrenal pathway, and a slow response mediated by the hypothalamic-pituitary-adrenal axis. As a result of the first, epinephrine (adrenalin) is released into the bloodstream; as a result of the second, cortisol is released into the bloodstream. This biological stress response is adaptive, but if it is activated for too long or too often it may have deleterious health effects. Because people from lower socioeconomic strata are more exposed to psychosocial stressors, they may suffer more from these deleterious health effects.[399,400]

Both epinephrine and cortisol have a wide range of effects on metabolism, the haemostatic and cardiovascular systems, immunity, and cognitive functioning. These effects have been documented in animal studies, and to some extent in human studies, but it is not yet clear what the quantitative contribution of such mechanisms is to the explanation of inequalities in health. Evidence encompassing complete pathways from socioeconomic status through neuroendocrine responses to ill-health is still rare.[446]

Some of it comes from the British Whitehall study, which found strong socioeconomic gradients in prevalence of the 'metabolic syndrome', that is, a combination of impaired glucose tolerance, lipid abnormalities, and central obesity. These gradients could only partly be explained by conventional risk factors such as smoking, obesity, and other behavioural factors, and were partly explained by socioeconomic differences in exposure to job stress. This suggests that there is a separate biological pathway running from low socioeconomic position through psychosocial stress and metabolic factors to heart disease, diabetes, and other chronic conditions.[446]

Allostatic load

The idea that chronic life stress, in various forms, leads to physiological dysregulation and thereby to poor mental and physical health has been more fully developed in the theory of 'allostasis' and 'allostatic load'. 'Allostasis' is the adaptive process that maintains stability or 'homeostasis' of the body during exposure to physical and psychological stressors, and while this is critical to survival it also carries a cost, that is, 'allostatic load' which is defined as the 'cumulative physiological burden exacted on the body through attempts to adapt to life's demands'.[447]

This is commonly operationalized with a battery of biological parameters, not only including indicators of neuroendocrine activity (e.g. epinephrine, cortisol) but also metabolic factors (e.g. cholesterol, glucose, obesity), cardiovascular factors (e.g. blood pressure, heart rate), and biomarkers relating to the immune system and inflammatory processes (e.g. interleukins, C-reactive protein).[448,449] Cumulative scores of these biomarkers appear to predict mortality, as well as declines in cognitive and physical functioning, independent of other factors.[449]

Socioeconomic gradients in allostatic load have been found in many countries, with lower socioeconomic groups having higher cumulative scores.[448] These gradients, together with the general rise of allostatic load with age, have been interpreted as indicating differences between socioeconomic groups in 'wear and tear' of their bodies, with lower socioeconomic groups accumulating allostatic load over their life course at a higher rate than lower socioeconomic groups.[450] In one study from the United States, allostatic load explained about a third of educational inequalities in mortality.[451] Of course, socioeconomic inequalities in allostatic load are themselves a result of differences between socioeconomic groups in material, psychosocial and behavioural factors.[452]

3.4 **Theories about the explanation of health inequalities**

Scientific explanation

The available evidence thus suggests that health inequalities can partly be explained by differential exposure over the life-course to a range of well-known health determinants, and that these factors are ultimately 'embodied' by various biological pathways. It would be useful if these insights could be integrated into a general scientific theory of how health inequalities arise, for example along the lines of the famous 'covering law model' of German philosopher Carl Hempel (1905–97). He proposed that scientific explanation should consist of creating a logical argument leading from a set of 'general laws' and 'initial conditions' to the 'phenomenon to be explained'. For example: Newton's general law of gravitation and the fact that the apple is cut loose from the tree, together explain why the apple falls towards the ground.[453]

This model suggests that we should try to find one or more 'general laws' and 'initial conditions' that help us to understand why people with a lower socioeconomic position tend to have more health problems and to die at an earlier age than people with a higher socioeconomic position. To give an example that we will encounter in a more elaborate form later on: health inequalities (the 'phenomenon to be explained') arise because all human beings are evolutionarily programmed to avoid illness and death (the 'general law') and because people with a lower socioeconomic position have less means of avoiding illness and death (the 'initial conditions').

In this section we will review a number of attempts at such a more general understanding of how health inequalities arise, including why they are so persistent. Although a single, comprehensive, and commonly accepted scientific theory of health inequalities does not exist, a number of theories have been proposed that try to explain health inequalities at a more general level of understanding than in terms of the distribution of a shorter or longer list of contributing factors (Table 3.1). None of these theories is mutually exclusive, and it may well be that several, or even all of them, capture a relevant part of reality.

The theories have been classified in four groups, depending on their main focus: selection into socioeconomic groups, differential health progress, social disadvantage, and social production of disease. The order in which the theories are presented is not entirely arbitrary: in this order they go from a more 'benign' attribution of health inequalities to social selection (e.g. 'health inequalities are mainly the result of differences in composition of socioeconomic groups, and have little or nothing to do with the extent of social inequality in a society') to a more 'conflictual' attribution to the social production of disease (e.g. 'health inequalities ultimately result from abuses of power and privilege by the higher socioeconomic groups').

In the column labelled 'proposed explanation for health inequalities' we have tried to summarize each theory in three statements: something resembling a general law (e.g. 'medical care helps to lower morbidity and mortality'), one or more initial conditions (e.g. 'due to market forces the supply of medical care is inversely proportional to need') and the phenomenon to be explained (, '[as a result,] higher socioeconomic groups have lower morbidity and mortality').

Theory focusing on selection into socioeconomic groups

The main thrust of this theory is that health inequalities are at least partly due to selection factors, either in the form of health-related selection or reverse causation (i.e. health determining entry into and/or exit from socioeconomic groups) or 'indirect selection' or confounding (i.e. personal characteristics such as cognitive ability and personality traits determining entry into and/or exit from socioeconomic groups).

As we saw in section 3.2 'Education, occupation, income, and health', these mechanisms do plausibly play a role in generating health inequalities by education, occupational class, and income,

Table 3.1 General theories explaining health inequalities

Group	Name of theory	Scientific origins, proponent(s), selected references	Proposed explanation for health inequalities
I. Selection into socioeconomic groups	Social selection	Michael Young[57] Patrick West[230] Johan Mackenbach[236]	Personal characteristics like cognitive ability and personality traits determine whether people can effectively use opportunities for health improvement. In modern societies, people are socially mobile, and 'sorted' into socioeconomic groups based on their personal characteristics. As a result, higher socioeconomic groups have better health.
II. Differential health progress	Diffusion of innovations	Eugene Rogers[454] Alan Lopez[455]	Health improvements often result from the adoption of new behaviours, and due to their tendency for earlier uptake of new ideas higher socioeconomic groups are usually the first to adopt new behaviours. As a result, the higher socioeconomic groups are also the first to benefit from most health improvements.
	Cultural capital	Pierre Bourdieu[456] Thomas Abel[457]	Cultural resources, such as beliefs, preferences and knowledge, affect health because health improvement is driven by lifestyle changes, and inequalities in such 'cultural capital' are still large in modern societies' socioeconomic groups. As a result, higher socioeconomic groups have better health.
	Inverse equity	Cesar Victora[458]	Health improvements often result from the introduction of new interventions, and due to a relative absence of cultural, geographical and financial barriers to the uptake of new interventions higher socioeconomic groups are usually the first to use them. As a result, the higher socioeconomic groups are also the first to benefit from most health improvements.
III. Social disadvantage	Inverse care law	Julian Tudor Hart[459]	Medical care helps to lower morbidity and mortality, but due to market forces the supply of medical care is still inversely proportional to need, i.e. lower in more disadvantaged areas. As a result, higher socioeconomic groups have lower morbidity and mortality.

(continued)

Table3.1 Continued

Group	Name of theory	Scientific origins, proponent(s), selected references	Proposed explanation for health inequalities
	Neo-materialism	Black Report[20] John Lynch[460] George Davey Smith[461]	Material resources, both at the individual and community level, are important for health, and due to the way material resources are distributed in society higher socioeconomic groups still have more of them. As a result, higher socioeconomic groups also accumulate less health-damaging exposures and experience over their life-course and have better health.
	Psychosocial environment	John Cassel[462] Michael Marmot[463] Richard Wilkinson[464]	A lower relative position in society, and the perception of the associated inequalities in prestige and access to resources, affects health by giving rise to psychosocial stress, and differences in relative social position are still large in modern societies. As a result, higher socioeconomic groups have better health.
IV. Social production of disease	Fundamental causes	Stanley Lieberson[465] Bruce Link[466] Jo Phelan[467]	A higher socioeconomic position provides the individual with flexible resources, such as knowledge, money, power, prestige, and beneficial social connections, which can be used to avoid disease risks or to minimize the consequences of disease once it occurs, regardless of the prevailing disease and risk factor profile. As a result, higher socioeconomic groups have better health.
	Political economy of health	Lesley Doyal[468] Vicente Navarro[469] Nancy Krieger[470]	Inequalities in political and economic power in society produce inequalities in the material and social conditions under which people live and work, and these conditions structure their exposure to health risks and opportunities for health improvement. As a result, higher socioeconomic groups have better health.

and what this theory claims is that trends and differences in the magnitude of health inequalities can also be understood in part from trends and differences in the rates of social mobility, or in the degree of selectivity on health or personal characteristics of social mobility, or both. To be more precise: that more social mobility, and more selectivity during social mobility, leads to larger health inequalities, all other things being equal.

The idea originates with British medical sociologist Patrick West, who 're-thinking the health selection explanation for health inequalities' emphasized the important role of education in determining intergenerational social mobility, and proposed a central role in the generation of health inequalities for the 'attitudes, experiences or behaviours [...] associated with different [educational] aspirations or orientations which […] have consequences for future mobility trajectories [and] are correlated with health.[230] (p. 380)

Social mobility and health inequalities

Building on these ideas, it has been proposed that selection during intergenerational social mobility might explain the persistence of health inequalities over time despite the inequalities-dampening effects of the welfare state, because intergenerational social mobility has increased over time, and has probably become more selective with regard to health-relevant personal characteristics, particularly in countries with generous welfare arrangements.[13]

Trends in social mobility have been studied extensively, and there is no doubt that intergenerational social mobility has increased in all European countries, in the sense that birth cohorts born around the middle of the twentieth century have been more socially mobile, particularly upwardly mobile, than earlier born birth cohorts. This applies to both education and occupational class, and is the result, quite simply, of changes in the overall distribution of education and occupational class in the population.[471]

Due to educational expansion and economic modernization, the proportion of people with a higher level of education and a non-manual occupational class has increased in all European populations, and this upward shift in educational and occupational levels has implied, and even required, substantial upward mobility of children as compared to their parents. Stratification sociologists call this 'absolute mobility', and it has increased between birth cohorts born in the beginning, and those born around the middle of the twentieth century in all European countries.[471]

It is also likely that intergenerational social mobility has become more selective with regard to individual characteristics that are relevant for health, but here the evidence is only indirect, and based on the weakening association between the socioeconomic position of parents and that of their children. It used to be the case that parents' socioeconomic position (in terms of education, occupational class, income) was a strong predictor of their children's socioeconomic position. This leaves little scope for selection on children's personal characteristics that may predispose them for illness later in their lives, or will keep them healthy.

However, this association has weakened over time, as is clear from studies which have shown that 'relative mobility', or 'social fluidity' (i.e. upward or downward mobility net of changes in the overall distribution of education and occupational class in the population) has increased over time. Although a famous study by Swedish sociologist Robert Erikson and John Goldthorpe found relative mobility rates to be more or less constant over time,[59] a more recent and more detailed study by British sociologist Richard Breen found an increase in social fluidity, in terms of both educational and occupational class mobility, for birth cohorts born between the 1920s and 1960s in many European countries (with stagnation thereafter).[472] This was probably facilitated by structural changes in the economy and educational expansion, but also helped by educational reforms aiming at an equalization of opportunities for higher education.[473]

Whereas trends in intergenerational social mobility may partly explain the persistence of health inequalities over time, differences between countries in social mobility may partly explain why some countries have larger health inequalities than others. Relative intergenerational mobility—whether classified by education, occupational class or income—has been lower-than-average in Southern Europe, France, and Germany, and higher-than-average in the Nordic countries, the Netherlands, and (post-)communist countries in Central-Eastern and Eastern Europe, with the United Kingdom in-between.[474,475] This may help to understand why the Nordic countries have larger health inequalities than expected on the basis of the magnitude of their inequalities in poverty and other material living conditions.[476] We will further investigate this mechanism in Chapter 4.

Meritocracy

To some extent, modern societies have become 'meritocracies', in which a person's educational and occupational achievement is no longer dependent on family background but on his or her own talents and efforts, and thus on personal characteristics like cognitive ability and personality.[477] Because these personal characteristics are also important for health, for example, because they influence health-related behaviour, inequalities in health probably have increased as a consequence. The tragedy thus is that in modern societies social inequality has found new ways to sustain and reproduce itself, and that old forms of disadvantage have partly been replaced by new forms of disadvantage, in the disguise of personal characteristics like cognitive ability and personality.

It is important to remind ourselves that the term 'meritocracy' was coined by British sociologist Michael Young 1915–2002), not to *celebrate* but to *criticize* the increasing dependence of educational achievement on intelligence, and the emergence of a new elite based on very narrow selection criteria.[57] However, although European societies have indeed become more meritocratic, the association between parental socioeconomic position and children's socioeconomic positions has not disappeared, and there is still intergenerational transmission of earnings and wealth, due to cultural transmission of savings behaviour, genetic inheritance of cognitive skills and other determinants of economic success, and direct bequests of money.[478]

Also, and paradoxically, educational achievement now explains more of the association between social origin and occupational class than in the past, due to the fact that parents in higher occupational classes are better able to let their children succeed in the educational system. In this way, meritocratization is actually amplifying inequality in occupational position by social origin.[472]

Theories focusing on differential health progress

The main thrust of these theories is that the persistence of health inequalities is due to the fact that health is continually improving, but at different speeds in lower and higher socioeconomic groups. According to American economist and Nobel laureate Angus Deaton 'inequality is the handmaiden of progress', and both economic and health progress are often accompanied by a widening of inequalities, both between and within countries.[479] The 'diffusion of innovations', 'cultural capital', and 'inverse equity' theories offer different but overlapping explanations for this phenomenon.

Diffusion of innovations

Studies of the 'diffusion of innovations' have found that people with a higher socioeconomic position often are early adopters of new behaviours in many fields, only later to be followed by people with a lower social position.[454] This also applies to many health-related behaviours, such as cigarette smoking. The higher socioeconomic groups were the first to take up the new habit, but also the first to stop, and as a result the declining phase of the smoking epidemic is often accompanied by widening inequalities in smoking. A 'model of the cigarette epidemic' has been proposed which describes the diffusion of smoking behaviour through populations in four stages.[455]

In stage 1, smoking is an exceptional behaviour and mainly a habit of men, particularly from higher socioeconomic groups. In stage 2, smoking becomes ever more common, and is now also picked up by women in higher socioeconomic groups and by men in lower socioeconomic groups. In stage 3, prevalence rates among men start to decrease since many men stop smoking, especially those who are better off, but women reach their peak rate only later during this stage.[455] In stage 4, smoking rates keep declining for both men and women, and smoking becomes concentrated in lower socioeconomic groups.[x]

This descriptive model more or less fits the European experience, including the reversal from a positive to a negative association between socioeconomic status and smoking found in many

European countries.[413,414,480] The underlying mechanism may indeed be a delay in the diffusion of new behaviour, but other factors, such as lack of effectiveness of health education efforts among lower socioeconomic groups, may also have played a role.

In the case of obesity the higher socioeconomic groups also historically were the first to become overweight, but as a clear decline has not yet set in we do not know whether a similar widening will occur.[132] In some developing countries, obesity is still more common among people of higher socioeconomic position, and with economic development the burden of overweight gradually shifts towards lower socioeconomic groups.[481] This illustrates that processes of diffusion of behaviour, such as dietary habits and physical exercise, may play a role here too, but that these are conditioned by the availability of food and the necessity of physical exercise.

Cultural capital

Another approach to the understanding of behaviour, and behaviour change, is to acknowledge the fact that behaviour, whether healthy or unhealthy, can act as a status symbol: the choice of a particular 'lifestyle' signals to others that one belongs to a particular social class. This may apply to eating habits, language use, leisure activities, musical preferences, and many other aspects of everyday culture.

French sociologist Pierre Bourdieu (1930–2002) has given a classic description of these differences in his book 'Distinction; a social critique of the judgement of taste', and was also the first to apply this idea to preferences with regard to body shape and size. He found that people with a higher socioeconomic position were more likely to consume lean and light food products, and viewed thinness as an image of success and willpower, whereas lower socioeconomic groups were more concerned with the strength of the body. He even saw the human body as 'the most indisputable materialization of class taste'.[456 (p. 190)]

Many differences in behaviour, and underlying differences in the social prestige of behaviour, show a distinct dynamic. Aspects of 'lifestyle' in modern societies are often first adopted by the higher social classes, and only later become more widely distributed. At that moment, however, they lose their distinctive character, and it becomes attractive for the higher social classes to abolish the behaviour and/or to search for new sources of distinction. This phenomenon is also known under various other names, such as 'sinking cultural goods' (a term popular in continental Europe that was introduced by German folklorist Hans Naumann (1886–1951)) and 'trickle-down effect' (a concept more popular in the English-speaking world).[482]

For example, until the end of the nineteenth century, eating too much and exercising too little were reserved for the wealthy, but they were taken over by the less privileged when food became available in abundance and the necessity for physical labour disappeared. The well-to-do then found a new source of distinction in a new cultural norm of paying attention to their weight and trying to remain slim.[132]

People from different socio-economic groups also differ in what they find 'tasty': the taste preferences of people from lower socio-economic groups have been characterized as a 'taste of necessity', instead of a 'taste of luxury'.[483] The higher socioeconomic groups try to distinguish themselves by emphasizing the health aspect in their diet, while the lower socioeconomic groups tend to attach more value to recently acquired luxury products such as white bread, meat, sweets, and snacks. This is not only a confirmation of Bourdieu's theories, but also a reminder of times that food abundance was not yet normal.[xi]

Such cultural differences also apply to preferences in body size, particularly among women who are more subject to these aesthetic standards than men.[132] The interaction between cultural differences and sex-specific aesthetic norms may explain why being overweight among women shows a stronger correlation with socio-economic status than among men (section 3.3 'Six groups of contributing factors').

Differences between socioeconomic groups in preferences do not only depend on their economic resources, but may also depend on their cultural resources or 'cultural capital'. The concept of cultural capital was introduced by Bourdieu to denote 'widely shared, high status cultural signals (attitudes, preferences, formal knowledge, behaviours, goods, and credentials) used for social and cultural exclusion'.[484]

In the context of health inequalities, this theory explains inequalities in health-related behaviour from differences between socioeconomic groups in attitude, knowledge, and competency which are transmitted from one generation to the next.[457] Empirical studies suggest that differences in cultural capital indeed partly explain socioeconomic inequalities in dietary patterns,[485] physical activity,[486] and body weight.[487]

Applying this perspective to the paradox of persisting health inequalities, two questions arise. Did the welfare state reduce inequalities in cultural capital? This seems unlikely,[488] and persistence of inequalities in cultural capital may then partly explain persistence of health inequalities. Did the welfare state have an effect on the need for 'social distinction' on the basis of health-related behaviour? Well, it may have had. Due to the decline in opportunities to distinguish oneself by outward signs of material prosperity, the need for distinction on the basis of non-material signals like leisure-time physical exercise, a slim body or eating quinoa may well have increased.

Inverse equity

The 'inverse equity' hypothesis postulates that 'new interventions will initially reach those of higher socioeconomic status and only later affect the poor [...] which results in an early increase in inequity ratios'. It predicts that after introduction of a new intervention, if there are cultural, geographical, or financial barriers to access, health inequalities will first increase and then decline when the intervention gradually reaches the most deprived groups, after the coverage among the most privileged groups has already reached 100%.[458]

It is based on a line of reasoning similar to that of the diffusion of innovations theory described above, but focuses on the emergence of inequalities in the use of preventive or curative health care during periods of introduction of new interventions or services, which may be due to differences in both access and uptake. Since its publication in 2000 this hypothesis has frequently been tested, mostly but not exclusively in low- and middle-income settings, and mostly with positive results.[489]

For example, in a worldwide analysis of the increase in hospital (instead of home) births, the magnitude of inequalities in hospital deliveries followed a striking curvilinear pattern: up to a national coverage rate of 50% socioeconomic inequalities increased, because of early adoption by the wealthy, and after this point had been passed inequalities declined again, because the poor also began to give birth in hospitals.[489]

The inverse equity hypothesis has less often been tested in a high-income setting, but it is easy to imagine that a combination of delayed access to new preventive and curative health care interventions, and delayed adoption of new health-promoting behaviours, partly explains inequalities in health improvements seen in so many European countries over the past decades.

Theories focusing on social disadvantage

The main thrust of theories focusing on social disadvantage is that health inequalities reflect, in a straightforward manner, inequalities in general living conditions which determine exposure to a wide range of disease risks, and that the persistence of health inequalities is due to the persistence of inequalities in living conditions. The theories differ, however, in the sort of living conditions which they claim to be the most important.

The 'inverse care law'

When in the United Kingdom it became obvious that the National Health Service had not elim-inated inequalities in mortality by occupational class, and people started to search for possible explanations, it soon became clear that inequalities in health care utilization had not disappeared at all. On the contrary, 'higher income groups know how to make better use of the service; they tend to receive more specialist attention; occupy more of the beds in better equipped and staffed hospitals; receive more elective surgery' etc.[490] (cited in 459,p. 405)

Although financial barriers to access had largely been removed, the availability of good medical care differed importantly between areas, with general practitioners in more disadvantaged areas where most sickness and death occurs 'having more work, larger lists, less hospital support, [...] and hospital doctors shoulder[ing] heavier case-loads with fewer staff and equipment, more ob-solete buildings, and suffer[ing] recurrent crises in the availability of beds and replacement staff'. This has since become known as the 'inverse care law': due to the fact that market forces still operate even in a National Health Service, 'the availability of good medical care tends to vary in-versely with the need of the population served'.[459] (p. 412)

This idea was a source of inspiration for the 'inverse equity' hypothesis described above, and could be generalized to include all services and benefits provided by the welfare state. Even when services and benefits are targeted to lower socioeconomic groups, those who are relatively better off, and thus are in less need, usually find it more easy to access the services and receive the benefits.

Neo-materialism

On various occasions we have already mentioned the Black report.[20] The writers of this report not only discussed the relative merits of 'causation' and 'selection' explanations, but also discussed the relative importance of various specific explanations, particularly behavioural and 'materialist' factors, concluding that the latter were the most important.[20]

The idea that material living conditions are still important determinants of health, and im-portant contributors to health inequalities, has sometimes been called a 'neo-material' or 'neo-materialist' interpretation.[460] In contrast to explanations of health inequalities in behavioural or psychosocial terms, neo-materialist explanations emphasize the role of negative exposures (such as occupational risks and unfavourable housing conditions) and lack of resources (such as money and power) held by individuals, as well as the macro-level determinants of material living conditions (such as underinvestment in public infrastructure and services) in generating health inequalities.[460]

Many of the factors contributing to health inequalities that we reviewed in the previous para-graph can be seen as at least partly determined by the material living conditions of people with lower and higher socioeconomic positions.

Psychosocial environment

Neo-materialist explanations were partly emphasized as a critique on psychosocial explanations, which during the 1990s and early 2000s had a lot of traction in the scientific literature. One strand of research, described in section 3.3 'Six groups of contributing factors', focused on the role of psy-chosocial stress and the behavioural and biological mechanisms converting stress into ill-health and premature death.

Another strand of research, already briefly mentioned in section 1.3 'The need for a broader picture', focused on the association between income inequality and average population health which was brought to the attention of a wide readership, both professional and lay, by Richard Wilkinson.[40,41,464] In the course of his research and writing Wilkinson has offered several possible explanations for this relationship, but in his widely sold book 'The Spirit Level; why greater equality makes societies stronger' as well as in his most recent book 'The inner level' (both written with Kate Pickett) his main explanations are psychosocial.[41,491]

In his view, wide income inequalities, and wide social inequalities more generally, lead to loss of self-esteem and social insecurity among the worse off, as well as to feelings of inferiority and shame, to status anxiety, and loss of social trust. A person's relative position in the hierarchy of society has a crucial effect on his or her psychosocial well-being, and these psychosocial effects may then generate a wide variety of health effects, from illicit drug use to obesity, and from mental ill-health to premature death.[41,491]

There is indeed some evidence that 'status anxiety', i.e. the degree to which people are concerned with their social status and with status competition, is higher in countries with more income inequality, not only among people with lower incomes but also among people with higher incomes,[492] which—as Wilkinson and Pickett speculate—could lead to higher levels of stress and a range of unfavourable health outcomes throughout society.[491]

In a similar vein of reasoning, but with a stronger focus on health inequalities, Michael Marmot in his book 'Status Syndrome; how social standing affects our health and longevity', has hypothesized that the main mechanism linking lower socioeconomic position to ill-health and premature death is lack of control. In his view, how much control people have over their lives is crucial for their well-being and longevity, and it is the inequality in degrees of autonomy, power, and control that ultimately generates health inequalities.[463]

Empirical studies have found some support for these psychosocial theories. For example, a lower perceived social rank is associated with higher allostatic load,[493] and inequalities in (perceived) control explain part of inequalities in mortality.[494] These psychosocial theories may also help to explain the persistence of health inequalities in modern welfare states: it is easy to imagine that the welfare state has been more effective in reducing inequalities in material living conditions, than in reducing inequalities in status and power within societies.

Theories focusing on the social production of disease

Theories of 'social production of disease' come in different forms, but in common they emphasize the social origin of health inequalities. Instead of focusing on the differences in exposure, or behavior, or care access between people with a lower and higher socioeconomic position, they focus on how these differences come about. These inequalities in exposure, or behavior, or care access are not regarded as natural phenomena, but are seen as 'produced' by human action.[470]

Fundamental causes

A popular, but very general, framework for integrating much of the evidence on the explanation of health inequalities is the 'fundamental causes' theory, proposed by American social epidemiologists Bruce Link and Jo Phelan. This theory is based on the idea that the social forces underlying social stratification are the ultimate causes of health inequalities, and that these provide a better explanation for health inequalities and their persistence, than differences in proximal risk factors such as smoking, working conditions, stressful life events, etc. The general idea is that as long as social inequality persists, health inequality will also persist.

According to the fundamental causes theory the persistence of health inequalities over time and across different national contexts is due to the fact that a higher socioeconomic status provides people with 'flexible resources'. These include 'knowledge, money, power, prestige, and beneficial social connections' which can be used 'to avoid disease risks or to minimize the consequences of disease once it occurs' regardless of the prevailing circumstances.[466] (p. 487) The association between socioeconomic status and health then 'is reproduced over time via the replacement of intervening mechanisms', and when opportunities for avoiding or treating disease continue to expand, as they have consistently done over the past decades, health inequalities will continue to exist.[467] (p. 629)

The fundamental causes theory thus gives a central role to the 'actionability' of health problems, and to purposive action or 'health-directed human agency'. Socioeconomic differences in the availability of the means to take advantage of this 'actionability' (by behaviour change, accessing health care, getting protection from occupational risks, applying road safety measures, ...) are the crucial factor on which the fundamental relationship between socioeconomic status and health rests.[495]

The mechanism posited in this theory thus emphasizes the role of the individual who disposes (or not, in the lower socioeconomic groups) over material and non-material resources which help him or her to protect and promote health. The theory is about purposive action with different means: the assumption is that all people, regardless of their socioeconomic position, pursue good health, but that they differ in their means to achieve this goal.[496]

This may well be true to some extent, but as others have argued 'differences in means among purposive agents do not account for all the [...] ways that socioeconomic status causes health'. For example, the fact that car drivers with a lower level of education less often put on their seat belts cannot be explained by differences in access to the 'resource' of seat belts, because all cars nowadays have seat belts.[496] (p. 72)

The suggestion has thus been made to expand the fundamental causes theory to include several other mechanisms: (i) 'Spill-overs within socioeconomic groups'. Even if they do not have the intention to pursue good health as an individual, people with a higher socioeconomic position will still benefit from the purposive action of other individuals in the same group, for example, because their neighbours campaign for a safer neighbourhood. (ii) Different preferences for health. People with a higher higher socioeconomic position 'may exhibit a stronger and more consistent preference for future good health than others', for example, because of different time horizons or as part of a common culture. (iii) Different treatment by institutions. Schools, medical care facilities and other public institutions may treat people from lower and higher socioeconomic status differently, which may result in different health outcomes, independent from the individual health-directed agency postulated in the original version of the fundamental causes theory.[xii]

Political economy of health

Nancy Krieger has criticized epidemiology for a lack of attention to theory, and has criticized the available epidemiological theories for a lack of attention to human agency. Of one well-known epidemiological model of the causes of disease, the so-called 'web of causation' which maps all known determinants of a disease as independent factors, she has rhetorically asked: 'where is the spider?', that is, where is the human agency that has created the exposure to all these health determinants?[497]

To some extent this criticism also applies to the theories discussed so far: these are silent on how inequalities in material and non-material resources are generated, and on who benefits from these inequalities. This is even true for the fundamental causes theory, which does not specify how the inequalities in 'flexible resources' come about. If we want to understand why health inequalities are so persistent, we also need to ask whose interests these health inequalities, and the inequalities in their determinants, serve.[470]

Several such theories have been proposed, and most have an explicitly Marxist perspective emphasizing the role of the economic and political context in generating health inequalities. For example, in an early attempt to identify the possible links between capitalism and health inequalities, several different pathways were explored and illustrated, such as the link between 'the imperatives of capital accumulation' and the need for shift work and use of dangerous chemicals in the workplace, the link between income and housing inequalities, and the 'contradiction between the pursuit of health and the pursuit of profits'.[468]

Spanish sociologist Vicente Navarro, a Marxist scholar of health and health inequalities, has published widely on the role of economic and political power relations in generating health inequalities. His empirical work has found that political parties with egalitarian ideologies tend to implement redistributive policies, and that policies aimed at reducing social inequalities, such as welfare and labour market policies, reduce (average) infant mortality and increase life expectancy at birth.[469,498]

In Chapter 5 we will return to Marxist and other viewpoints on the ultimate causes of social inequality.

Key points

- Research into the explanation of health inequalities has advanced rapidly over the past decades, but recent methodological advances have created uncertainty about the validity of some of the results. This applies particularly to applications of the counterfactual approach to causality (where quasi-experimental studies have tended to cast doubt on the causality of the relationship between socioeconomic position and health) and to advances in mediation analysis (which have cast doubt on the validity of previous estimates of the contribution of specific determinants to health inequalities).

- At the current state of our knowledge, it seems highly likely that there is a causal effect of education on health, and that the observed association between education and health is therefore partly (but not wholly) due to such a causal effect. It is also likely that there is a causal effect of parental income on children's health, and while there is no evidence for an effect of modest changes in income on adult health, it is plausible that larger changes in income, particularly at the low end of the income distribution and particularly in countries with lower average incomes, do have an effect on adult health. It is unclear whether there is a causal effect of occupational class on health.

- Six groups of specific health determinants play a role in the explanation of health inequalities, by linking the 'social' to the 'biological' throughout an individual's life-course in mutually reinforcing ways: genetics, childhood environment, material living conditions, social and psychological factors, health-related behaviours, and health care.

- Nine theories propose a more general explanation of health inequalities and their persistence: 'social selection', 'diffusion of innovations', 'cultural capital', 'inverse equity', 'inverse care law', 'neo-materialism', 'psychosocial environment', 'fundamental causes' and 'political economy of health'. While all theories are likely to cover at least part of reality, only the last two emphasize the social origin of health inequalities.

Chapter 4

Patterns of health inequalities explained

4.1 Set-up of the analyses

Three mechanisms

In this chapter we will have another look at the macro-level patterns of health inequalities in Europe. Building upon the insights gained in Chapter 3, we will show that three interrelated mechanisms play a role in the persistence of health inequalities: changes in social stratification, social mobility, and composition of socioeconomic groups (section 4.2 'Changes in social stratification'); health improvements occurring at a faster speed in higher socioeconomic groups (section 4.3 'Rapid but differential health improvements'), partly due to 'differential' effects of the factors driving national health improvement (section 4.4 'Differential effects of factors driving population health change'); and continued social patterning of individual-level health determinants (section 4.5 'Continued social patterning of health determinants'). In a final section we will apply our findings to explain why health inequalities are larger in some European countries than in others (section 4.6 'Understanding the European experience').

Macro-level analyses and their pros and cons

The data sources and analytical methods used in this chapter are briefly explained in Box 4.1. Whereas Chapter 3 was a review of the literature, which mainly consists of 'microscopic' studies with individuals as units of observation, this chapter is based on 'macroscopic' studies in which we exploit variations in the magnitude of health inequalities between European countries.

Macro-level studies have some obvious drawbacks, but also some unique advantages. A first drawback is that what can be studied is limited by the availability of comparable data in a large number of countries—and that therefore many potentially important factors remain out of sight. A second drawback is that these are 'ecological' studies in which whole populations are the units of observation—and that therefore no firm conclusions can be drawn on what drives health inequalities at the individual level.[511]

However, these 'macroscopic' studies also have unique advantages. The first is that they use a much wider range of variation in health inequalities and their determinants than individual-level studies, which are usually conducted within one circumscribed population. The second advantage—mirroring the second drawback—is that they are directly geared to answering a crucial question: what drives health inequalities at the population level? Answering this question helps us to answer the central question of this book: why do health inequalities persist in modern welfare states? Although macro-level studies cannot meet the rigorous standards for establishing causality that individual-level studies can aspire to, they are indispensable for addressing some of these wider questions.

Box 4.1 Set-up of the analyses in chapter 4

Data sources

1. Mortality

We collected and harmonized data on inequalities in mortality for 17 European countries, covering varying points in time between ca. 1980 and ca. 2014 and including around 10 million deaths. Most data stemmed from a longitudinal mortality follow-up after a census, in which socioeconomic information of the population-at-risk and of the deceased was recorded in the census, but for some countries in Central and Eastern Europe data were collected in a cross-sectional unlinked format. Most data covered complete national populations with the exceptions of England and Wales, and France (1% representative samples) and Spain and Italy (Barcelona and Turin only). More information on the mortality data can be found in recently published papers.[197,499,500]

2. Self-reported morbidity

We collected and harmonized data on self-reported health problems from various surveys: National Health Interview Surveys (NHIS; self-assessed health, long-standing health problems; 23 European countries; varying points in time between ca. 1970 and ca. 2012), the European Social Survey (ESS; self-assessed health and activity limitations; 30 European countries; bi-annual waves between 2002 and 2014) and the European Union Statistics on Living Conditions survey (EU-SILC; self-assessed health and activity limitations; 28 European countries; annual waves between 2004 and 2014). More information on the self-reported morbidity data can be found in recently published papers.[181,501]

3. Individual-level determinants

We collected and harmonized data on health and social determinants at the individual level from the same surveys as self-reported morbidity (NHIS, ESS, EU-SILC; same countries, same time-points). Determinants used in explanatory analyses in this chapter include smoking (current daily smoking, mainly from NHIS), obesity (body mass index above 30, calculated from self-reported height and weight, mainly from NHIS), material deprivation (inability to pay for at least three out of nine items deemed to be necessary for a normal life; mainly from EU-SILC), and social mobility and clustering of socioeconomic disadvantage (mainly from ESS). More information on these data can be found in recently published papers.[502–504]

4. National-level determinants

We collected data on national level determinants of population health for the same countries and points in time from international harmonized data sources, including the World Health Organization Health for All Database (WHO-HFA; national income, health care expenditure), Standardizing the World Income Inequality Database (SWIID; income inequality[505]), Quality of Government Dataset (QoG; democracy, cultural values[506]), Comparative Political Dataset (CPDS; left party government[507]), OECD Social expenditure database (OECD-SOCX; social transfers[24]), International Smoking Statistics (ISS; tobacco sales[508]), and various publications on tobacco control.[509,510] These datasets were all accessed in 2017.

Box 4.1 Set-up of the analyses in chapter 4 (*continued*)

Analytical methods

All health outcome data (mortality, self-reported morbidity, smoking, overweight, and obesity) were directly age-standardized using the European Standard Population. For descriptive purposes, we used both relative and absolute measures of health inequalities (see Box 2.2). In regression analyses we only used rates by socioeconomic group (mainly defined by level of education, because of the wider availability of data by this indicator) as dependent variable, and tested for the significance of interaction terms to assess whether effects of national-level determinants differed between socioeconomic groups. We applied country- and period-fixed effects to remove, as far as possible, confounding by unobserved country characteristics and by common time-trends. We often also controlled for national income, to further reduce the likelihood of false-positive results. All regression analyses were done with the SPSS 24 routine for linear mixed models. This allowed us to apply a multilevel framework and thus to take into account dependency of data within countries. We also used an autoregressive model of order 1 (AR(1)) to take into account the serial autocorrelation in the mortality and morbidity rates. In order to take into account heteroskedasticity, analyses of mortality were weighted by the square root of the number of deaths, and analyses of survey data by the number of respondents in the survey. More details on some of these methods can be found in recent papers.[175,504]

4.2 **Changes in social stratification**

Broader changes in society

Chapter 3 gives us good reasons for thinking that changes in social stratification, social mobility and composition of socioeconomic groups play a role in the persistence of health inequalities: when health inequalities are the result of causation processes, their magnitude will depend on the relative social (dis)advantage attached to different socioeconomic positions, and when health inequalities are the result of selection processes or confounding, their magnitude will depend on how social mobility has determined the composition of socioeconomic groups.

The findings that we present below confirm this, and show that broader changes in society have, to some extent, undone the inequalities-reducing effects of the welfare state, by partly substituting older mechanisms linking social inequality to health inequalities for new mechanisms. The greater importance of education as a social stratification variable has strengthened the association between socioeconomic position and personal characteristics that are important for health, and higher rates of intergenerational social mobility have created more opportunities for social selection on the basis of health and health determinants. Furthermore, because these changes have occurred earlier in countries with more advanced welfare states, these countries now have larger-than-expected health inequalities.

Educational expansion

Since World War II, the proportion of the population with a lower level of education (primary school, or lower secondary school only) has declined massively in all European populations, and the proportion of the population with a higher level of education has correspondingly increased. This shift in educational distribution continues to the present day. Around 1980, the proportion of low educated men still ranged between 40% and 90% in the 17 countries covered by our data, and declined to between 15% and 60% around 2015. In the same period, the proportion of high educated men increased from between 5% and 20% to between 15% and 30%.[512]

This expansion of schooling ('educational expansion') has occurred in all European countries, but has started earlier in some countries than in others, which has resulted in important differences between countries in the current proportion of low and high educated people. The proportion of high educated people is generally higher in Northern and Western Europe than it is in Southern, Central-Eastern, and Eastern Europe.[512] Corresponding changes have occurred in the proportions of people in unskilled manual and higher non-manual (e.g. professional) occupations, with similar differences between countries.

These changes in the relative size of lower and higher socioeconomic groups have been accompanied by changes in the relative health status of these groups, as compared to each other and to the national average. This is particularly clear for the low educated and for those in manual occupations: while lower socioeconomic groups became smaller, their relative health disadvantage became larger. However, the reverse (i.e. a smaller relative health advantage when the group becomes larger) is not seen for higher socioeconomic groups. This is illustrated for educational inequalities in all-cause mortality in Figure 4.1.

Reading panel A of this figure (unconventionally) from right to left, we see that when the population share of the lowest education group gets smaller, its relative excess mortality goes up. This is shown by the rise of the Rate Ratio from just above 1.0 to around 1.5, the latter indicating an excess mortality of 50% for the low educated as compared to the national average. However, reading panel B (conventionally) from left to right, we see that when the population share of the highest education group becomes larger, as it does when the population share of the lowest educated group goes down, its mortality advantage does not diminish at all, as indicated by the Rate Ratio still hovering around 0.7. This difference between lower and higher socioeconomic groups in how their relative health (dis)advantage responds to changes in their size is also found for occupational class and mortality, as well as for education and self-assessed health and GALI limitations.[i]

This asymmetry, which is also found in multivariate analyses with country-fixed effects, implies that educational expansion is accompanied by increasing relative inequalities in mortality: when the mortality disadvantage of the low educated goes up while the mortality advantage of the high educated remains the same, the gap between the two widens.[513] It also implies that the effects of educational expansion may have undone some of the inequalities-reducing effects of the welfare state—particularly in countries with advanced welfare states, where educational expansion has progressed further than elsewhere, such as the Nordic countries.

But why is the effect of educational expansion on the relative (dis)advantage of socioeconomic groups asymmetrical? It is easy to think of reasons why the relative health disadvantage of the low educated goes up when group size goes down, for example, because a smaller group will be more socially marginalized, or there will be a more adverse selection on cognitive ability or other personal characteristics from the birth cohort from which it originates. But why does the relative health advantage of the high educated not go down when group size goes up, despite the fact that the high educated will have lost some of their prestige in society because of their larger numbers, and despite the fact that they will have become more heterogeneous in terms of social background?

Increased clustering of advantage among high educated

A first explanation suggested by our data is that the social advantages accruing to higher levels of education have increased over time. Two examples are shown in Figure 4.2. Because regular European surveys with data on different indicators of socioeconomic position have only been

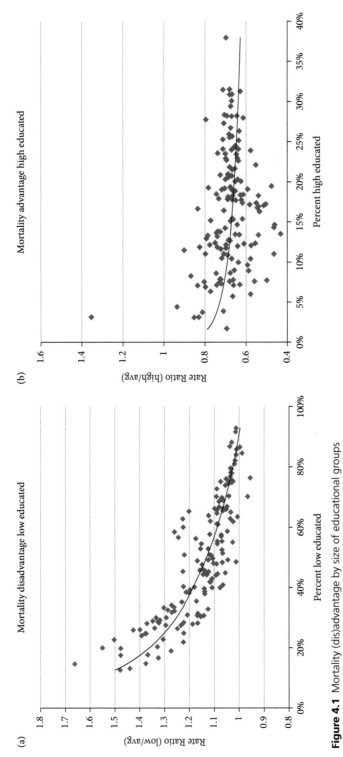

Figure 4.1 Mortality (dis)advantage by size of educational groups

Notes: Graphs show Rate Ratio of all-cause mortality comparing low and high educated each with average in whole population. Dataset of 17 European countries, ca. 1980–ca. 2010. Men; women similar.

Source: dataset constructed in DEMETRIQ/LIFEPATH projects, with harmonized data from national/regional mortality registers.

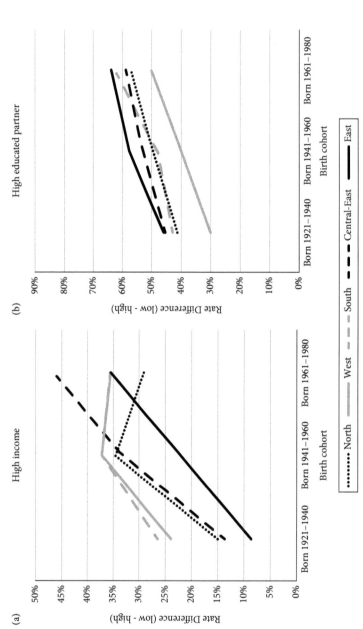

Figure 4.2 Educational inequalities in household income and partner's education

Notes: Graphs show absolute difference between low and high educated in percent having a net household income in the highest quintile of the national income distribution (panel A) and having a tertiary educated wife (panel B). Men; women similar. Pooled dataset of 25 countries. Regions: see Figure 3.4.

Source: data from European Social Survey cumulative data file 2002–14 (https://www.europeansocialsurvey.org/data/, accessed 2 April 2017).

established recently, it is impossible to assess time trends over many decades. What we have done in Figure 4.2, therefore, is compare different birth cohorts, in this case birth cohorts born in 1921–40, 1941–60 and 1961–80. Because inequalities between low and high educated arise in young adulthood, and then remain in place during people's lifetimes, changes between birth cohorts give us an idea of the changes that have occurred over a much longer time.

Panel A of Figure 4.2 shows that the difference between low and high educated in having a high income has increased substantially in more recently born, as compared to earlier born, birth cohorts. In other words, a high level of education has become much more important for earning a high income, or as economists say: the 'monetary returns to education' have increased importantly.[514] To the extent that a high income contributes to better health, this may have helped to strengthen the health advantage of the high educated. And even if income is not the main factor driving the health advantage of the high educated, the widening of income inequalities between education groups illustrates the more general trend of education becoming more important as a social stratification variable.

Among men, the advantages of a higher education have been further strengthened by increasing 'homogamy', that is, the likelihood of two partners having the same level of education. This has resulted in increased inequalities between low and high educated men in having a highly educated wife (panel B of Figure 4.2). This trend towards greater educational homogamy has been found in many countries, and is explained by a diminished shortage of high educated women for highr educated men seeking a partner.[515] Because having a highly educated wife is protective for health, independent of one's own level of education,[126] this may have helped high educated men to retain their health advantage despite their larger share in the population.

More scope for direct and indirect selection

A second explanation for the asymmetry between low and high educated in the effect of a shrinking or growing group size can be found in the operation of selection mechanisms during intergenerational social mobility.

The decline in the size of lower, and the increase in the size of higher socioeconomic groups presuppose substantial intergenerational social mobility. Because of educational expansion and expansion of professional and other service occupations, many sons and daughters have had to be upwardly socially mobile as compared to their parents' generation. As we have seen in Chapter 3, this increase in 'absolute' social mobility has been accompanied by an increase in 'relative' social mobility, also known as 'social fluidity', weakening the link between parents' and children's level of education.

This is illustrated in Figure 4.3, which shows that this increase in 'fluidity' has been observed throughout Europe, but more so, or earlier so, in some countries than in others. Clearly, fluidity has risen earlier and is considerably larger in Northern Europe than in other European regions, implying that the link between fathers' and children's educational level has become much less strong in Northern Europe than in other European regions. Eastern Europe (i.e. the countries of the former Soviet Union) also has high levels of fluidity, probably due to the introduction of more open schooling systems in the communist era.[472,475]

This increase in intergenerational social mobility has also increased the scope for selection on personal characteristics like cognitive ability, personality, and mental health, and may through that mechanism have contributed to the persistence of the association between socioeconomic position and health. It may also explain the asymmetry, if increasing numbers of downwardly mobile people in lower educated groups further strengthen the mortality disadvantage of those groups, and if increasing numbers of upwardly mobile people in higher educated groups compensate for the reduced mortality advantage of those groups when they become larger (section 3.2 'Education, occupation, income, and health').

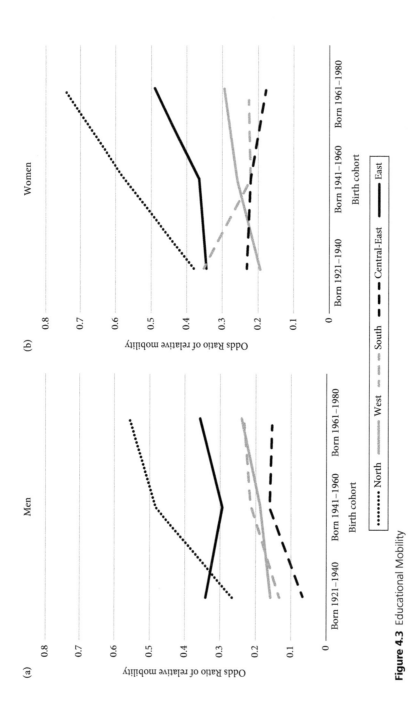

Figure 4.3 Educational Mobility

Notes: Graphs show relative mobility ('fluidity', i.e., odds ratio measuring likelihood of being mobile taking into account changes in marginal educational distributions) in intergenerational educational mobility, comparing education level of sons and daughters with education level of their fathers, averaging mobility between low and mid, and between mid and high education. Pooled dataset of 25 countries. European regions: see Figure 3.4.

Source: data from European Social Survey cumulative data file 2002–14 (https://www.europeansocialsurvey.org/data/, accessed 2 April 2017).

Greater 'absolute' and 'relative' mobility in Northern Europe, and the associated social selection mechanisms, may also contribute to larger inequalities in mortality in Northern Europe as compared to other European regions, including Southern Europe where intergenerational social mobility and social 'fluidity' have been much lower (Figure 4.3).[476]

4.3 **Rapid but differential health improvements**

Changes in population health

A second mechanism contributing to the persistence of health inequalities is that health improvements have generally been faster in higher than in lower socioeconomic groups. As we have seen in section 3.4 'Theories about the explanation of health inequalities', this phenomenon has been widely recognized, and has given rise to several theories about the explanation of health inequalities (i.e. diffusion of innovations, cultural capital, inverse equity), whereas the fundamental causes theory has proposed a general explanation in terms of the 'flexible resources' that higher socioeconomic groups can use as soon as health problems become 'actionable'.

In this section we will study differential health improvements in European countries in more detail, starting with a closer look at the predictions of the fundamental causes theory. We then proceed by studying two examples of health improvement (smoking and mortality from amenable causes), but also two examples of health deterioration (obesity and excessive alcohol consumption). Our main finding for this part of the analyses is that higher socioeconomic groups benefit more from opportunities for health improvement, and are better protected against new health risks. Because countries with more advanced welfare states have generally experienced massive health improvements over the past decades, this is another mechanism contributing to their larger-than-expected health inequalities.

Increased actionability, mathematical artefacts, and fundamental causes

Over the past decades, the health landscape has changed rapidly, due to the fact that many health problems have declined, whereas some others have risen in frequency to only partly replace them. These improvements were the result of favourable trends in background factors such as prosperity, and of progress in the prevention and treatment of health problems, including cardiovascular disease, several cancers, and road traffic injuries. In other words, many more health problems have become 'actionable' than in the past.[516]

However, the resulting progress in population health has been uneven, with declines usually being faster, in relative terms, in higher than in lower socioeconomic groups. The resulting, almost universal rise of relative health inequalities has even been called a 'mathematical artefact'.[89,517] Relative risks for mortality and morbidity generally tend to be higher when average mortality and morbidity are lower,[518] which suggests that increasing relative inequalities in health outcomes are inevitable when the overall level of the outcome falls.[89,517,519]

However, a mathematical regularity does not equal a mathematical necessity. It has been shown that in practice mathematical constraints play no role in determining relative inequalities in health,[520] and that it is perfectly possible for the Rate Ratio to go down when the average rate of morbidity or mortality goes down—it just requires relative declines to be a little bit faster in lower than in higher socioeconomic groups.[521] It is more fruitful, therefore, to search for substantive explanations of why declines are faster in higher socioeconomic groups when the frequency of health problems declines.

As we have seen in Chapter 3, several factors conspire to create larger relative declines in health problems in higher socioeconomic groups. One is the frequent dependence of health improvement on behaviour change, and thus on health literacy and on living conditions facilitating behaviour change—circumstances which are generally better in higher than in lower socioeconomic groups. Another is subtle differences in access to, or quality of, prevention and treatment facilities, such as smoking cessation support, treatment of ischaemic heart disease, and cancer screening programmes.

Also, when population health deteriorates, as it sometimes does when new health hazards arise, it takes time before these new hazards can effectively be tackled collectively, and in the meantime those with higher education or income are usually less exposed or are better able to protect themselves on an individual basis. It is this combination of increased 'actionability' and differential progress (or delayed 'actionability' and differential protection) that plays an important role in the persistence of health inequalities.

The concept of actionability of health problems is also central to the theory of 'fundamental causes'. As illustrated in Box 4.2, our data are generally (although not perfectly) in agreement with predictions based on this theory.

Box 4.2 The fundamental causes theory and inequalities in cause-specific mortality

The 'fundamental causes' theory, which was introduced in section 3.4 'Theories about the explanation of health inequalities', asserts that the persistence of health inequalities arises from the fact that as new opportunities for health improvement arise, persons with a higher socioeconomic status use their larger resources to derive more, or earlier, benefits from these new opportunities.

This is indeed what we see in our European dataset, both in analyses of inequalities in mortality from various causes of death at one point in time, and in analyses of changes in mortality from various causes over time. When we look at the magnitude of inequalities in mortality at one point in time, and classify causes of death into four groups based on their actionability (amenable to behaviour change, amenable to medical intervention, amenable to injury prevention, and non-preventable) we find the largest inequalities for causes of death amenable to behaviour change, such as alcohol- and smoking-related conditions. Inequalities in mortality are generally larger for causes amenable to behaviour change, medical intervention, and injury prevention than for non-preventable causes.[522] We already noted this when studying Figure 2.4 in Chapter 2.

Figure 2.4, however, also shows that not all our findings are in correspondence with the predictions of the fundamental causes theory. It is not immediately clear, for example, why inequalities in mortality from road traffic accidents are so small among women. This has been attributed to the fact that among low educated women, higher injury incidence and/or higher case fatality are compensated by lower traffic exposure, for example, because of lower access to motorized transport.[156]

Other 'anomalies' relate to the historically higher rates of breast cancer mortality among high educated women, which is due to the fact that modern patterns of child-bearing behaviour (delayed child bearing, smaller numbers of children, less breast feeding, ...) have been adopted by high educated women first,[143,523] and the higher rates of lung cancer mortality among high educated women in Southern Europe, which is due to the fact that women in these countries have taken up smoking relatively recently.[413]

These exceptions suggest a need to more explicitly consider the introduction of new health risks. Because the core of the 'fundamental causes' theory is based on the notion that 'as

<hr>

Box 4.2 The fundamental causes theory and inequalities in cause-specific mortalit (*continued*)

opportunities for avoiding disease expand so health inequalities continue to exist',[524] (p. 265) it does not explain what happens when new health risks, such as those of motorized transport, modern patterns of child-bearing or smoking are introduced. These risks often manifest themselves first among those with a higher income (because new products or behaviours are expensive) or higher education (because information on new products or behaviours reaches them first).

Only when the new products or behaviours have diffused towards the lower socioeconomic groups, and when the health risks of these products or behaviours have become known and 'actionable', can 'health-directed human agency' and differential access to resources start to produce an inverse association between socioeconomic status and mortality. While these exceptions may only be temporary deviations from the relationships stated by the fundamental causes theory, they underline the importance of other mechanisms such as 'diffusion of innovation'[525,526] or 'status pursuit': adopting behaviour that is bad for health but helps to maintain or increase social status.[527]

If the 'fundamental causes' theory is correct, one should also expect to find that as opportunities for lowering mortality arise, declines in mortality will be larger among those with a higher socioeconomic position. This is indeed what the data generally show: inequalities in cause-specific mortality decline are larger when mortality declines faster.[528] This could already be gleaned from Figure 2.6 in chapter 2, although this graph also shows that the association between speed of mortality decline and gap in mortality decline is rather weak.

Figure 2.6 also showed that mortality from some conditions has increased over time, as in the case of alcohol-related mortality among men and women, and lung cancer among women. One would expect the increase to be less in higher educational groups, because they are supposed to be better able to protect themselves against these new dangers.[529] This is indeed what we see in Figure 2.6, although the relationship is far from consistent, probably because of 'countervailing mechanisms' such as 'diffusion of innovations' and 'status pursuit'.[528]

<hr>

Differential behaviour change: smoking

The smoking epidemic

In many European countries, smoking is not only the most important cause of premature mortality in the population as a whole,[530] but also the single most important contributor to socioeconomic inequalities in mortality, at least among men.[261,262,531] We will discuss the evidence supporting this claim in more detail in section 4.4 'Differential effects of factors driving population health change', but will first look at trends in smoking behaviour in a selection of European countries (Figure 4.4).

Among men, trends in smoking have been almost uniformly downwards over the last decades, both among the low and the high educated. Because percentage declines have been faster among high than among low educated men, relative inequalities in the prevalence of smoking have exploded. This rise of relative inequalities in smoking has occurred nearly everywhere, but it has been particularly strong in Northern Europe (represented by Denmark in Figure 4.4) and in England and Wales.

Among women, trends in smoking have been more variable between countries and between socioeconomic groups. Sometimes a clear pattern of rise and fall can be discerned, for example among high educated women in Denmark, the Netherlands, and Spain, and among low educated

(a)

Men

Men, low

Men, high

Men, Rate Ratio

Age-adjusted prevalence

Age-adjusted prevalence

Rate Ratio (low/high)

70%   60%   50%   40%   30%   20%   10%   0%
1978 1982 1986 1990 1994 1998 2002 2006 2010

70%   60%   50%   40%   30%   20%   10%   0%
1978 1982 1986 1990 1994 1998 2002 2006 2010

3.5   3.0   2.5   2.0   1.5   1.0   0.5   0.0
1978 1982 1986 1990 1994 1998 2002 2006 2010

·····Denmark   ·····England & W   ——— Lithuania   ━━━ Netherlands   ●━●Poland   ━ ━ ━Spain

(b)

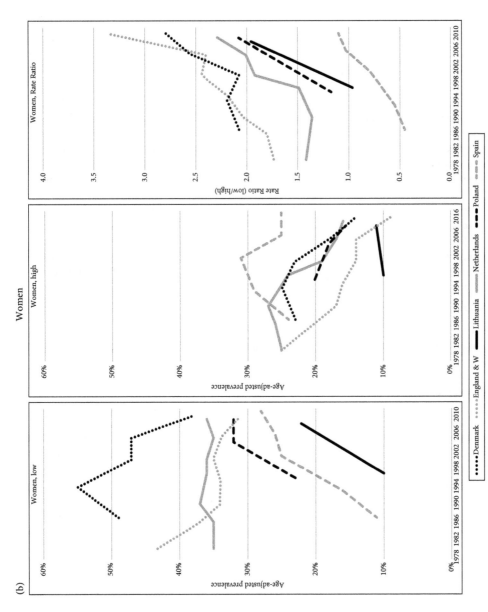

Figure 4.4 Trends in smoking by education

Notes: Smoking = current smoking.

Source: dataset constructed in DEMETRIQ/LIFEPATH projects, with harmonized data from National Health Interview Surveys.

women in Denmark. Among low educated women there are also many countries where smoking is still increasing. As a result, inequalities in smoking have often risen even more steeply among women than among men.

As we discussed in section 3.4 'Theories about the explanation of health inequalities', the 'model of the cigarette epidemic' is a good starting-point for understanding how inequalities in smoking have arisen.[455,532] European countries differ substantially in the stage of progression of the smoking epidemic, as shown by time series data of cigarette sales. Countries in which cigarette sales rose early and reached their peak in the 1970s can mainly be found in the North and West of Europe, whereas countries which reached their peak in the 1980s or later can mainly be found in the South and East.[533]

Some of the countries with an early peak, for example, Finland, Sweden, the United Kingdom, Ireland, and the Netherlands also had very strong declines in cigarette sales since the peak level was passed, whereas countries which peaked later, such as Spain, Italy, and the Baltic countries, usually had more modest declines in cigarette sales, simply due to the fact that less time has passed since the peak was reached. This also means that the scope for inequalities in smoking to emerge is larger in countries with an early peak (and more declines) than in countries with a later peak (and less declines).

Differences between countries in progression of the smoking epidemic indeed offer a partial explanation of current differences in the magnitude of inequalities in smoking, particularly among women. This is evident from the fact that inequalities in smoking among women are larger in countries where the smoking epidemic started earlier, such as Finland, Sweden, the United Kingdom, and Ireland, and smaller in countries where smoking was adopted later, such as the Mediterranean countries (see Figure 3.5).

Tobacco control policies

However, the progression of the smoking epidemic is not the only factor involved: tobacco control also plays a role. Dissemination of information about the health-damaging effects of smoking started shortly after these effects became widely known in the 1960s, but more structured policies to reduce smoking in the population were implemented much later, usually long after smoking had already passed its peak.

Among European countries Finland was the first, starting systematic tobacco control policies in the second half of the 1970s, with Sweden and Italy starting in the 1980s, and most other countries starting in the early or late 1990s.[509] As a result of differences in implementation of tobacco control policies European countries currently differ substantially in how much they do to curb smoking. For example, the United Kingdom, Ireland, Sweden, and Norway are much more active than Germany, Austria, and Denmark.[510]

There is not much doubt about the effectiveness of tobacco control policies, but whether these policies have had differential effects by socioeconomic position is less clear. Only one type of policy has more consistently been shown to have a larger impact on smoking in lower than in higher socioeconomic groups, that is, an increase in the price of tobacco products by raising taxation. Findings for most other policies have been inconsistent, and include larger impacts on higher socioeconomic groups.[534,535]

Studies relating inequalities in smoking at the country level to the intensity of national tobacco control efforts have not produced consistent findings,[536–538] but when we limit the analysis to Northern and Western European countries where the tobacco epidemic started and peaked early, we do find a negative correlation between the intensity of tobacco control efforts and smoking, at least among men (Figure 4.5). In countries with more intensive tobacco control efforts smoking rates tend to be lower, both among low and high educated men, and also, although less clearly so, among high educated women.

Figure 4.5 also suggests that, in this limited set of countries, more intensive tobacco control efforts are associated with larger inequalities in smoking. Because the effects of intensifying tobacco control efforts seem to be equally large, in absolute terms, among low and high educated men, more intensive tobacco control efforts are associated with constant absolute but widening relative inequalities in smoking among men. Among women, more intensive tobacco control efforts are associated with widening absolute and relative inequalities in smoking. These correlations suggest an unfortunate side effect of tobacco control efforts.

Please also note the exceptionally low smoking rates among low educated Swedish men, which cannot be explained by the intensity of Sweden's tobacco control efforts (we will further discuss this anomaly in section 4.6 'Understanding the European experience').

Differential behaviour change: obesity

Trends in obesity

Trends in obesity have been unfavourable: its prevalence has risen everywhere, both among men and women. Absolute increases in prevalence were generally larger among the low than among the high educated, and as a result, absolute inequalities in obesity have increased, whereas in many countries relative inequalities in obesity have remained more or less stable.[503]

Figure 4.6 illustrates these trends for a small number of European countries. In Denmark, Ireland, France, Italy, and Hungary the prevalence of overweight and obesity among men in the manual occupational class rises ahead of that among men in the non-manual occupational class. Only in Lithuania do men in the non-manual class seem to be ahead, but their disadvantage is decreasing over time, as shown by the Rate Ratio which, coming from far below 1, is rising.

Remarkably, whereas in the case of smoking the lower socioeconomic groups have followed the higher socioeconomic groups, in the case of obesity the reverse seems to be happening, at least within the time frame of this analysis. Since the early 1980s, and in contrast to what the theory of 'diffusion of innovations' would predict, rates of obesity among the low educated seem to be ahead of those among the high educated. This is more in line with the 'fundamental causes' theory: the high educated have until recently been able to mostly avoid obesity, but the risks of becoming obese are now rising so fast that even the high educated are losing control.

The rise in the prevalence of obesity has been attributed to societal and environmental changes resulting in more 'obesogenic' environments, characterized by abundance of food and lack of necessity for physical exercise. Whereas differential exposure to obesogenic environments was once thought to contribute to socioeconomic inequalities in obesity, it is unclear whether lower socio-economic groups are indeed more exposed to a food environment in which healthy food is available less abundantly and at higher costs.[539–542]

It is more likely that lower socioeconomic groups are more *vulnerable* to the effects of an obesogenic environment. One possible explanation is that financial hardship and other stressful living conditions consume mental resources and reduce cognitive capacity, thereby interfering with decision making, long-term planning and risk avoidance.[543] Another is that obesity spreads through people's social networks,[544] and cultural capital and need for social distinction play a role in keeping the higher educated slim.[457]

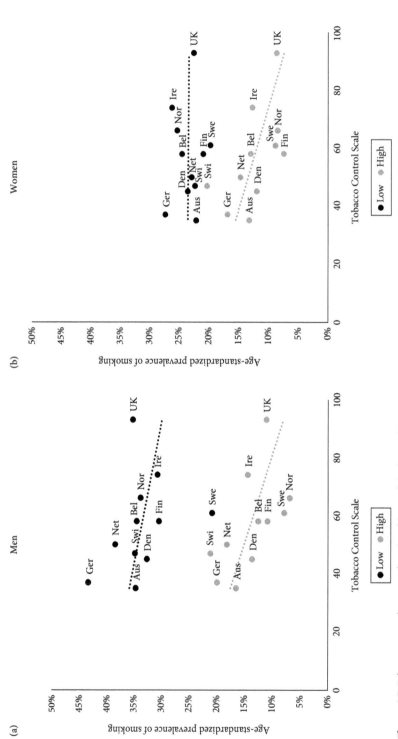

Figure 4.5 Tobacco control versus educational inequalities in smoking

Notes: Dotted lines respresent regression lines of smoking prevalence on Tobacco Control Scale score. Correlation between Tobacco Control Scale and smoking: low educated men r = −0.41; high educated men r = − 0.45; low educated women r = 0.15; high educated women r = −0.20. Current smoking ca. 2010, Tobacco Control Scale 2007. Aus = Austria, Bel = Belgium, Den = Denmark, Fin = Finland, Ger = Germany, Ire = Ireland, Net = Netherlands, Nor = Norway, Swe = Sweden, Swi = Switzerland, UK = United Kingdom.

Source: dataset constructed in DEMETRIQ/LIFEPATH projects, with harmonized data on smoking from National Health Interview Surveys; data on tobacco control from Joossens L, Raw M. 'Progress in Tobacco Control in 30 European Countries, 2005 to 2007'. Bern: Swiss Cancer League, 2007.[510]

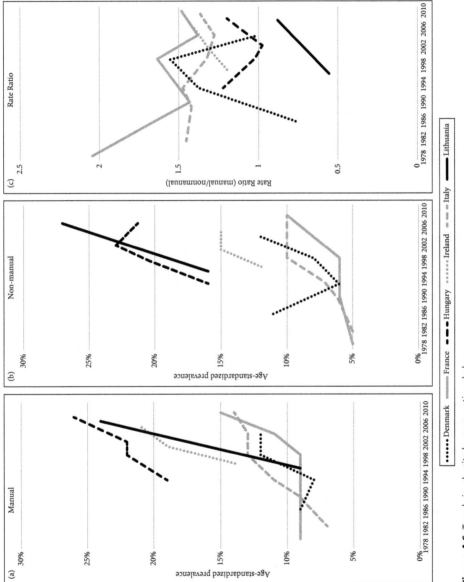

Figure 4.6 Trends in obesity by occupational class

Notes: Obesity = Body mass index > 30 kg/m2, calculated from self-reported weight and height. Men.

Source: dataset constructed in DEMETRIQ/LIFEPATH projects, with harmonized data from National Health Interview Surveys.

Differential behaviour change: excessive alcohol consumption

Trends in alcohol-related mortality

Trends for excessive alcohol consumption have also been unfavourable, and as a result mortality from alcohol-related conditions like alcoholic psychosis and liver cirrhosis has increased in many European countries. These unfavourable trends have hit the lower socioeconomic groups more than the higher socioeconomic groups, and like obesity this is therefore an example of an emerging health problem to which the higher socioeconomic groups have been better able to protect themselves.

Figure 4.7 shows large differences between European countries in the rise of mortality from alcohol-related conditions, and in the widening of the gap in mortality between educational groups. Mortality from alcohol-related conditions has risen dramatically among the low educated in Central-Eastern and Eastern Europe (represented by Hungary and Estonia) and in some Northern European countries (represented by Finland), has remained stable in Southern Europe (represented by Italy), and has declined in France and Switzerland. Although mortality from alcohol-related conditions has also risen among the high educated in several of the same countries, these rises have been much more modest. As a result, absolute inequalities in alcohol-related mortality have gone up markedly in Central-Eastern and Eastern European countries and in some Northern European countries.[197]

These trends partly reflect the increasing affordability of alcohol, due to a combination of rising incomes and stable or declining costs of alcoholic drinks. Because lower income groups are more responsive to price changes, increased affordability of alcohol leads to larger increases in consumption in lower socioeconomic groups. Between 1996 and 2004 affordability of alcohol has increased strongly in many European countries, including Lithuania, the United Kingdom, and Finland.[545] Finnish studies have shown that the impact of these changes in affordability has been largest in the lowest socioeconomic groups.[546,547] Inequalities in alcohol-related mortality have increased most in countries in which affordability has increased most.[197]

Alcohol control policies

Some of these changes in the affordability of alcoholic drinks are the effect of reduced taxation, as a consequence of harmonization of excise tax rates within the European Union. More generally, policy changes play an important role in trends in alcohol-related mortality. Between 1950 and 2000, alcohol control has become less strict in Northern Europe, partly as a result of harmonization of national laws and regulations following membership of the European Union, but more strict in Southern Europe, and also France.[548]

This may help to explain the relatively favourable trends in countries like France, Spain, and Italy,[549–551] where tightening of alcohol control policies appears to have had a greater beneficial effect on alcohol-related mortality among the low than the high educated. However, it does not explain our findings for all the Nordic countries. Loosening of alcohol control policies coincided with a rise of mortality from alcohol-related causes among low educated men in Finland, but not in Sweden or Norway, whereas the rise of mortality from alcohol-related causes among low educated men in Denmark coincided with a slight tightening of alcohol control policies.[552]

In Central-Eastern and Eastern Europe excessive alcohol consumption surged around 1990 when cheap alcohol flooded the market.[553] The strong increases of alcohol-related mortality seen in these countries reflect the economic crisis following the collapse of the Soviet Union and the resulting stress in the population, and the extreme liberalization of alcohol markets with a breakdown of control measures in the chaotic first years after the political changes.[554–556] More recently, rising income and increased affordability of alcohol may also have played a role.[557]

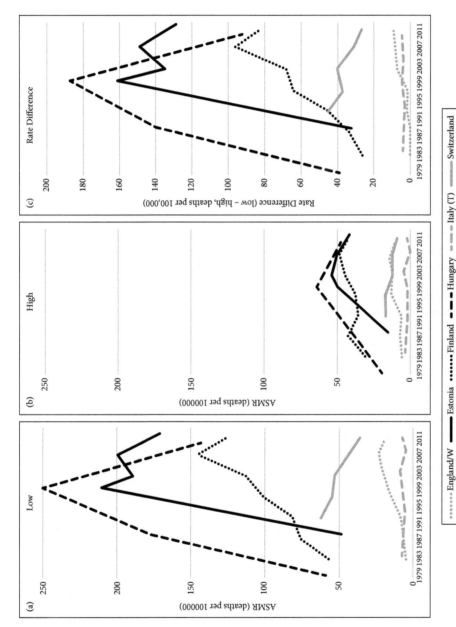

Figure 4.7 Trends in alcohol-related mortality by education

Notes: ASMR = Age-Standardized Mortality Rate. Alcohol-related mortality = mortality from alcoholic psychosis, dependence and abuse; alcoholic cardiomyopathy; alcoholic diseases of the liver; and accidental poisoning by alcohol. Men; pattern of differences between education groups and countries similar for women, but absolute rates much lower among women than among men.

Source: dataset constructed in DEMETRIQ/LIFEPATH projects, with harmonized data from national/regional mortality registers.

Differential benefits from health care

Over the past half century, health care has become an important determinant of population health, as the introduction of effective methods for preventing and treating disease has contributed substantially to mortality decline.[558,559] Although the causes of health inequalities must ultimately be sought outside of the health care system, inequalities in access to new prevention and treatment methods, or inequalities in the quality with which these are delivered, may therefore have aggravated health inequalities.[ii]

Trends in amenable mortality

In the 1970s, 'avoidable' or 'amenable' mortality has been proposed as a measure of the effectiveness of health care services, and causes of death included in this category range from infectious diseases such as tuberculosis and pneumonia to preventable or curable cancers such as cervical cancer and Hodgkin's disease, and from cerebrovascular disease and appendicitis to asthma and perinatal mortality.[49] Since then many studies have shown remarkable declines in amenable mortality over time, probably reflecting gradual improvements in quality and/or accessibility of health care services.[52]

Our European data show that substantial declines in mortality from amenable causes have occurred in both lower and higher socioeconomic groups (Figure 4.8). That there have apparently been substantial improvements among lower socioeconomic groups in prevention and treatment of these conditions is a major achievement of European health systems, but a closer look at the data reveals that relative declines have been faster in higher socioeconomic groups.[500]

On average, over the past decades annual mortality decline for amenable causes was 3.5% for high educated men, against 2.2% for low educated men, and 3.3% among high educated women, against 2.1% among low educated women. This may be due to inequalities in access or quality of medical care, but may also be due to other factors, such as inequalities in compliance with treatment, or a higher frequency of aggravating co-morbidity in lower socioeconomic groups. Whatever the explanation, relative inequalities in amenable mortality have increased in all European countries.[500]

Although this is in line with other results presented in this paragraph, all suggesting differential benefits from population health improvements, it is useful to have an even closer look at the data. When we compare inequalities in relative mortality decline from amenable causes with inequalities in relative decline of all-cause mortality, we see that the second are larger than the first. In other words, comparatively stronger declines in mortality from amenable causes among the low educated have dampened the widening of relative inequalities in all-cause mortality.[499]

This is even more clear when we look directly at absolute declines in mortality from amenable conditions. In Western European countries absolute declines of amenable mortality have been greater in lower socioeconomic groups, resulting in a substantial narrowing of absolute inequalities in mortality, despite a widening of relative inequalities in mortality from these conditions (Figure 4.8).[500] This has contributed to the more favourable development of absolute inequalities in all-cause mortality, which have remained stable or have declined in many countries.[499] We will come back to the role of health care in aggravating or alleviating health inequalities in section 4.4 'Differential effects of factors driving population health change'.

Trends in ischemic heart disease and breast cancer mortality

Ischemic heart disease is sometimes included in selections of causes of death amenable to medical intervention.[52] Not one single cause of death is completely determined by whether or not adequate medical care is delivered. This is a matter of degree, and in our analyses of amenable mortality we

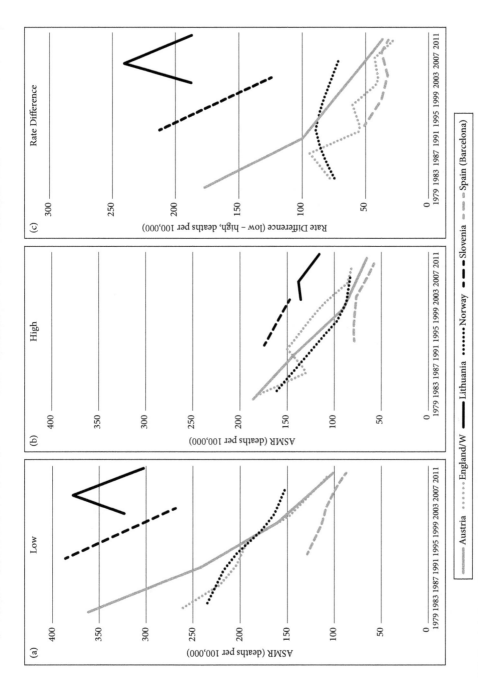

Figure 4.8 Trends in amenable mortality by education

Notes: ASMR = Age-Standardized Mortality Rate. Women; men similar. The following conditions were included in amenable mortality: a number of infectious diseases (tuberculosis, pneumonia/influenza, HIV/aids, other infectious and parasitic diseases), a number of cancers (cervix uteri, testis, colorectum, Hodgkin's disease, leukaemia), a number of cardiovascular diseases (cerebrovascular disease, rheumatic heart disease, hypertensive disease, selected other heart diseases), and a number of other diseases (asthma, appendicitis/hernia/cholelithiasis/cholecystitis, peptic ulcer, prostate hyperplasia, maternal deaths, congenital heart disease, and conditions originating in the perinatal period).

Source: dataset constructed in DEMETRIQ/LIFEPATH projects, with harmonized data from national/regional mortality registers.

have not included ischemic heart disease, because trends in mortality from this disease are also strongly determined by other factors. Declines in mortality from ischemic heart disease have been attributed to a combination of risk factor changes (less smoking, modest improvements in diet, more physical exercise, …) and improvements in prevention and treatment (hypertension detection and treatment, statins, surgical interventions, thrombolytic therapy, …).[560–562]

Nevertheless, for ischemic heart disease mortality we observe similar trends as for mortality from amenable causes: with the exception of countries in Central-Eastern and Eastern Europe, mortality has declined strongly over the past decades in both lower and higher socioeconomic groups. Because relative declines were faster among the high educated, relative inequalities in ischemic heart disease have increased. This illustrates our general point that when new opportunities for health improvement arise, higher socioeconomic groups usually benefit more. However, absolute declines were larger among the low educated, and as a result absolute inequalities in ischemic heart disease mortality have declined. Amenable causes and ischemic heart disease have been the main contributors to stable or narrowing absolute inequalities in total mortality in Western Europe.[499]

The fact that absolute declines in lower socioeconomic groups have exceeded the declines in higher socioeconomic groups, implies that risk factor changes or improvements in prevention and treatment of ischemic heart disease (or both) have also reached many people in lower socioeconomic groups. The only countries for which this has been studied in more detail are England and Scotland, in which the narrowing of absolute inequalities in cardiovascular disease mortality has been attributed to an even distribution of treatment benefits rather than to risk factor changes,[563,564] again suggesting that the health care sector has had a dampening effect on health inequalities.

Breast cancer is another cause of death from which mortality has generally declined over the past decades, but here the underlying incidence and case fatality trends are more mixed than in the case of ischemic heart disease where both incidence and case fatality have declined. Mortality from breast cancer has declined despite increasing incidence, partly as a result of the introduction of breast cancer screening and partly as a result of improvements in breast cancer treatment, which have both helped to improve survival from breast cancer.[565]

Mortality from breast cancer has declined among low and high educated women, but much more so among high educated women. In the 1980s it was still quite common for breast cancer mortality to be higher among high educated women, but because of the stronger mortality declines among high educated women these 'reverse' gradients are disappearing and turning into 'normal' gradients in more and more European countries.[143]

Whether the weaker declines in breast cancer mortality among low educated are due to less favourable trends in incidence (e.g. because modern reproductive behaviours are only now taking their toll among low educated women) or to inequalities in preventive or curative health care is unknown. Whatever the underlying causes, this is yet another example of higher socioeconomic groups benefiting more from new opportunities for health improvement.

4.4 Differential effects of factors driving population health change

Overall results of the analyses

The previous section has shown that the persistence of health inequalities is partly due to the fact that health improvements have been faster in higher than in lower socioeconomic groups (and that health deteriorations, when they occurred, have been faster in lower than in higher socioeconomic groups). This paragraph will show that this can often be understood from differences between socioeconomic groups in the effect of the factors driving population health change at the national level.

In support of this paragraph we systematically explored the role of a number of 'upstream' factors that had previously been found to influence average population health in Europe: two economic variables (national income[566] and income inequality[567]), two cultural variables (secular-rational and self-expression values[568]), two political variables (level of democracy[569] and years of left party government[498]), and two policy variables (percentage of national income spent on social security transfers[570] and health care[571]).

Only four of these factors had *differential* health effects leading to a widening or narrowing of health inequalities: national income, income inequality, level of democracy, and health care expenditure (Table 4.1). In general, the strongest and most consistent effects were found for mortality; for self-reported health problems statistically significant results were rare, again illustrating the more idiosyncratic nature of inequalities in these health outcomes. Data and methods have been introduced at the beginning of this chapter in Box 4.1, and further details can be found in the endnotes.[iii]

Table 4.1 Differential effects of country characteristics on mortality

A. Men

Determinant	Trend	Effect on all-cause mortality				
		Education		Inequalities	
		Low	High	Absolute	Relative
National income	**up**	**down**	**down**	no change	**widen**
Income inequality	**up**	**up**	down	**widen**	**widen**
Level of democracy	**up**	**up**	**down**	**widen**	**widen**
Health care expenditure	**up**	down	**down**	**narrow**	no change

B. Women

Determinant	Trend	Effect on all-cause mortality				
		Education		Inequalities	
		Low	High	Absolute	Relative
National income	**up**	**down**	**down**	no change	**widen**
Income inequality	**up**	up	**down**	**widen**	**widen**
Level of democracy	**up**	up	**down**	**widen**	**widen**
Health care expenditure	**up**	down	**down**	no change	no change

Notes: In bold: statistically significant effects (p<.05). For definition of independent variables, see following sections of section 4.4. Country- and period-fixed effects analyses, controlling for GDP. Effect on mortality among low and high educated determined in analyses stratified by education level. Effect on absolute and relative inequalities in mortality determined in analyses in a pooled dataset with interaction terms between level of education and the variable of interest.

Economic growth

The health improving and mortality lowering effects of growing prosperity are well known, and the level of national income is a powerful predictor of mortality and morbidity rates, not only historically and in worldwide comparisons, but also currently and within Europe.[566,572]

Over the past decades, national income has increased gradually in most European countries, but not in a smooth pattern. Central-Eastern and Eastern European countries went through an economic crisis in the early 1990s, as did Finland and Sweden to a much lesser extent, and all countries experienced the Great Recession that started after the 2008 financial crisis.

Our findings show that when national income goes up, mortality goes down among both the low and the high educated. However, what we are interested in is whether the effect differs between socioeconomic groups, and our regression results show that it indeed does (Table 4.1). Percentage or relative declines of mortality are stronger among the high than among the low educated, and as a result relative inequalities in mortality go up when national income rises. This is unfortunate, but absolute inequalities remain roughly the same, because rising national income is not associated with different absolute declines in mortality among the high and low educated (Figure 4.9).

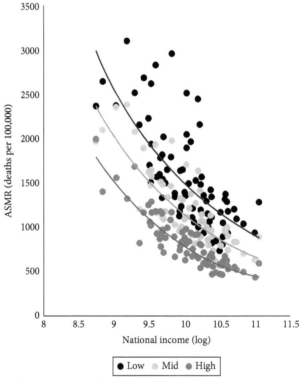

Figure 4.9 National income and mortality by education

Notes: ASMR = Age-Standardized Mortality Rate. National income = natural logarithm of Gross Domestic Product per capita (in $1000, purchasing power adjusted). All-cause mortality, men. Pooled dataset of mortality by level of education in 17 European countries, ca. 1980–ca. 2014.

Source: dataset constructed in DEMETRIQ/LIFEPATH projects, with harmonized data from national/regional mortality registers; data on GDP from World Health Organization Health for All Database (WHO-HFA)(https://gateway.euro.who.int/en/datasets/european-health-for-all-database/, accessed April 2017).

That these effects are found in a country- and period-fixed effects analysis, suggests that what we see is a causal effect of rising prosperity on mortality and mortality inequalities. Differential effects favouring the high educated are seen for most specific causes of death.[iv] Underlying these differential effects of national income on mortality must be specific determinants of mortality whose prevalence declines more among the high than the low educated when national income goes up. Poverty does not seem to be involved, because in our analyses rising national income is accompanied by stronger declines of poverty among the low than among the high educated. Smoking and obesity are more likely candidates, because rising national income is accompanied by stronger declines in smoking among the high than the low educated, and by stronger rises of obesity among the low than the high educated. However, many other determinants, mentioned in section 3.3 'Six groups of contributing factors', may be involved as well, because rising national income is usually accompanied by favourable changes in many material and non-material living conditions.

This widening of (relative) inequalities in mortality with rising national income was first noticed in a study of low and middle income countries by British economist Adam Wagstaff, who compared this to 'swimming against the tide'.[573] This also appears to be one of the explanations for the persistence of health inequalities in modern welfare states. The build-up of the modern welfare state has gone hand in hand with rising prosperity, and countries with a more highly developed welfare state tend to also have a higher national income. The inequalities widening effects of rising national income are therefore likely to have offset some of the inequalities reducing effects of the welfare state.

Rising income inequality

Income and wealth are still highly unequally distributed within European societies, and there is good evidence that these inequalities are on the rise again in many countries, after they had been substantially reduced in the middle decades of the twentieth century as a result of income redistribution and the rise of the welfare state.[37] This renewed rise since the 1980s was partly due to policy changes (e.g. less income redistribution and lower welfare benefits), partly due to autonomous changes in society, and the economy (e.g. changes in household composition and increased globalization).[574]

Although a rise of income inequality has been observed in all European countries, even in the Nordic countries, it has not been equally strong everywhere, and the timing has also been different. In the United Kingdom, income inequality rose strongly during the 1980s, but then stabilized at a high level during the 1990s and into the twenty-first century. In Central-Eastern and Eastern Europe, income inequality rose strongly after the collapse of the Soviet Union in the early 1990s, but despite a strong rise, income inequality in the Czech Republic remained comparatively low while it reached very high levels in the Baltic countries.[574]

This implies that we can use differences between countries and over time to study the effect of income inequality on the magnitude of health inequalities. The literature on this topic is scarce, so it is not exactly clear what we should expect. If there is a causal effect of income on health—an issue we discussed extensively in section 3.2 'Education, occupation, income, and health'—one would expect larger income inequalities to go together with larger health inequalities. There is some evidence that larger income inequalities go together with larger inequalities in self-assessed health by income level,[310] but studies of the effects of income inequality on health inequalities along other socioeconomic dimensions, such as level of education or occupational class, have produced mixed results.[575,576]

In our European dataset we do, however, find that larger income inequalities go together with larger educational inequalities in mortality. The association is rather weak, and mainly rests on the rise of both income inequality and inequality in mortality in Central-Eastern and Eastern Europe after 1990, but it holds up in country- and period-fixed effects analyses. We actually find that rising income inequality goes together with declining mortality among the high educated, and rising mortality among the low educated (Table 4.1).

We found an inequality-widening effect of rising income inequality for many specific causes of death (Figure 4.10), but not for self-assessed health. Rising income inequality is also associated with rising inequality in material deprivation, suggesting that the effect of income inequality on inequality in mortality is due to its effect on rates of poverty.

More generally, these results suggest that some of the widening of inequalities in mortality seen over the past decades, particularly in Central-Eastern and Eastern Europe, can be attributed to the rise of income inequality in these countries. Whether this has also contributed to the persistence of health inequalities in advanced welfare states is uncertain, in view of the lack of evidence of a causal effect of income on adult health in high-income countries. In other words, the co-occurrence of widening income inequalities and widening health inequalities in Western Europe may also have been a co-incidence.

As we mentioned in section 1.3 'The need for a broader picture', the interest of health researchers in income inequality as a determinant of population health has not been limited to the effects on health inequalities—on the contrary, inspired by Wilkinson's work it has mostly focused on the effects of income inequality on average population health.[40,41,491] Some studies have found clear associations between income inequality and higher average rates of mortality and self-reported ill-health, even after controlling for individual income levels.[577] This has been

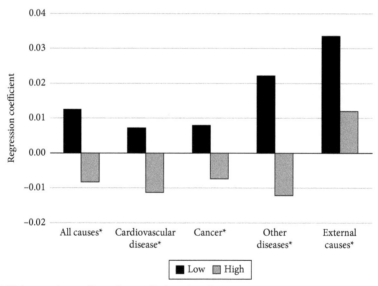

Figure 4.10 income inequality and mortality by education

Notes: Results of country- and period-fixed effects regression of natural logarithm of mortality on income inequality, controlling for national income. Income inequality = Gini coefficient for net equivalized household income. * indicates a statistically significant interaction on mortality between education and income inequality. Men; results for women similar. Pooled dataset of mortality by level of education in 17 European countries, ca. 1980–ca. 2014.

Source: dataset constructed in DEMETRIQ/LIFEPATH projects, with harmonized data from national/regional mortality registers; income inequality data from Standardizing the World Income Inequality Database (SWIID).[505]

interpreted as indicating a 'contextual effect' of income inequality, which may increase health risks for everyone, perhaps through social comparisons and the resulting psychosocial stress,[41,491] or through erosion of social capital.[578] However, the evidence is far from unambiguous, and more strictly controlled studies tend to find less or no effects of income inequality on mortality,[314] so a fair judgement is that the jury on the average population health effects of income inequality is still out.

Nevertheless, it is possible that even in the absence of an effect of income inequality on average health, there is an effect on health inequalities, because a widening of the income gap between rich and poor may well increase disparities in various health risks and opportunities for health improvement.

Political disruption

As European countries differ a lot in the political composition of their governments over the past decades, one would expect that if left-party government is effective in reducing health inequalities, countries with more of it in the past would have smaller health inequalities now. However, that is not what the data tell us. We find no evidence that left-party government has reduced inequalities in mortality or self-reported health problems.[v] This is in line with previous findings for average population health, which also found no effects of left-party government.[579]

This is not to say that politics have had no effect on health inequalities at all. After 1989, countries in Central-Eastern and Eastern Europe made a transition from communist rule to various grades of democracy. Democracy has generally been found to have positive effects on population health, perhaps because democratic governments make decisions in accordance with their voters' interests, and are more inclined to promote the public good than authoritarian governments.[580]

However, it has also been shown that the transition to democracy in Central and Eastern Europe was temporarily associated with lower life expectancy, particularly among men.[581] Our data show that the rise of mortality during democratization in Central-Eastern and Eastern Europe was limited to low educated men (Table 4.1). Among high educated men, mortality quickly started to decline, as it did among high educated women. As a result, inequalities in mortality widened considerably.

Widening of inequalities in mortality occurred for many specific causes of death, of which a few examples are shown in Figure 4.11. Alcohol-related mortality rose in all groups, but more so among the low than among the high educated. Mortality from amenable causes started to decline immediately among the high educated, but not among the low educated. The prevalence of smoking increased, but self-assessed health began to improve.

The rise of mortality during the transition to democracy in Central-Eastern and Eastern Europe has been attributed to the disruption of these societies that accompanied the abrupt political changes. This was a double transition (not only political, also economic, with a change from a communist to a capitalist economy), and in some cases even a triple transition (with an additional dissolution of old states and the formation of new ones, as in the case of the Czech and Slovak Republics and the former Yugoslav republics).

The disruptions were particularly clear in the case of road injuries, which soared as a result of increased access to cars and inadequate road infrastructure.[582] Economic restructuring was accompanied by declining national income, rising unemployment and widening of income inequalities, so in the case of Central-Eastern and Eastern Europe there is likely to be considerable overlap between the effects of national income (Figure 4.9), income inequality (Figure 4.10), and democratization (Figure 4.11).

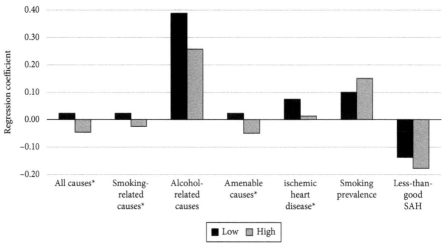

Figure 4.11 Democratization and health outcomes by education

Notes: Results of country- and period-fixed effects regression of natural logarithm of mortality, smoking and self-assessed health on level of democracy, controlling for national income. Because levels of democracy in Western Europe were uniformly high, the effect of level of democracy seen in these analyses reflects temporary rises or declines accompanying the transition to democracy in Central and Eastern Europe. Level of democracy: combined Freedom House—Polity 2 democracy score (ranging from 0, for no democracy, to 10, for complete democracy). * indicates a statistically significant interaction on mortality between education and level of democracy. Men; results for women similar. Pooled dataset of mortality by level of education in 5 Central and Eastern European countries, ca. 1980–ca. 2014.

Source: dataset constructed in DEMETRIQ/LIFEPATH projects, with harmonized data from national/regional mortality registers; level of democracy data from Quality of Government Dataset:.[506]

Health care expansion

One of the reasons why the persistence of health inequalities is considered a paradox is that the higher levels of social expenditure in more advanced welfare states are expected to reduce the gap in material living conditions between lower and higher socioeconomic groups, and thus to decrease health inequalities.

This paradox is also present in our European dataset: a simple comparison of Figure 1.2 (level of social expenditure in different European countries) with Figure 2.1 (magnitude of inequalities in mortality in different European countries) already showed that there is little relationship between the two. We also find no evidence for differential health effects of social expenditure in more sophisticated analyses, regardless of the measure of social expenditure used. Higher levels of social expenditure are in some analyses associated with lower rates of mortality and less-than-good self-assessed health, but not more so among the low than among the high educated. These 'negative' results do not exclude the possibility of more subtle effects as found in individual level studies,[583] but at the macro-level patterns of health inequalities do not appear to be influenced by levels of social expenditure.

In contrast, we do find clearly differential effects of levels of health care expenditure. As we discussed in section 4.3, 'Rapid but differential health improvements', some of the persistence or widening of health inequalities may be due to differential uptake by lower and higher socioeconomic groups of advances in health care. Over the past decades, health care has expanded in all European countries to accommodate a combination of greater demand and enlarged opportunities for intervention, but this increase has not moved as quickly everywhere, and current levels of spending are also very different between countries.[584]

That the expansion of health care has likely contributed to the decline of mortality follows from the observation that increases in health care expenditure are associated with declines in mortality from causes amenable to medical intervention.[585] Our data show that when health care spending increases, mortality from amenable causes decreases among both the low and high educated (Figure 4.12). Higher health care expenditure is not associated with lower mortality from non-amenable causes.[500]

Remarkably, and in contrast to what we observed for national income, the effect of health care expenditure on amenable mortality is equally strong, in relative terms, among the low and the high educated. In absolute terms, the effect is stronger among the low than the high educated, which implies that rising health care expenditure goes together with a narrowing of absolute inequalities in amenable mortality (Table 4.1 and Figure 4.12). The good news therefore is that in this European context—with universal access to health care in most countries—rising health care expenditure has had a dampening effect on absolute inequalities in mortality.[500]

As more advanced welfare states usually also have higher levels of health care expenditure, this does not explain their larger-than-expected health inequalities, but it does help to understand some of the large health inequalities in Central-Eastern and Eastern Europe, where health care expenditure is comparatively low.

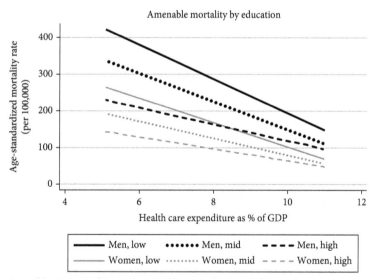

Figure 4.12 Health care spending and amenable mortality by education

Notes: Lines represent regression lines obtained in country- and period-effects analyses controlling for national income. Pooled dataset of mortality by level of education in 17 European countries, ca. 1980–ca. 2014. For causes of death included in amenable mortality, see Figure 4.8.

Source: data from ref. [500]

4.5 **Continued social patterning of health determinants**

Overall results of the analyses

The third factor contributing to the persistence of health inequalities is persistence of social disadvantage, as emphasized in theories focusing on access to welfare state institutions (inverse care law), material living conditions (neo-materialism), and non-material living conditions (psychosocial environment). As a result of the persistence of social disadvantage, plus other circumstances including selection effects and differences in cognitive ability and other personal characteristics, there are persistent social inequalities in practically all health determinants: poverty, working and housing conditions, psychosocial stressors, health-related behaviours, use of health care, etc. (see section 3.3 'Six groups of contributing factors').

Our analyses show that inequalities in some of these health determinants, that is, material deprivation, smoking and obesity, also partly explain the patterns of health inequalities that we observe at the macro-level. Admittedly, these determinants cover only a few of the many that are known to play a role in generating health inequalities. The reason why our analysis focused on these three is practical: data are available by level of education in many countries for many points in time. This allows us to quantify their contribution to inequalities in health using country- and period-fixed effects analyses, which remove, as far as possible, confounding by other factors. For other determinants the available data do not permit such analyses, but some qualitative evidence will be reviewed at the end of this paragraph.

Details on data and methods have been presented in Box 4.1, and some key results from the analyses can be found in Table 4.2. In short, these analyses show that both material deprivation and smoking play a role in determining macro-level patterns of inequalities in all-cause mortality, whereas both smoking and obesity partly determine patterns of inequalities in self-assessed health.[vi]

Inequalities in material deprivation

All European countries still have substantial inequalities in material deprivation, as we saw in Figure 3.2 in Chapter 3. These inequalities are smaller than average in social-democratic welfare states (Finland, Sweden, Norway, and Denmark) and some Christian-democratic welfare states (the Netherlands and Switzerland), than they are in liberal welfare states (the United Kingdom and Ireland) and in countries with a Mediterranean welfare regime (Spain and Italy), and are much larger than average in Post-communist countries in Central-Eastern and Eastern Europe.

Cross-sectionally, there are strong correlations between the prevalence of material deprivation and mortality: levels of mortality tend to be higher when the level of material deprivation is higher, particularly among the low educated.[504] These cross-sectional associations are confirmed in country- and period-fixed effects analyses, but only among men (Table 4.2). In our dataset the aggregate level Relative Risk of mortality for material deprivation is 1.50 (95% CI: 1.23–1.82), indicating a small but statistically significant mortality-increasing effect of the level of deprivation. Among women, the Relative Risk is only 1.20 (95% CI: 0.95–1.51), and not statistically significant. For self-assessed health, no associations with material deprivation are found in these analyses.

Variations between countries and over time in the prevalence of material deprivation also explain some of the variations in mortality among the low and high educated. The aggregate level Relative Risk of mortality comparing the low with the high educated is 2.00 (95% CH: 1.84–2.17) among men and 1.68 (95% CI 1.56–1.81) among women. When we adjust this effect of low education for the level of material deprivation, the Relative Risk goes down from 2.00 to 1.86, implying

Table 4.2 Contributions of poverty, smoking and obesity to inequalities in health

			RR	95% CI		RR	95% CI		RR	95% CI		RR	95% CI	
Mortality	Men	Low education	**2.00**	1.84	2.17	**1.86**	1.72	2.01	**1.58**	1.46	1.70	**1.59**	1.40	1.81
		Mid education	**1.43**	1.31	1.57	**1.38**	1.30	1.46	**1.26**	1.19	1.34	**1.25**	1.15	1.36
		Material deprivation				**1.50**	1.23	1.82				**1.45**	1.15	1.84
		Smoking							**2.98**	2.15	4.14	**2.04**	1.25	3.32
	Women	Low education	**1.68**	1.56	1.81	**1.72**	1.58	1.87	**1.52**	1.44	1.61	**1.47**	1.28	1.69
		Mid education	**1.26**	1.16	1.37	**1.25**	1.18	1.33	**1.19**	1.13	1.25	**1.15**	1.06	1.25
		Material deprivation				1.20	0.95	1.51				**2.15**	1.29	3.58
		Smoking							**2.07**	1.53	2.79	1.25	0.96	1.62
			RR	95% CI		RR	95% CI		RR	95% CI		RR	95% CI	
SAH	Men	Low education	**2.07**	1.90	2.26	**2.33**	1.98	2.73	**1.91**	1.67	2.19	1.14	0.81	1.59
		Mid education	**1.51**	1.39	1.64	**1.61**	1.44	1.80	**1.46**	1.31	1.63	1.10	0.90	1.34
		Smoking				0.53	0.25	1.12				**3.52**	1.30	9.58
		Obesity							**5.41**	1.05	27.93	**22.92**	3.00	175.24
	Women	Low education	**1.93**	1.77	2.10	**1.80**	1.61	2.01	**1.85**	1.54	2.22	**1.33**	1.00	1.76
		Mid education	**1.34**	1.23	1.46	**1.29**	1.18	1.42	**1.34**	1.19	1.50	**1.16**	1.00	1.36
		Smoking				**1.90**	1.00	3.62				**7.49**	3.00	18.71
		Obesity							2.25	0.41	12.29	1.79	0.31	10.17

Notes: RR = Relative Risk. 95%CI = 95% Confidence Interval. SAH = less-than-good Self-Assessed Health. In bold: statistically significant effects (p<.05). Multilevel country- and period-fixed effects analyses. For mortality, results are shown for material deprivation and smoking only, because no statistically significant effects were found for obesity. For self-assessed health, results are shown for smoking and obesity only, because no statistically significant effects were found for material deprivation. Rate Ratios for material deprivation, smoking, and obesity can be interpreted as the ratio of health problems in a population with 100% exposure compared to a population with 0% exposure.

Source: analyses on dataset constructed in DEMETRIQ/LIFEPATH projects, with harmonized data from mortality registers and national and international surveys.

that a small part of the excess risk of the low educated as compared to high educated is explained statistically by inequalities in the prevalence of material deprivation (Table 4.2).[vii]

This effect is found for many specific causes of death. The effects are strongest for mortality from tuberculosis—a disease known to be strongly related to poverty.[586] Among the larger groups of causes of death (cardiovascular disease, cancer, other diseases, and external causes) the effect is strongest for mortality from external causes. In country- and period-fixed effects analyses we found no clear evidence for a role of material deprivation in determining patterns of inequalities in self-assessed health or activity limitations.

These findings suggest that between-country variations in the magnitude of inequalities in mortality are partly determined by variations in inequalities in material deprivation, or to be more specific: that larger inequalities in mortality in Central-Eastern and Eastern Europe are probably partly due to larger inequalities in material deprivation. In view of the high levels of material deprivation seen in this region—the result of low levels of national income, large inequalities in market income, and a rudimentary welfare state—this is perhaps not very surprising.

However, what do these results tell us about the persistence of health inequalities in advanced welfare states, such as the Nordic countries? Thanks to their generous welfare states and low levels and small inequalities in material deprivation, mortality inequalities are probably smaller in these countries than they would otherwise have been. Whether the residual inequalities in material deprivation play a role in the persistence of health inequalities in these countries is perhaps plausible, but cannot be directly inferred from our data.

Inequalities in smoking and obesity

Smoking

Inequalities in smoking are an even more important driver of the magnitude of inequalities in mortality than inequalities in material deprivation. Countries differ in the magnitude of inequalities in smoking, and large inequalities in smoking occur in countries with both small and large inequalities in material deprivation, and vice versa, as can be seen in panel A of Figure 4.13). For example, Sweden and Norway both have small inequalities in material deprivation, but Sweden has small, and Norway has large inequalities in smoking. On the other hand, Portugal and Estonia both have large inequalities in material deprivation, but Portugal has small, and Estonia has large inequalities in smoking.

In fact, there is no correlation between the two, which implies that inequalities in smoking can be expected to explain another dimension of the pattern of between-country variations in health than inequalities in material deprivation, which, as we saw above, mainly appears to drive larger inequalities in mortality in Central-Eastern and Eastern Europe.[viii]

As shown in Table 4.2, in our European dataset the aggregate level Relative Risk of smoking for all-cause mortality is 2.98 (95% CI: 2.15–4.14) among men, and 2.07 (95% CI: 1.53–2.79) among women. These are strong effects, obtained in country- and period-fixed effects analyses and therefore relatively robust against confounding by other factors.[ix]

Adjustment for smoking reduces the Relative Risk for mortality of low educated groups from 2.00 to 1.58 among men, implying that higher rates of smoking statistically explain almost half of the excess mortality rates of low as compared to high educated groups, which is considerably more than the part explained by their higher prevalence of material deprivation. Among women, the contribution of inequalities in smoking to inequalities in mortality at the macro-level appears to be smaller, as adjustment for smoking reduces the Relative Risk for mortality of low education by around a quarter, from 1.68 to 1.52.

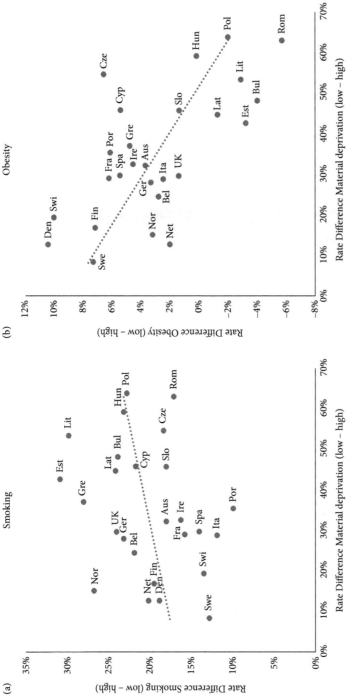

Figure 4.13 Educational inequalities in material deprivation, smoking, and obesity

Notes: Correlation between inequalities in material deprivation and smoking: r = 0.29. Correlation between inequalities in material deprivation and obesity: r = −0.67. Dotted lines respresent regression lines of inequalities in material deprivation. Rate Differences between low and high educated, in percentage of population. Obesity = Body mass index > 30 kg/m2. Smoking = current smoking. Men only; results for smoking among women similar; results for obesity among women different (i.e., no correlation). Data for ca. 2010. Aus = Austria, Bel = Belgium, Bul = Bulgaria, Cyp = Cyprus, Cze = Czech Republic, Den = Denmark, Est = Estonia, Fin = Finland, Fra = France, Ger = Germany, Gre = Greece, Hun = Hungary, Ire = Ireland, Lat = Latvia, Lit = Lithuania, Net = Netherlands, Nor = Norway, Pol = Poland, Por = Portugal, Rom = Romania, Slo = Slovenia, Spa = Spain, Swe = Sweden, Swi = Switzerland, UK = United Kingdom

Source: dataset constructed in DEMETRIQ/LIFEPATH projects, with harmonized data on smoking and obesity from National Health Interview Surveys, and data on material deprivation from EU Statistics on Income and Living Conditions).

This effect of smoking, and the attenuation of inequalities in mortality upon adjustment for smoking, are seen for many specific causes of death. Despite the fact that the relatively short period captured by our smoking and mortality data does not allow us to take into account lag-times, we find strong macro-level effects of the prevalence of smoking on mortality from lung cancer mortality, COPD and other directly smoking-related causes, and—less surprisingly, given the shorter lag-times—on mortality from ischemic heart disease. Among the larger groups of causes of death (cardiovascular disease, cancer, other diseases, and external causes) the strongest effect was found for mortality from cardiovascular disease.

These findings indicate that the social patterning of smoking plays an important role in generating the patterns of inequalities in mortality that we observe at the national level. Other macro-level estimates of the contribution of inequalities of smoking to inequalities in mortality also show that this contribution is substantial (Box 4.3). Inequalities in smoking also partly drive inequalities in self-assessed health, particularly among women (Table 4.2).

Box 4.3 Quantifying the contribution of smoking to inequalities in mortality

Recently, three methods have been applied to quantify the contribution of inequalities in smoking to inequalities in mortality at the aggregate or population level.

Smoking-related causes of death

The simplest method consists of calculating the contribution of causes of death for which we know that a large fraction can be attributed to smoking, such as lung cancer, laryngeal cancer, and COPD. Because of its ease of application, this method has repeatedly been used with European data.[144,273,499] Inequalities in these three smoking-related causes account for around 20% of inequalities in all-cause mortality among men, and around 10% among women, with large variations between countries, the range going from 13 to 32% among men and from –5 to 30% among women.[144] Because smoking causes many more diseases than lung cancer, laryngeal cancer, and COPD, this method will tend to underestimate the contribution of smoking to inequalities in mortality. On the other hand, because there is a decades-long delay between smoking and these causes of death, mortality from smoking-related causes reflects historical smoking behaviour, and if smoking has been more prevalent in the past than it currently is, this method will overestimate the contribution of smoking.

Lung cancer mortality and the Preston-Glei-Wilmoth method

Several methods have been developed that extrapolate lung cancer mortality rates to all smoking-attributable mortality, for example by using the observed associations between lung cancer mortality and all-cause mortality at the aggregate level, as in the Preston-Glei-Wilmoth method[530] This method suggests that in European countries inequalities in smoking account for around 30% of inequalities in all-cause mortality among men, and around 15% among women, but, again, with huge variations between countries, the range in this case going from 20% to 55% among men, and from –10% to 15% among women.[589] This method solves some of the problems of the first method, and in principle captures the effect of life-time smoking exposure on current mortality, but relies on several tenuous assumptions, for example, that

> **Box 4.3 Quantifying the contribution of smoking to inequalities in mortality** (*continued*)
>
> lung cancer among never smokers is stable over time and across countries, and that the effect of smoking on mortality is similar across socioeconomic groups.[589]
>
> ### *Survey data on smoking and population-attributable fractions*
>
> The contribution of smoking to inequalities in mortality can also be estimated directly from smoking rates as measured in health interview and other surveys. Using the prevalence of smoking by socioeconomic group and Rate Ratios of mortality for smoking as reported in the literature, one can use population-attributable fractions to estimate the proportion of deaths, and the proportion of inequalities in mortality, due to smoking.[261,262,264] Using this method it has been estimated that inequalities in smoking account for around 15% of inequalities in all-cause mortality among men, and for around 8% of inequalities in all-cause mortality among women, with values ranging between 4% and 26% among men, and between 1% and 20% among women.[262] The main limitation of this method is the mirror image of the main limitation of the first method: it measures the effect of current smoking only, and ignores the past and time-lags. For example, because smoking has declined among men, this method likely underestimates the full impact of smoking on inequalities in mortality among men.[262]
>
> Despite the differences between these methods, they all indicate a substantial contribution of inequalities in smoking to inequalities in mortality. They also indicate similar patterns of geographical variation, for example substantial contributions of smoking to inequalities in mortality among women in the North and West, and small contributions in the South of Europe.

Here we have a factor that clearly helps to understand the persistence of health inequalities in advanced welfare states: more advanced welfare states do not have smaller inequalities in smoking than less advanced welfare states—on the contrary, some, such as Norway, have larger inequalities in smoking.

Obesity

Obesity is more frequent among the low educated, but countries differ substantially in the magnitude of these inequalities. In contrast to smoking, there is a correlation between inequalities in material deprivation and inequalities in obesity, as can be seen in panel B of Figure 4.13. Among men, inequalities in obesity are smaller in countries where inequalities in material deprivation are larger. They are even 'reverse' in Central-Eastern and Eastern European countries where inequalities in material deprivation are very large, suggesting that high levels of material deprivation in lower socioeconomic groups are a barrier for becoming obese. Inequalities in obesity are largest in countries where inequalities in material deprivation are smallest, i.e., in the Nordic countries, as if low levels of deprivation facilitate obesity. This may even be an example of a paradoxical effect of the welfare state: by reducing material deprivation, it may have removed a barrier for becoming obese.

Obesity is a much weaker determinant of mortality than smoking at the individual level, so it is unsurprising that it also plays a less important role in generating inequalities in mortality at the aggregate level (Table 4.2). Inequalities in obesity partly explain inequalities in mortality from some causes of death, including diabetes: inequalities in diabetes mortality are larger where inequalities in obesity are larger, particularly among men.[590]

For men, a higher prevalence of obesity is also associated with a higher prevalence of less-than-good self-assessed health (and with a higher prevalence of long-standing health problems, not shown in Table 4.2). Adjustment for obesity reduces the Relative Risk of less-than-good self-assessed health for the low educated from 2.07 to 1.91. Similar results, but with smaller effects, are found for women.

Nevertheless, population-attributable risk analyses suggest that among women, obesity is often more important as a determinant of inequalities in mortality than smoking, particularly in the South of Europe, but this is a larger share in smaller inequalities in mortality.[261, 591] Whereas smoking makes a substantial contribution to inequalities in ischemic heart disease mortality among men in Northern and Central-Eastern Europe, obesity makes a substantial contribution to inequalities in ischemic heart disease mortality among women in Southern Europe.[592,593]

Inequalities in other health determinants

Of course, material deprivation, smoking, and obesity are not the only health determinants that are socially patterned, and that contribute to the persistence of health inequalities in modern welfare states. For a small number of other factors we also have evidence that they play a role in generating variations between countries in the magnitude of health inequalities.

As we have seen in Figure 2.4, alcohol-related mortality is very much more frequent among the low educated, and as we have seen in Figure 4.7, these inequalities are particularly large in Central-Eastern and Eastern Europe and some Northern European countries. The contribution of alcohol-related mortality to inequalities in all-cause mortality therefore also varies substantially between countries, and is around 10% or more among both men and women in some Northern, Central-Eastern, and Eastern European countries.[146,594]

This is likely to be an underestimate, because excessive alcohol consumption raises the risk of many more causes of death, including ischemic heart disease and injuries. For example, excessive alcohol consumption often plays a role in homicide, by reducing problem-solving capacity and increasing impulsivity, which increases the probability of disputes and the use of violence in drinking situations.[595,596]

Large inequalities have also been found in mortality from conditions amenable to medical care. These inequalities are much larger in some countries than in others: inequalities are largest in Central-Eastern and Eastern Europe, smaller in Northern and Western Europe and smallest in Southern Europe. Inequalities in mortality from amenable conditions contribute between 11% and 24% to inequalities in partial life expectancy between the ages of 30 and 64.[151] Although these inequalities do not correlate with inequalities in doctor visits,[597] the international pattern is somewhat similar to that of inequalities in unmet need (Figure 3.7), suggesting that they arise from socioeconomic inequalities in quality and/or accessibility of health care services.

Turning to less tangible factors, we have seen in Figure 3.4 that all European countries, including those with advanced welfare states, have substantial inequalities in non-material resources. Whereas countries in Northern Europe do have smaller inequalities in material living conditions, they do not necessarily have smaller inequalities in social, cultural, and psychological conditions. For example, inequalities in living without a partner, frequent TV watching, and the traditional cultural value of 'security seeking' are actually larger, not smaller, than elsewhere. Also, inequalities in cultural values have remained largely constant between earlier and later born birth cohorts in Northern Europe—again an illustration of the refractory nature of inequalities in non-material conditions.[x]

4.6 **Understanding the European experience**

'Nordic paradox'

†We can now try to understand more fully why health inequalities are larger in some countries than in others. What explains the 'Nordic paradox (i.e. large health inequalities in Northern Europe despite egalitarian policies), the 'Southern miracle' (small health inequalities in Mediterranean countries despite lack of egalitarian policies), and the 'Eastern disaster' (explosion of health inequalities in Central and Eastern Europe after the collapse of communism)?[598]

The persistence of substantial inequalities in mortality in the Nordic countries—and in continental-European countries with similarly advanced welfare states—has puzzled researchers ever since the first rigorously conducted comparative study shattered the illusion that health inequalities in these countries were smaller than elsewhere.[26]

Since that first study, published in 1997 and based on data from the first half of the 1990s, the situation has become even worse: over the past decades, inequalities in mortality have widened more in the Nordic countries than in other European countries (Figure 2.5), and Norway and Denmark now rank as the European countries with the largest relative and absolute inequalities in mortality among women (Figure 2.1).

This has sometimes been interpreted as indicating that Nordic welfare policies do not help to reduce health inequalities. However, this is a mistake, and the contrary is likely to be true. The correct interpretation is that in the Nordic countries the inequalities-narrowing effects of welfare policies are over-ridden by the inequalities-widening effects of *other* factors:

◆ Further advanced changes in social stratification, social mobility and composition of socioeconomic groups. Educational expansion has happened earlier and has advanced further than elsewhere, and intergenerational mobility is more 'fluid' than elsewhere, which has created more scope for selection into and out of socioeconomic groups on the basis of personal characteristics such as cognitive ability, personality, and mental health (section 4.1 'Set-up of the analysis').

◆ Further advanced changes in population health, which—as elsewhere—have been more favourable in higher than in lower socioeconomic groups. The smoking epidemic is further advanced in the Nordic countries, and due to that and to more intensive tobacco control efforts inequalities in smoking are larger than elsewhere. Some of the Nordic countries have also been severely hit by a rise in alcohol-related mortality, which was stronger in lower than in higher socioeconomic groups (section 4.3 'Rapid but differential health improvements'). Larger relative inequalities in health in the Nordic countries are also partly a by-product of their higher levels of prosperity (section 4.4, 'Differential effects of factors driving population health change').

◆ Continued inequalities in social disadvantage, with continued social patterning of health determinants. Inequalities in material living conditions are smaller in the Nordic countries than elsewhere, but inequalities in non-material living conditions are not systematically so. As a result, inequalities in important risk factors for morbidity and mortality, such as smoking, obesity, excessive alcohol consumption and other health-related behaviours are often not smaller in the Nordic countries than elsewhere (section 4.5, 'Continued social patterning of health determinants').

These factors apply to all four Nordic countries, but Sweden does better than the other three countries, particularly in terms of relative and absolute inequalities in mortality among men (Figure 2.1).

---

† Text from section 4.6 has been expanded and adapted with permission from Mackenbach J.P. 'Nordic paradox, Southern miracle, Eastern disaster: persistence of inequalities in mortality in Europe'. *European Journal of Public Health*, Volume 27(suppl. 4): pp. 14–17. Copyright © 2017, Oxford University Press. https://doi.org/10.1093/eurpub/ckx160.

One could even say that the 'Nordic paradox' does not really apply to Swedish men, although it does to Swedish women. The likeliest explanation is that the comparatively low mortality rates among low educated Swedish men are due to their exceptionally low smoking rates. These are not the result of Sweden's superior tobacco control policies (Figure 4.5), but of the use of 'snus', a form of smokeless tobacco which is particularly prevalent among low educated Swedish men.[599]

Smoking is also important for understanding Norway's disadvantage, which is of recent date and due to the fact that inequalities in mortality among Norwegian men and women have widened rapidly over the past decades.[174] Inequalities in smoking-related conditions (e.g. lung cancer) have also risen substantially in Norway, and if one removes the effect of smoking from inequalities in mortality, inequalities in mortality are no longer larger in Norway than elsewhere.[589] Norway is further advanced in the smoking epidemic than many other countries, particularly among women, which may be related to the high levels of gender equality in this country.[600] Norway's stricter tobacco control policies may also have contributed to a wider gap in smoking (Figure 4.5).

Similar comments can be made about Denmark, where smoking rates among low educated women are appallingly high (Figure 4.4), as are lung cancer mortality rates. Here again, gender equality may have put Danish women at a disadvantage, but in this case stricter tobacco control policies are not to blame (Figure 4.5).

'Southern miracle'

Southern European countries have small inequalities in mortality—this does not only apply to Spain and Italy but also to Portugal, Malta, Greece, and Cyprus.[166] Their favourable profile has emerged over the past three or four decades, due to the fact that no widening of inequalities in mortality occurred in Southern Europe.[499]

Several of the explanations for the Nordic paradox are likely to play a role again—but now in a reverse direction. During the twentieth century, economic, social, and cultural modernization occurred later in Southern Europe than in other European countries—a situation that was aggravated by the general stagnation under the military dictatorships that ruled Portugal, Spain, and Greece until the middle of the 1970s.[581] This delayed modernization has miraculously helped to avoid a widening of inequalities in mortality, via two pathways.[601]

First, the delay in expansion of the service sector and of higher education implies that, particularly among older generations which dominate current mortality rates, the low educated are still numerous and less socially marginalized than in other European countries, and that a larger and better advantaged high educated group has not yet emerged. In Southern Europe, education is also less important as a predictor of occupational class than in other European regions.[602]

Second, the social and cultural modernization that usually accompanies economic modernization, in the form of changes in, for example the position of women, cultural values, and dietary, drinking, and smoking patterns, also occurred later in Southern Europe. The best documented example is the delay between Southern Europe and other European regions in timing of the smoking epidemic. For example, among women in Spain smoking-related mortality is still higher among high educated than among low educated women, which keeps inequalities in all-cause mortality very low.[409]

That traditional values do not protect against all inequalities is clear from the large inequalities in obesity among Southern European women, which are probably related to traditional gender roles (i.e. greater numbers of children and less leisure time physical exercise among low educated women, and more labour force participation and stronger social norms for thinness among high educated women).[149] However, because obesity is a much weaker determinant of mortality, this does not compensate the near absence of smoking as a determinant of mortality among the low educated in Southern Europe.

In addition to smoking and obesity, other culturally determined factors also play a role. Smaller inequalities in cardiovascular disease mortality in the South are partly due to the persistence of the Mediterranean diet, and a delay in shift towards a more western-style diet, in lower socioeconomic groups. The persistence of these traditional dietary patterns among the low educated in Spain, Italy, and other Mediterranean countries is helped by the abundant availability and low costs of healthy dietary items like fruits, vegetables, and olive oil in Southern Europe. Also, when the ischemic heart disease epidemic finally reached Southern Europe, therapeutic advances that had been made elsewhere plus reasonably good access to health care helped to keep mortality rates low, and to avoid large inequalities in ischemic heart disease mortality.[601]

'Eastern disaster'

As we have seen many times in this book, the biggest contrast in the magnitude of mortality inequalities within Europe is that between Central-Eastern and Eastern Europe and the rest of the subcontinent. Inequalities in mortality in countries like Slovenia, the Czech Republic, Hungary, Poland, and Lithuania are huge for most causes of death, and although health inequalities were already present under communist governments (Box 4.4), these exceptionally large inequalities

---

Box 4.4 Health inequalities under communism

At the end of the World War II, countries in Central-Eastern Europe, such as Czechoslovakia (now split into the Czech Republic and Slovakia), Hungary, Poland, Romania, and Bulgaria, were occupied by the Soviet Union, and following the Yalta agreement between Stalin, Churchill, and Roosevelt fell under Soviet influence, which meant that within a few years they all had communist governments.[604]

In a first phase, these communist governments were strongly committed to abolishing social inequality, and there is little doubt that they were highly effective in doing so, often by taking draconic measures. They reduced income inequality, increased access to education, reduced differences in prestige between manual and non-manual occupations, and reduced the intergenerational transmission of social advantage, for example, by abolishing wealth inheritance. However, after the 1950s this commitment gradually faded out, and in a second phase of communist government structural social inequalities re-emerged, now partly along party membership lines.[605]

Data on health inequalities in European countries under communism are rare and of uncertain quality, and most data we have date from the latter parts of this second phase, that is, from the 1970s and 1980s when communism was no longer the successful motor of social change that it was in the first decades after the World War II. Quite clearly, health inequalities along lines familiar from capitalist countries already existed in the 1970s and 1980s, for example, in the form of inequalities in infant mortality by mothers' education in Hungary [606] and Yugoslavia,[607] and of large inequalities in life expectancy by adult education in Russia, of at least the same magnitude as those observed in Western Europe.[608]

Hungary is a country with extraordinarily long time-series data on inequalities in mortality by (adult) level of education, spanning forty years between 1970 and 2010. Because over the

Box 4.4 Health inequalities under communism (*continued*)

years the design of the data collection did not change, these data allow robust trend analyses and comparison with a few Western European countries with similarly long time-series data, such as Finland, England and Wales, and Italy (Turin).[174]

Trends in all-cause mortality by educational level in Hungary were presented in Chapter 2 (Figure 2.5). In the 1970s and 1980s, trends and patterns of mortality in Hungary were remarkably different from those in Western Europe. Mortality among men was on the rise, but particularly so among low educated men, and whereas mortality among women was stable, it was on the rise among high educated women. Among men, mortality was higher among the low educated, such as in Western Europe, but among women mortality was higher among the high educated.

In Figure 4.14 we show trends in mortality from selected specific causes of death by educational level in Hungary. These show that the relatively small inequalities in all-cause mortality among men in the communist period, that is, the 1970s and 1980s, were partly due to reverse inequalities for ischemic heart disease mortality—a phenomenon also seen in some Western European countries in earlier time-periods.[152]

The figure also shows that the inverse inequalities in all-cause mortality among women in the communist period were due to higher mortality among the high educated from ischemic heart disease, lung cancer, breast cancer, suicide, and road traffic injuries—again patterns that are not completely unique, but are much more outspoken than anywhere in Western Europe during this period. In the post-communist period, mortality declined among men and women, but much more so among the high educated, and as a result several inequalities in cause-specific mortality reversed and inequalities in all-cause mortality rose dramatically.

One factor that contributed to inequalities in mortality among men in the communist period was the lack of effective tobacco and alcohol control measures, combined with heavy tobacco and alcohol consumption due to economic, cultural, and social conditions. Smoking tobacco was an accepted part of Hungarian lifestyle under communism, and there was little attention to its negative health effects when these became more widely known only in the 1990s and 2000s, although higher education groups had already partly given up smoking earlier.[609]

Heavy drinking was also common in all social groups. This has been explained by a combination of four factors: the general state of 'anomie' under state socialism, migration from rural to urban areas with loss of old social networks, rising income with lack of other opportunities for spending money, and a strong cultural tradition of wine-growing and spirit-distillation.[610] This happened against the background of the state's attempt at rapidly modernizing Hungarian society. After 1985 alcohol consumption started to decline as a result of gradual tightening of alcohol control and diminished tolerance for heavy drinking[611]—however, mortality from alcohol-related conditions did not start to decline much later (Figure 4.14).

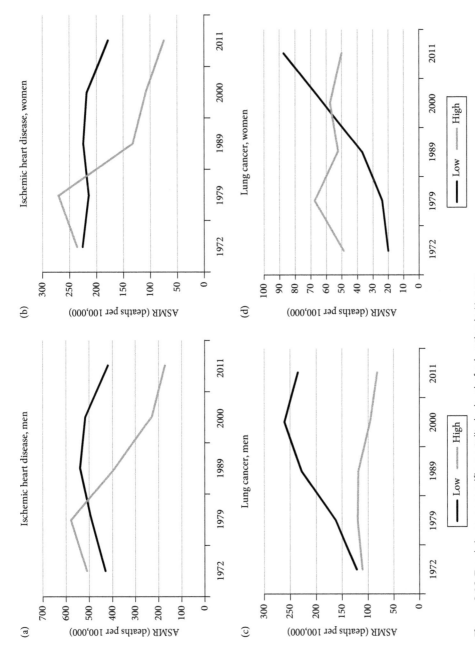

Figure 4.14 Trends in cause-specific mortality by level of education in Hungary

Notes: ASMR = Age-Standardized Mortality Rate.

Source: dataset constructed in DEMETRIQ/LIFEPATH projects, with harmonized data from Hungarian national mortality register.

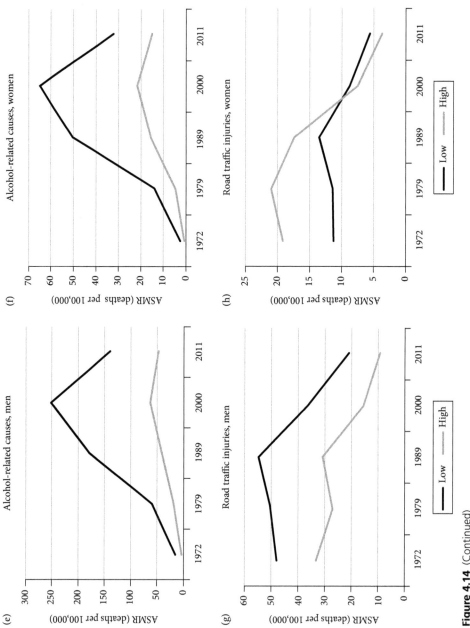

Figure 4.14 (Continued)

have arisen relatively recently, during the profound political and economic changes that followed the collapse of the Soviet Union around 1990.[603]

The political transition towards liberal democracy and the economic transition towards capitalism were accompanied by a temporary rise of mortality in many Central-Eastern and Eastern European countries, which was due to a rise in unemployment and poverty, a breakdown of protective social, public health, and health care institutions, and a rise in excessive drinking and other risk factors for premature mortality.[556,612]

As we have seen above, this rise of mortality was not equally shared within the population, and mainly occurred among those with a lower level of education. Apparently, people with a higher level of education were better able to protect themselves against increased health risks, and even to benefit from new opportunities for health gains, for example, the introduction of new cardiovascular drugs from the West.[176]

As a consequence, inequalities in mortality exploded in Central-Eastern and Eastern Europe. In-depth analyses have shown that the larger inequalities in mortality which emerged after 1990 can be explained by a combination of large inequalities in poverty, excessive alcohol consumption, and lack of access to good quality health care.[504]

The recent reversal of the mortality trend among the low educated in several Central-Eastern and Eastern European countries is equally remarkable, and of course very welcome (Figure 2.1). The declines in mortality among the low educated are due to declines in mortality from smoking-related causes, amenable causes, and ischaemic heart disease, and sometimes also from alcohol-related causes and suicide.[175]

For the total population these changes have been attributed to a combination of long-term declines in smoking, improvements in health care, dietary changes, road traffic safety measures, and alcohol control policies.[613] Apparently, these mortality-lowering policies have finally also reached the low educated. The fact that the European Commission supported massive investments in these countries' infrastructure may also have helped. However, despite the welcome trend reversal, levels of mortality among lower socioeconomic groups remain extremely high.

Key points

◆ This chapter reports on the results of a series of in-depth analyses of determinants of health inequalities at the macro-level, focusing on what might explain the persistence of health inequalities in modern welfare states.

◆ Health inequalities are partly driven by changes in social stratification, such as educational expansion, social fluidity, and changes in the size and composition of socioeconomic groups. These have contributed to the persistence, and sometimes widening of health inequalities over time.

◆ Widening of health inequalities is also partly driven by differential health improvement, particularly by differential mortality decline which often benefits higher socioeconomic groups more (in relative terms) than lower socioeconomic groups. Higher socioeconomic groups have benefited more from rising prosperity and rising health care expenditure, and have suffered less negative health impacts from rising income inequality and the transition towards liberal democracy in Central and Eastern Europe.

◆ Persisting and sometimes increasing social inequalities in health determinants also play an important role in the persistence and sometimes widening of health inequalities, as illustrated by the substantial contribution of inequalities in poverty and smoking to patterns of health inequalities in Europe.

- The same forces that have played an important role in the persistence of health inequalities over time—remodelling and persistence of social inequality, and a rapidly changing health landscape—also explain why countries with highly developed welfare states still have such large health inequalities. These countries are in the forefront of changes in social stratification and improvements of population health, and these have undone some of the health inequalities reducing effects of the welfare state.

Chapter 5

A broader picture

5.1 Why social inequality persists in modern welfare states

The causes of the causes

‡After having identified the factors underlying the persistence of health inequalities in modern welfare states, it is time to address the more fundamental question why social inequality as a more general phenomenon is so durable, and to ask ourselves how the persistence of health inequalities fits into the broader picture of persistence of social inequality.[614]

It has been argued that, in order to understand health inequalities, we must search for 'the causes of the causes'. For example, we should not be satisfied with tracing back the determinants of health inequalities to smoking, psychosocial stress, or lack of access to health care, but should open our eyes to the fact that inequalities in smoking, stress, and health care are themselves caused by the unequal distribution of advantage and disadvantage in society.[615] True, but should the next question then not be for the 'causes of the causes of the causes', in other words, for what causes social inequality?

Most of the theories of health inequalities that we have reviewed in Chapter 3 take the existence of social inequality as a given, and explain how the unequal distribution of resources over social positions 'gets under the skin'.[444] Some theories focus on selection into different social positions, and others on differential health improvement or continued social disadvantage, but with the exception of the 'political economy of health' theory they do not explain why valuable resources are unequally distributed, and why this unequal distribution is so persistent.

Explaining social inequality has been at the heart of the discipline of sociology since its very beginnings, and this has led to an abundance of theories of social inequality, including those of Rousseau, Marx, Weber, Durkheim, Pareto, Parsons, Davis, Bourdieu, Wallerstein, Elias, Tilly, and many others. Two main strands of thinking can be distinguished: a more 'conservative' tradition, which emphasizes the function of social inequality for society as a whole, and a more 'radical' tradition, which emphasizes conflict over scarce resources and 'rent-seeking' of social elites.[54]

This range of views resembles the one we encountered reviewing theories on the explanation of health inequalities: 'social selection' fits within wider 'functionalist' theories of social inequality, and 'political economy of health' within wider 'conflict' theories of social inequality. As we will see, the other theories of health inequalities also have borrowed various elements from sociological theories of social inequality.

Functionalist theories

The more 'conservative' line of reasoning is based on the premise that social stratification has a useful function for human societies, because hierarchy improves group functioning. For example,

‡ Text from section 5.1 has been expanded and adapted with permission from Mackenbach J. P. 'Persistence of social inequalities in modern welfare states: Explanation of a paradox.' *Scandinavian Journal of Public Health*, Volume 45, Issue 2: pp.113–120. Copyright © 2017, © SAGE Publications. https://doi.org/10.1177/1403494816683878.

hierarchy has been suggested to improve collective decision-making, to facilitate the coordination of individual action (e.g. in the form of a division of labour), and to increase motivation of members to act in the group's interest.[616]

These functionalist theories, as articulated by Parsons, Davis, and others, argue that social stratification benefits society as a whole, because it gives monetary and non-monetary rewards to those who are most useful to society, and therefore provides indispensable motivation for those with talent and a taste for enterprise, whose efforts will then ultimately benefit everyone.[33,34]

The idea that social inequality may have benefits for society as a whole is supported by insights from the related discipline of sociobiology. Humans are not the only species with social inequality—on the contrary many nonhuman species, from ants to chimpanzees, have dominance hierarchies, that is, a form of group organization whereby animals of higher rank dominate those of lower rank, for example, in the distribution of food and sexual partners.[617] Among nonhuman primates a higher social rank is associated with better health and a longer lifespan, as it is among humans.[618i]

These social hierarchies are thought to have resulted from evolutionary pressures, in the sense that they have provided reproductive or survival advantages for the species as a whole, for example, by increasing the efficiency of cooperation within the group and by minimizing hostile exchanges.[617] The fact that forms of social inequality exist in animals with less complex behaviour than humans, suggests that these hierarchies are to some extent the outcome of universal, perhaps even biologically programmed processes.[619]

It is important to note that, even if such 'natural' explanations for social inequality are true, they do not tell us that social inequality is good from a normative standpoint. The idea that 'natural behaviours' are inherently good or inevitable has been called the 'naturalistic fallacy'.[620] Humans have often been able to transcend their natural tendencies, but it is nevertheless important to understand why things are as they are.

At first sight, functionalist theories have good papers for explaining the persistence of social inequality, because they posit that all societies need a certain degree of social inequality, for example to provide an adequate reward system. As long as there are differences between individuals in 'human capital', for example, in the form of cognitive ability or motivation to work, and as long as society gives higher rewards to those who are perceived to have more value to society, some individuals will end up in social positions with more access to valued resources.

Functionalist explanations of social inequality have parallels in economic explanations for rising income inequality: because of rising demand for highly educated labour on the one hand, and restricted supply due to scarcity of talent on the other, wage inequality between high and low educated people has risen strongly.[514] Globalization, with its enhanced opportunities to employ unskilled labour in countries with lower levels of income, also plays a role.[39]

Other more or less 'benign' accounts for the persistence of social inequality in spite of counter-measures point to changes in demographic behaviour, which have contributed to an accumulation of advantage or disadvantage in the same families. As we have seen in section 4.2, 'Changes in social stratification', there is increased educational 'homogamy': partners in marriage increasingly have the same level of education.[515,621] Also, due to higher life expectancy there is more overlap between the lifetimes of grandparents and grandchildren, which may strengthen multigenerational transmission of (dis)advantage.[622]

Conflict theories

The second, and more 'radical' tradition of sociological theorizing on the origins of social inequality suggests that other explanations are more important. In this tradition, competition or conflict within societies is seen as the ultimate basis of social inequality. For example, according to classical Marxism the exploitative nature of capitalism is the main motor of social inequality, as those who own the means of production use their power to exploit those who are dependent on selling their labour in the labour market.[35]

Since the nineteenth century, the nature of the economy and the occupational structure have changed considerably, and differences in access to resources between different groups of employees have become at least as important as those between the owners of the means of production and their employees.[623] Neo-Marxists therefore recognize a more finely graded distinction between social groups in modern societies on the basis of their ability to extract 'rents', that is, earnings in excess of their investments in education or the value of their efforts for society.[624]

For example, although CEOs of large companies are formally employees, their salaries and other benefits far exceed those of other employees, without any apparent justification in terms of their value for the company. The recent explosion of income inequalities in many countries cannot be explained from market forces alone: managers of large companies have increasingly reached a position in which they determine their own earnings, thereby increasing their opportunities for rent-seeking.[39]

These material advantages naturally create an interest among the beneficiaries in the protection of their advantages, both for themselves and for their children. This interest is protected in subtle and less subtle ways: according to Marxism, it has led to the structural embedding of social inequality in institutions (e.g. laws that protect property, and an educational system that is more easily accessible to the children of the rich) as well as in society's dominant culture (e.g. religious beliefs that legitimize social inequality).[625]

Like functionalist theories, conflict theories go a long way in explaining the ubiquity of social inequality across species borders and throughout human history—not by pointing to the usefulness of social inequality, but by pointing to a universal tendency to compete for resources and to seek prestige in the eyes of others, and therefore to dominate others whenever possible. According to some scholars, social inequality is the normal throughout human history, and it is egalitarianism that needs to be explained.[626]

It is not difficult to see many examples of such competition, some more subtle than others. The pursuit of self-interest by the better-off often directly or indirectly harms the less well-off, sometimes in unintended ways. For example, many high educated people do not send their children to socially mixed schools, but choose to maximize the opportunities of their children by sending them to socially homogeneous schools with better educational outcomes, thereby reducing the educational opportunities for children from less advantaged parents.[627]

Although countries differ in their degree of intergenerational transmission of disadvantage, social origin is still very much a determinant of cognitive ability, educational achievement, and subsequent social position and life trajectory, partly as a result of the active striving of well-off parents to transmit their advantages to their children.[628]

Once a hierarchy is established, it is also reinforced by psychological processes. Power transforms individual psychology so that the powerful think and act in ways that lead to the retention and acquisition of power. Status also generates expectations for behaviour and opportunities for advancement that favour those with a status advantage.[629]

Although the durability of the individual-level mechanisms mentioned above may explain part of the persistence of social inequality, structural factors also play a major role. People entering the labour market mostly do not themselves create their jobs, but, in Schumpeter's terms, enter a 'hotel room' that for them is a given, as part of the occupational structure in which the economy operates. The distribution of rewards over these occupations is not decided on a case-by-case basis, but part of long-standing conventions and regulations.[53]

Over the past decades there has been a clear shift in the balance between labour and capital, to the advantage of the latter, and as a result wages have risen much less than company profits.

This shift in power relations is partly due to the fact that ideological changes have led to declining union membership, and to less income redistribution by governments.[37]

Residential segregation is another structural factor that helps to perpetuate social inequality. Children growing up in poor neighbourhoods have less school readiness and achievement, and more behavioural and emotional problems, through a range of pathways including institutional deficiencies, less supportive social relationships, and less favourable social norms and collective efficacy.[627]

A middle ground

Ecological-evolutionary theory

Although these two sociological traditions hold contradictory views on the origins of social inequality, they have to some extent been integrated in Lenski's 'ecological-evolutionary theory'. American sociologist Gerhard Lenski (1924–2015) combined elements from both traditions, and based his theory on the premise that humans are driven by self-interest, that most objects of their striving are in short supply, and that therefore a struggle for rewards is present in all societies. Also, because humans are unequally endowed, genetically or otherwise, some are more successful in this struggle for resources than others.[54]

However, because human societies need cooperation, there is a limit to the resulting material inequality in that resources necessary for basic functioning will generally have to be distributed on the basis of need—this is in the interest of all. But according to Lenski's theory the surplus will often be distributed on the basis of power, that is, on the basis of social class membership, only to be mitigated by egalitarian policies when humans consciously choose to transcend their individual interests.[54]

Lenski's theory explicitly recognizes that even though social inequality in its generic sense is durable, its specific characteristics (such as the nature of the social positions that determine the distribution of resources, and the skewedness of the distribution of resources over these positions) may change over time.[54]

For early human history, trends in social inequality have been assessed in archaeological research, for example by studying burial gifts, that is, the valuables that were buried with the dead in their graves. Because these were given to only a small fraction of the dead, the distribution and size of burial gifts are seen as an indicator of the extent of social inequality in prehistorical societies. The archaeological evidence suggests that social inequality was limited in hunter-gatherer societies, but rose substantially during the Neolithic period (between 11,000 and 3,000 BCE) with the invention of agriculture.[630]

This finding has been confirmed in anthropological research among current hunter-gatherer groups, and has given rise to the idea that, although the human tendency to compete for resources and to seek prestige may be universal, egalitarian behaviour is certainly not exceptional. An egalitarian ethos is widespread among hunter-gatherers, perhaps because opportunities for accumulating resources are less than in agricultural and industrial societies, but also because human beings dislike being dominated.[631,632] In later phases of history, egalitarian tendencies have been strengthened by the development and propagation of religious and ideological beliefs emphasizing equality.[54]

For more recent periods, direct information is available on the extent of social inequality, and this shows that during the early stages of industrialization social inequality (indicated by inequalities in income and wealth) first rose even further, but then started to decline in the early twentieth century. This reversal is due to a whole range of factors, both economic and sociocultural: massively increased productivity making it easier for the upper class to share resources with the lower classes; expansion of knowledge and the increased importance of education for highly specialized jobs; the rise of democratic ideologies and the greater bargaining power of lower classes when organized in labour unions; and the expansion of the role of government and the rise of bureaucracy.[54,633]

Neo-weberian theories

It is important to note that in both the conservative and radical sociological traditions, as well as in Lenski's synthesis, the emphasis is on social inequality in economic resources, and this is indeed a central element of social inequality. However, other theories have also acknowledged the importance of non-material resources. For example, as briefly mentioned in section 2.1 'Measurement issues', Weber's theory of social stratification makes a distinction between economic, political, and symbolic (or cultural) resources, allowing for the possibility that social stratification systems are not uni- but multidimensional.[634]

Neo-Weberians have taken this a step further by recognizing the important role of social and cultural capital in reinforcing economic capital, by creating exclusionary processes that support the 'social closure' of groups that have managed to access the most resources.[635] Bourdieu and others have argued that in post-industrial societies education is the gateway to higher paid occupations, and that because the education system reflects the culture of the higher classes, the cultural capital of parents determines their children's success, so that higher education remains relatively closed to the lower classes.[456,636]

Ambition and other tastes for educational and occupational advancement are dependent on cultural factors like time preferences and role models. Children from lower class families may have self-fulfilling beliefs due to discrimination, and may be discouraged by negative expectations of teachers and other elements in the dominant discourse.[637]

Ultimately, the durability of social inequality should then be understood from the persistence of its underlying fundamental mechanisms and processes: (i) Humans are driven by self-interest, while most objects of their striving are in short supply, and therefore a struggle for rewards is present in all societies. (ii) Humans are unequally endowed, therefore some are more successful in this struggle for resources than others. (iii) The inequalities resulting from these individual level actions are structurally fixated through the intergenerational transmission of (dis)advantage, various societal institutions, and cultural factors.

This probably also explains why the modern welfare state has not been able to eliminate social inequality—it has softened some of the sharper consequences, for example, by reducing the prevalence of absolute and relative poverty,[638] but has only marginally affected the many other underlying mechanisms and structural factors.

Links between social inequality and health inequalities

From social inequality to health inequalities

If social inequality is so difficult to eradicate, readers may wonder how feasible it is to ever eradicate health inequalities. It is easy to see how health inequalities almost follow automatically from social inequality: humans have an innate drive for survival and for avoiding illness, and thus will inevitably use some of the resources that their social position provides to pursue these goals.[466] In other words, as long as social inequality persists, and as long as health is seen as a goal worth striving for, health inequalities will persist.

However, social inequality is not the only driving force behind health inequalities. The 'Nordic paradox' shows that it is possible for less social inequality to go together with more health inequality, whereas the 'Southern miracle' shows the reverse (section 4.6 'Understanding the

European experience'). This is because health inequalities are also generated by other mechanisms, such as processes of 'selection' or 'reverse causation', and 'confounding' by personal characteristics that are independent from the socioeconomic conditions in which people have been raised.

From health inequalities to social inequality

An equally intriguing question is whether health inequalities are just a consequence of social inequality, or also play a role in the generation and persistence of social inequality. There are several reasons to suspect the latter.

First, health certainly plays a role in the allocation of individuals to social positions, one of the three central elements of social inequality. Although the contribution of health-related selection to total health inequality remains uncertain, health-related social selection has been shown to operate over the life-course: children with physical or mental health problems have worse educational outcomes than their healthy peers, adults with health problems are less likely to be upwardly socially mobile and more likely to experience a loss of income, and elderly who have experienced health problems during their lives are less wealthy than those who have not.[228,230,315] Thus, whereas social disadvantage may cause health disadvantage, the latter may in its turn aggravate social disadvantage, creating vicious circles.[639]

Second, if social inequality helps society to function smoothly, as functionalist theories stipulate, one may wonder whether health inequality also has some usefulness for society. Is receiving a few extra years of life and having to spend less years of life with disease and disability not an enormous bonus on top of the other rewards for perseverance in education and excelling at one's job? Of course, to be effective as an incentive these health benefits would have to be widely known to the general public, either consciously or unconsciously, but some recent studies suggest a fairly widely diffused awareness of health inequalities among the general public.[640]

Third, if social inequality is the outcome of competition for scarce resources, as conflict theories imply, health inequality is among its most dramatic outcomes, with disease and premature death being the losers' fate. This is certainly part of the story, as the examples of tobacco and junk food show: it is in the interest of those who have invested their wealth in the tobacco and food industries, to continue to sell unhealthy products to people who do not have the knowledge or the self-directedness or the money to buy healthier products. Health inequality then indeed is the ultimate outcome of power relations, as Marxist scholars suggest.[498]

But could health inequality somehow also strengthen these power relations? For example, because ill-health of the poor and low educated helps to further shift the balance of power towards those who already have more of everything? Or because ill-health leads to social exclusion through loss of work and the necessity of remaining ill, in order to avoid loss of one's disability benefit? Also, the higher prevalence of depression in lower socioeconomic groups has been interpreted as a form of adaptive behaviour that strengthens social inequality, by making lower status people refrain from competition.[641,642]

Thus, there are reasons to think that health inequality is more than a consequence of social inequality, and plays a more profound role by amplifying social inequality in various ways that deserve further study.

5.2 Health inequalities and welfare state reform

Factors driving welfare state reform

As mentioned above, the persistence of health inequalities does not imply that the welfare state has been a failure. The welfare state has achieved a lot, particularly in terms of reducing poverty.

It has recently been estimated that welfare systems reduce the risk of poverty by 38% on average across the EU, but this impact varies from under 15% to over 60% across the member states, due to variations in transfers and taxes and other institutional factors such as minimum wages, collective bargaining, and active labour market programmes.[643]

Universal welfare states, such as those in the Nordic countries, redistribute the most, and are better in reducing poverty than welfare states that target resources towards the poorest, probably because universal welfare states create a coalition between the least well-off and the middle classes, which in the long run increases the total amount of money available for redistribution.[644]

However, since the 1970s the welfare state has come under pressure in many European countries, and it is by no means certain that the welfare state as we currently know it will continue to exist. Initially, the main issue was economic competitiveness: countries which spent a large fraction of their national income on social transfers and other welfare programmes, felt the need to reduce their public expenditure and started to reform their welfare arrangements, leading to various degrees of 'welfare retrenchment', that is, restrictions of benefit entitlement and reductions of benefit levels.[17]

But this was not the only factor behind the drive for welfare state reform. Extensive welfare arrangements had been introduced in all countries in Western Europe and North America after the World War II, partly as an expression of solidarity between rich and poor in the face of the shared ordeals of the war, partly as a safety measure against the threat of communism, which in the immediate post-war years seemed to find increasing support among workers in Western democracies. When the memories of the war started to fade, and the failures of communism in providing a good life to citizens in Eastern Europe started to become apparent, support for the welfare state became less, and inequality again became more acceptable.[45]

While this suggests that welfare state reform since the 1970s was at least partly driven by economic and ideological factors, there were also more intrinsic factors that necessitated a re-think of the aims and instruments of the welfare state. The old social risks which the welfare state had been designed to buffer, were gradually and to some extent replaced by new social risks for which the welfare state did not have a good solution.

This included increased life expectancy (which threatens to make pension systems unsustainable), the de-standardization of employment relations (undermining unemployment benefit schemes which protect employees), and widening inequalities between family types (particularly between two-earner households with both partners having a high education and income, and single low educated parents with children).[645,646]

These trends have all contributed to shifting attention from the traditional objectives of the welfare state (i.e. reducing risks of poverty for lower class single-earner families) to the need to find solutions for other problems. However, as these other problems have important health dimensions, the need to avoid and/or alleviate health inequalities should be central to welfare state reform. This will be illustrated with two examples: pension reform and active labour market policies.

Pension reform

In section 2.2 'Generalized but uneven', we briefly mentioned inequalities in total and disability-free life expectancy and their potential relevance for retirement policies. In order to reach the statutory retirement age in good health, people should have a disability-free life expectancy of at least that age (currently around 65 years in most countries,[169]) but there is no European country where this is currently the case for the average low educated man.

While this is already problematic, many countries are now considering raising their statutory retirement age to well over 65 years. Taking all high-income countries together, life expectancy at age 60 has increased from 18 to 23 years since 1970, and is expected to rise to 28 years by 2050. If retirement ages remain at the same level as today, expenditure on public pensions will rise enormously, and the costs will have to be carried by a relatively smaller working population. A possible solution is to gradually raise the pension age in parallel with rising average life expectancy, as has already been decided in countries like Denmark, Finland, Italy, the Netherlands, and Portugal. Based on current projections of life expectancy, this implies that by 2050 statutory retirement age will be above 70 years in Denmark, Italy, and the Netherlands.[169]

If this is not to lead to even bigger inequalities in reaching retirement in good health than already exist today, it requires strong and parallel improvements in disability-free life expectancy in all socioeconomic groups. This implies that pension policies should be aligned with health policies: the more successful we are in improving health of lower socioeconomic groups, and in reducing inequalities in health between socioeconomic groups, the more likely it will be that ambitions for raising pension age, without dramatic increases in sickness and disability benefits, can be attained. Otherwise it will be necessary to allow workers with lower levels of education and in lower occupational classes to retire at a younger age.[647]

Active labour market policies

Apart from varying degrees of 'welfare retrenchment', the main direction of change for welfare states has been a shift towards 'social investment' policies, that is, a move away from passive transfers towards the maximization of employability and employment. Some European countries have introduced 'flexicurity' systems, which are based on minimal job protection compensated by decent standards of income protection for the unemployed. At the same time, many European countries have turned towards activation and reintegration measures to stimulate self-reliance of the unemployed.[648]

There are important health dimensions both to job and income protection and to activation and reintegration. As we briefly mentioned in section 3.3 'Six groups of contributing factors', unemployment represents a health risk, and job and income protection likely help to reduce those health risks. On the other hand, ill-health is also a risk factor for becoming unemployed and for leaving the labour force through other channels, such as early retirement,[649] as well as for being unable to obtain work.[650] A higher prevalence of physical and mental ill-health in lower socioeconomic groups is one among many reasons why people in lower socioeconomic groups have a higher probability of being out of paid work.

This nexus between socioeconomic position, health, and employment implies that not only do labour market policies have potential effects on health inequalities, but also that improving the health situation of lower socioeconomic groups may help to increase their employment rates. Seen from this angle, policies to reduce health inequalities should form an integral part of active labour market policies and other attempts to improve the effectiveness of the welfare state.

In the meantime, it is unclear yet what the impact of flexicurity systems and other social investment policies will be on health inequalities. Analyses of flexicurity systems in European countries have revealed large variations in how these have been designed, without clear associations between degrees of flexibility and/or security on the one hand, and the likelihood of return-to-work for people in lower socioeconomic groups with health problems on the other hand.[651,652] Whatever the potential benefits of active labour market policies may be, maintaining sufficient levels of 'passive' income support remains essential for avoiding a widening of health inequalities.[646].

5.3 **Health inequalities and social justice**

Common intuitions

The intuition of many of those engaged with health inequalities is that because health is important and social inequality is unfair, health inequalities are a particularly troubling form of social injustice. Are health *inequalities* not by definition health *inequities*?

Perhaps the strongest expression of this idea can be found in the WHO Commission on Social Determinants of Health's 2008 report 'Closing the gap': 'Where systematic differences in health are judged to be avoidable by reasonable action they are, quite simply, unfair. [...] Putting right these inequities [...] is a matter of social justice. [...] Social injustice is killing people on a large scale'.[653] (executive summary)

Several attempts have been made to formalize and underpin the intuition that health inequalities are inequitable,[ii] for example, by elaborating explicit criteria to judge health inequalities,[227] or by applying a formal theory of justice to health inequalities.[656,657] Clearly, if health inequalities are inequitable, we have a collective duty to try to remedy them. It has even been proposed to formalize this duty in a 'human rights' framework.[658]

However, building a convincing case for the inequitableness of health inequalities is less straightforward than it seems. In this paragraph we will systematically discuss possible viewpoints with regard to the inequitableness of health inequalities, acknowledging from the outset that whether one sees health inequalities as inequitable is not a purely scientific, but also a normative question. Different viewpoints can be taken, both in the selection of a particular theory of justice and in its application to the available evidence, so that we will have to make some difficult choices based on our own values and beliefs.

Because philosophers disagree on what the best theory of justice is, it may come as a relief that there are also other compelling reasons to reduce health inequalities. For example, we may on a more voluntary basis want to act in accordance with a spirit of solidarity, or we may on a more calculating basis want to improve the health of the disadvantaged in order to promote economic growth or reduce the costs of health care. We will discuss these other viewpoints at the end of this paragraph.

A simple starting-point: Margaret Whitehead's principles

Principles of equity in health

A widely used set of criteria to judge the inequitableness of health inequalities is the one developed by Margaret Whitehead, and published in the early 1990s.[43,654] It was based on discussions within a working group convened by the Regional Office for Europe of the World Health Organization, and took as its starting point that 'health inequities' are 'differences which are [...] avoidable, but in addition are considered unfair [...]'.

Based on these two criteria, 'avoidability' and 'unfairness', seven main determinants of health inequalities were classified into whether the resulting health inequalities should be labelled a 'health inequity' or not:

- 'Natural, biological variation.' Not potentially avoidable, and not commonly considered unfair, and therefore not a health inequity.
- 'Health-damaging behaviour if freely chosen, such as participation in certain sports and pastimes.' Potentially avoidable, but not commonly considered unfair, and therefore not a health inequity.

- 'The transient health advantage of one group over another when that group is first to adopt a health-promoting behaviour (as long as other groups have the means to catch up fairly soon).' Potentially avoidable, but not commonly considered unfair, and therefore not a health inequity.
- 'Health-damaging behaviour where the degree of choice of lifestyles is severely restricted.' Potentially avoidable, and commonly considered unfair, and therefore a health inequity.
- 'Exposure to unhealthy, stressful living and working conditions.' Potentially avoidable, and commonly considered unfair, and therefore a health inequity.
- 'Inadequate access to essential health and other public services.' Potentially avoidable, and commonly considered unfair, and therefore a health inequity.
- 'Natural selection or health-related social mobility involving the tendency for sick people to move down the social scale.' Low income as a result of sick people moving down the social scale is potentially avoidable and commonly considered unfair, and therefore a health inequity.[43,654]

While this framework is useful as a first guide to identifying 'health inequities', it also has some weaknesses that become apparent upon further reflection.

Weaknesses

The first problem relates to the first criterion: how should 'avoidability' be defined? That this is not entirely straightforward, is already clear from Whitehead's use of the ambiguous term 'potentially avoidable'. This suggests that, even if we lack the money and manpower to tackle health inequalities, these should still be considered inequitable if effective intervention methods do in principle exist. On the other hand, it would seem reasonable to take the level of available resources into account—are health inequalities due to lack of access to expensive medical interventions not more inequitable in high-income than in low-income countries?

And what about health inequalities for which effective intervention methods do not yet exist, but might be developed in the future? Or health inequalities for which we know that they are caused by social inequality, but for which we can imagine no practical remedy, for example because human nature predisposes human beings to create hierarchies of power and advantage which can never be eliminated, as suggested by some theories of social inequality (section 5.1, 'Why social inequality persists in modern welfare states')? Does a lack of effective intervention methods really make health inequalities less inequitable?

These ambiguities of the criterion of 'avoidability' suggest that it is problematic to put so much emphasis on whether health inequalities can be reduced by human action, and that it may also be risky to apply this criterion as a first filter before the 'unfairness' of health inequalities is assessed.[659]

The second problem relates to the second criterion: when should differences in health be 'considered unfair'? This would appear to be *the* crucial question, but when applying this criterion to the seven determinants of health inequalities mentioned above, the report only says that its conclusions reflect 'the consensus view from the literature listed in the reference section', that is, that 'the crucial test of whether the resulting health differences are considered unfair seems to depend to a great extent on whether people chose the situation which caused the ill health or whether it was mainly out of their direct control'.[654 (p. 6)]

As no formal theories of justice are cited in the report, we are left in the dark with regard to why 'free choice' should have such a central role in determining whether health inequalities are 'unfair' or not. Furthermore, the fact that this criterion is not applied consistently suggests that other factors should also be taken into account. For example, 'a transient health advantage' of the higher educated is said to be 'not commonly considered unfair', despite the fact that delays in the adoption of new health-promoting behaviours are out of the direct control of people in lower socioeconomic groups, that one 'transient' advantage usually follows another, and that all these advantages are based on structural factors like access to new information and cultural capital carefully transmitted from one generation to the next.

The criterion of 'free choice' is also hard to operationalize. It makes intuitive sense that health inequalities resulting from 'health-damaging behaviour if freely chosen' do not qualify as health inequities, but when it comes to giving examples the report can only mention the proverbial skiing injuries suffered more frequently by higher socioeconomic groups, which do 'not arouse [a] sense of injustice, since the cause—skiing—is widely viewed as a voluntary activity chosen by those who accept and insure against the risks involved'.[654] (pp. 6/7) If it is impossible to give an example of a health problem that is more frequent in lower socioeconomic groups and that can be attributed to the exercise of 'free choice', this criterion loses its discriminatory power.

One wonders whether the judgement of fairness should not instead be based on whether health inequalities can be attributed to human actions, in which the socially advantaged benefit at the expense of the socially disadvantaged. After all, in the words of John Rawls (whom we will encounter further on in this section) the term 'fairness' refers to 'right dealing between persons who are cooperating with or competing against one another', and 'a practice will strike the parties as fair if none feels that, by participating in it, they or any of the others are taken advantage of'.[660] (p. 178)

More generally, and as already mentioned in section 1.3 'The need for a broader picture', Whitehead's framework does not explicitly take into account whether inequalities in health are generated by social inequality, that is, inequalities in access to resources along socioeconomic lines, or by differences along some other social dimension, such as gender, marital status, migrant status, urban versus rural location, etc. According to others, it does matter that we are dealing with health differences along a socioeconomic dimension.

For example, American social epidemiologist Paula Braveman has proposed a definition of 'health inequity' as 'systematic disparities in health [...] between social groups who have different levels of underlying social advantage/disadvantage'. Therefore, 'a health disparity is inequitable if it is systematically associated with social disadvantage in a way that puts an already disadvantaged social group at further disadvantage'.[44] (p. 254) This implies that whether or not health inequalities should be considered inequitable, partly depends on whether the broader social inequalities generating them are considered inequitable—which may then depend on whether one takes a more benign 'functionalist' or a more 'radical', 'conflict'-oriented view of the origins of social inequality.

Because of these problems, this section will take a detour around formal theories of justice that focus on the conditions under which social inequality can be considered inequitable, and we will then again try to classify different categories of health inequalities according to their inequitableness.

Egalitarian theories of justice and their application to health inequalities

Four groups of theories

There is no agreement among philosophers about what the best theory of justice is: each theory has been championed by some and criticized by others.[661] Box 5.1 describes some of the most common theories of justice which argue for some kind of equality, and which therefore fall under the broad heading of 'egalitarianism'.

Box 5.1 Egalitarian theories of justice

The term 'egalitarianism' is used in everyday language to refer to a political belief in favour of income redistribution and greater equality in other policy outcomes such as access to health care. However, in political philosophy 'egalitarianism' refers to a broad family of theories of justice, which differ importantly in what they would like to see equalized. We list them here according to their central principle, and in increasing order of orientation towards equality of final outcomes.

1. *Equality of opportunity*

This principle requires that social positions that confer superior advantages (e.g. jobs providing higher incomes) are open to all applicants, and that applications are assessed on their merits (i.e. applicants' talents and ambitions, and not their family connections or other characteristics irrelevant for the proper execution of the job). This is a widely shared ideal in liberal democracies that will, if fully implemented, lead to a 'meritocracy', that is, a society in which advantages are distributed according to people's merits. It is important to note, however, that this ideal has several important limitations. First, formal equality of opportunity at the point of recruitment is not sufficient to bring about actual equality of opportunity, because there may still be substantial inequality in the opportunity to become qualified (e.g. because talented children of poorer families experience financial barriers to higher education). Second, this ideal does not specify how unequal the distribution of advantages is allowed to be. Theoretically, nothing in the theory prohibits a society to let those who do not have sufficient 'merit' (e.g. because they have cognitive impairments) to live in destitute poverty. Recognition of these problems has given rise to the idea that this principle should be combined with other principles, such as that of a decent minimum amount to which everyone regardless of merit is entitled.[662]

2. *Equality of resources*

In response to the shortcomings of theories based on the principle of (formal) equality of opportunity American philosopher John Rawls (1921–2002) has proposed another theory of justice, 'Justice as fairness', which combines an attempt to create substantive (as opposed to merely formal) equality of opportunity with rules to restrict inequality in the distribution of advantage. In Rawls's theory, 'fair equality of opportunity' is satisfied if individuals who have the same native talent and the same ambition have the same prospects of success—which requires public policy to offset inequalities between families in child development and upbringing (e.g. by offering pre-school education) in order to restore their 'normal opportunity range'. Rawls's theory limits inequality in the distribution of advantage by stipulating that all persons should have the same basic rights and liberties (i.e. there should be an equal distribution of 'primary social goods') and that social and economic inequalities are permitted only to the extent that they are to the greatest benefit of the least advantaged members of society (this has been called the 'Difference Principle'; for example a certain degree of income inequality is permitted if this is necessary to stimulate economic growth, and if this economic growth then maximally raises the incomes of the least advantaged).[655] Rawls's theory is probably the most popular liberal theory of justice, but according to its critics does not provide sufficient equality in opportunity for welfare.[661]

Another theory of justice which tries to overcome some of the limitations of formal equality of opportunity is 'luck egalitarianism'. This theory, which was originally developed by American

Box 5.1 Egalitarian theories of justice (*continued*)

philosopher Ronald Dworkin, sees the point of distributive justice as equalizing individuals' opportunities for welfare. It therefore sees all inequalities in access to advantage that result from factors over which the individual has no control ('brute luck') as unfair and thus as warranting rectification by public policy, whereas inequalities in access to advantage which result from choices the individual made ('option luck') are not unfair and do not require rectification. Examples of bad 'brute luck' include the negative consequences of a lack of native talents, and those of a disability arising from health problems which the individual cannot reasonably be expected to avoid. Examples of bad 'option luck' include the negative consequences of a lack of desire to work hard and of a decision to engage in risky sports. According to this theory individuals have the right to be compensated for the first but not for the second.[663] This theory, when applied in practice, will achieve greater equality of resources than Rawls's theory, but it has been criticized because it is too harsh for those suffering from bad 'option luck', for example, by legitimizing the withholding of publicly funded medical care for smokers with lung cancer.[661]

3. Equality of capabilities

All the above theories aim for equality of 'opportunity', but this can be criticized as not going far enough in creating 'real freedom' to lead a flourishing life. For this, more is needed (e.g. good health), and we also need to take into account that people's preferences as to what constitutes a flourishing life differ, and that we therefore must avoid imposing one particular condition as the yardstick of equality and/or the objective of public policy (e.g. equality in income or in welfare). Indian economist and Nobel laureate Amartya Sen and American philosopher Martha Nussbaum have developed these ideas into a theory of equality of 'capabilities', that is, the capabilities that one needs for basic functioning. The core capabilities include, among others, bodily health, being able to move freely, being able to think, being able to love, being able to participate in political choices, etc. The theory claims that a society can only be considered decent if it secures at least a threshold level of these essential capabilities to all inhabitants.[664,665] Because of its explicit inclusion of good health as one of the core capabilities, this is the most popular normative framework in the health inequalities field, but it has been criticized for largely ignoring personal responsibility, and for implicitly including a vision of what constitutes a flourishing life, but avoiding an explicit discussion of the normative basis for that vision.[661]

4. Equality of welfare

In one indirect way or another, all theories of justice aim for a fair distribution of human good, so why not explicitly choose equality of 'welfare' as the yardstick of justice and the aim of public policy? This is indeed what theories of equality of welfare do, and these come in different forms that mainly differ in the way welfare is conceptualized. One way is to see welfare in terms of conscious states, such as pleasure or happiness; another is to see welfare in terms of success in fulfilling one's goals, for example by looking at the degree to which one's preferences are satisfied.[666] Despite their intuitive appeal, these theories have been criticized, not only (as some of the theories described above) for ignoring personal responsibility and inter-individual differences in conceptions of welfare, but also for being too radical, that is, for setting unrealistic goals and for risking serious conflict with other societal goals such as civil and political liberties.[661]

(Partly based on Richard Arneson's entries on 'Egalitarianism' and 'Equal opportunity' in the Stanford Encyclopaedia of Philosophy [661,662].)

We leave aside some other theories of justice which, on the contrary, argue *against* attempts to achieve equality of opportunity or condition, such as libertarian theories based on the supremacy of property rights. For example, the 'entitlement' theory of American philosopher Robert Nozick stipulates that everyone is entitled to his or her possessions provided they were acquired through earnings, inheritance, or other legal means, and that any attempt by government at redistribution is an injustice.[667] This implies a rather harsh viewpoint with regard to health and health inequalities, because even the creation of equal access to health care, by shifting resources from the rich to the poor, would be out of the question.[668]

We leave these non-egalitarian theories aside not because they are intellectually inferior—on the contrary, they are based on a plausible starting-point and are perfectly internally consistent—but because they accept health inequalities as an inevitable consequence of a higher good, that is, each person's fundamental liberty to pursue his or her own interests. If you would adhere to such a conception of justice, you would probably have stopped reading this book many pages ago.

As can be seen from this box, when equality of condition (particularly of welfare, but also of capabilities and resources) is chosen as the yardstick of justice, one will have to deal with the thorny issue of personal responsibility. The idea behind this issue is that some differences in, for example, happiness will be the result of differences in the life choices people make. The same applies to inequalities in income, which may partly be the result of differences in how hard people are prepared to work. Do we have a moral obligation to reduce these inequalities and/or their consequences? Those who answer this question negatively, will prefer theories of justice that aim for equality of opportunity only, or that exclude the consequences of voluntary choice from the resources to be equalized.

Ideology

These disagreements are not only a matter of conflicting technical-philosophical arguments, but also reflect differences in ideological position, with 'equality of opportunity' being more popular among those leaning towards the political right, and 'equality of welfare' being more popular among those leaning towards the left.

Ideological differences may also colour the application of theories of justice. Like Whitehead's framework, several formal theories of justice make a distinction between, on the one hand, the negative consequences of 'freely chosen' behaviour for which people should be held responsible themselves and which therefore cannot be seen as inequitable, and, on the other hand, the negative consequences of unfavourable living conditions over which people have no control and which therefore are often seen as inequitable.

Although such distinctions can sometimes be made on the basis of empirical evidence, many determinants of health inequalities do not neatly fall into either one of these categories. For example, smoking may, at some point in some intelligent adolescent's life, be a deliberate choice based on at least some knowledge of the long-term health consequences, but may, at other points and/or in other people's lives, also be an addiction. Whether we decide for one or the other perspective will then inevitably be influenced by our personal beliefs.

We can also see in Box 5.1 that some of these theories appear to articulate an ideal of positive equity. For example, luck egalitarians would like to see all inequalities in access to advantage that result from factors over which the individual has no control (i.e. 'brute luck', such as genetic differences that give rise to inequalities in talent), rectified by public policy. These inequalities cannot necessarily be blamed on anybody, but nevertheless lack of compensation for inequalities in native talent is seen as an inequity—or perhaps more accurately: a deviation from an ideal of positive equity.

What do these theories imply for the (in)equitableness of health inequalities? We will elaborate this starting with the most radical conception of equality, 'equality of welfare', and then work our way back to the least radical, 'equality of opportunity'.

Health inequalities versus equality of welfare

If deviations from equality of welfare are inequitable, then health inequalities are also inequitable, because health indisputably is a very important determinant of happiness, well-being and other dimensions of welfare. This is sometimes called a 'direct' approach, and represents a rather common normative position in the health inequalities field which simply holds that all health inequalities—to the extent that they are avoidable—are inequitable.[669]

For example, this is the position taken by Michael Marmot, not only in his role as chair and author of the WHO CSDH report (see the quotation at the start of this section), but also and very explicitly in his book 'The Health Gap'. In this book he reviews—like we are doing in this section— several theories of justice. Because these do not agree—as we have seen above—on what should be equalized, he proposes 'to help the philosophers' and to choose the 'approach to social justice [which] is most likely to increase health equity'.[47] (p. 80)

In other words, Marmot already knows that all avoidable health inequalities are inequitable, and can therefore turn the reasoning on its head by trying to find the formal theory of justice which comes closest to his intuitions. Although this turns out to be Sen's 'equality of capabilities' approach, the implicit theory underlying Marmot's viewpoint must be equality of welfare.

However, are all avoidable health inequalities really inequitable, regardless of how they are generated? Other authors on this issue take the view that it does matter how they are generated, as illustrated by Whitehead's criteria for assessing whether health inequalities are health inequities.[43] This implies that some health inequalities may be inequitable, whereas others are not or less so.

Some health inequalities are generated by inequalities in material and non-material living conditions over which individuals have little or no control—like Marmot, many people will probably tend to consider these inequitable. But are health inequalities inequitable which arise from differences in health-related behaviour over which individuals do have some degree of control? In Marmot's view, inequalities in smoking, alcohol consumption, diet, and other health-related behaviours are entirely due to the more severe constraints people in lower socioeconomic groups face,[47] but while such constraints certainly exist, it is by no means certain that there is not an element of choice as well.

Marmot does not explicitly discuss the normative evaluation of health inequalities that arise from differences in personal characteristics (such as cognitive ability, personality traits, etc.), some of which are transmitted genetically, or of health inequalities that arise from 'reverse causation', because he does not believe these to be important mechanisms. But to the extent that these mechanisms play a role, they would have to be considered 'inequitable' under the principle of 'equality of welfare'.

Health inequalities versus equality of capabilities

The 'capabilities' approach has led to some of the most articulate applications to the field of health inequalities.[658,659] This is unsurprising given the fact that health is one of the core capabilities that this theory distinguishes. In applications of this theory one will find statements such as the following: 'All human beings have a moral entitlement to the capability to be healthy.' 'It is unfair if social arrangements reduce capability to be healthy in some people.' 'The responsibility of governments is to create conditions that enable individuals to be as healthy as possible. This demands such a distribution of social determinants of health—to the extent that they can be controlled by human beings—that every individual has the same possibility to lead a healthy life'.[658] (p. 6)

This may seem almost as radical as 'equality of welfare', but there are some notable differences. The most apparent difference is that justice according to the 'equality of capabilities' approach does not label all health inequalities arising from differences in health-related behaviour as inequitable. People are left free to use their capabilities to lead the lives they value. Justice 'only' requires governments to create conditions that enable individuals to behave in a healthy way, and to eliminate 'social arrangements' that work the other way. This is a clever twist that increases the acceptability of the 'equality of capabilities' approach in societies emphasizing personal responsibility.

Because applications of the 'equality of capabilities' approach to health inequalities have focused on 'social causation',[658,659] it is not immediately clear how it would regard health inequalities generated by differences in personal characteristics, such as cognitive ability. However, as its central concern is to ensure that all individuals have the capability to be healthy, it could be argued that it does require such differences to be compensated by public policy.

A similar reasoning applies to health inequalities generated by downward social mobility among those who are ill: in this case ill-health itself is a barrier for leading an otherwise flourishing life, and it could be argued that the capabilities approach does require this to be counteracted by public policy.

Health inequalities versus equality of resources (justice as fairness)

Theories of 'equality of resources' have also been applied to health inequalities. American philosopher Norman Daniels has developed extensions of Rawls's theory of justice to health care, and to health and health inequalities. Health is not one of Rawls's 'primary social goods' (Box 5.1) and does not lend itself to direct redistribution, but Daniels argues that 'health is special ... because disease and disability, by impairing normal functioning, restrict the range of opportunities open to individuals'.[670 (p. 2)]

According to Daniels, Rawls's principle of 'fair equality of opportunity' implies that we have a collective obligation 'to restore the fair opportunity range for individuals to what they would have if social arrangements were more just and less unequal'. This obligation does not only encompass equality of access to health care, but also implies that we have to eliminate the social determinants underlying health inequalities, including where these give rise to inequalities in health-related behaviour.[670]

Somewhat optimistically, Daniels then goes on to argue that full application of Rawls's principles of justice would go a long way towards eliminating health inequalities. For example, 'the fair equality opportunity principle assures access to high quality public education, early childhood interventions aimed at eliminating class or race disadvantages, and universal coverage for appropriate healthcare. Rawls's "Difference Principle" permits inequalities in income only if the inequalities work (e.g. through incentives) to make those who are worst off as well off as possible.' This implies, as in the case of Whitehead's principles, that a transient health advantage may be acceptable, but Daniels emphasizes that 'making those who are worst off as well off as possible' goes beyond a simple 'trickle down' idea.[656 (p. 8)]

According to Daniels, 'a society complying with [Rawls's] principles of justice would probably flatten the socioeconomic gradient even more than we see in the most egalitarian welfare states of northern Europe. The implication is that we should view health inequalities that derive from social determinants as unjust unless the determinants are distributed in conformity with these robust principles.'[656 (p. 8)] We note in passing that Daniels appears to be unaware of the fact that the Nordic countries do not have particularly small health inequalities.

Like most applications of the 'equality of capabilities' approach, this incarnation of Rawlsian justice assumes that health inequalities are generated by 'social causation'. It is therefore silent on whether health inequalities that are due to inequalities in personal characteristics, or health inequalities generated by downward social mobility of those with health problems, are inequitable. However, because its central concern is with restoring the 'normal opportunity range' of individuals, it would probably consider such health inequalities to be inequitable.

Health inequalities versus equality of resources (luck egalitarianism)

Dworkin's 'luck egalitarianism', with its distinction between 'choice' ('option luck') and 'circumstance' ('brute luck'), has been applied to health (care) by Israeli political scientist Shlomi Segall. He sees 'the luck egalitarian view on health policy as one according to which society ought to fund biomedical treatment for any condition that is disadvantageous, could be fixed by biomedical intervention, and it would be unreasonable to expect the individual to avoid'.[671] (p. 348) Read 'prevention' for biomedical treatment or intervention, and it is clear how this can be applied to health inequalities.

Interestingly, this is the only theory of justice that not only labels health inequalities due to unfavourable living conditions as partly inequitable, but also explicitly considers inequalities due to (innate) personal characteristics as inequitable. It therefore requires compensation for inequalities in advantage generated by differences in cognitive ability and other personal attributes.[672]

By contrast, 'luck egalitarians' tend to see health inequalities resulting from differences in health-related behaviour as 'option luck', and therefore do not consider these inequitable. It is precisely on this point that luck egalitarianism has been rather widely criticized. For example, one can legitimately ask why the difference between 'choice' ('option luck') and 'circumstance' ('brute luck) should have such a weight, when some people are much better in making good choices than others.[673] The difference may also lead to rather futile distinctions, such as between someone being killed by a racing car when using a marked crosswalk ('brute luck') and someone being killed when crossing the street one metre beside the marked crosswalk ('option luck').[45]

Nevertheless, defenders of luck egalitarianism have argued that 'any account of justice in health would have to resort to some sort of mechanism for allocating scarce resources, and it is not obvious why considerations of personal responsibility should be precluded from performing that role'.[671] (p. 350) Luck egalitarianism has gained a certain popularity, as illustrated by attempts to quantitatively apportion health inequalities to those that arise from 'effort' and those that arise from 'circumstance'.[674]

Luck egalitarianism would probably see health inequalities generated by ill-health-related downward social mobility as at least partly unfair, that is, to the extent that the health problems involved are a matter of bad 'brute luck'.

Health inequalities versus equality of opportunity

We finally arrive at the application of (formal) 'equality of opportunity' to health inequalities. This theory requires the allocation of social positions and their related benefits to be based on 'merit' only. In a radical interpretation, this theory accepts that there are inequalities in advantage between social positions, even if these have consequences for the length and quality of life, as long as access to these positions is based on 'merit' only.

Although modern societies have become more 'meritocratic' over time, it is easy to see that even in the most socially and economically advanced countries a complete 'meritocracy' has not been realized (section 3.4 'Theories about the explanation of health inequalities'). This implies that health inequalities caused by social inequalities in material and non-material living conditions are at least partly inequitable under this theory of justice. The same goes for inequalities in health-related behaviour that follow from inequalities in living conditions. However, health inequalities arising from the fact that people in different social positions have different personal characteristics, or arising from health-related selection, would be seen as inevitable in meritocratic societies.

A comparison between theories

We summarize the results of this discussion in Table 5.1, which compares Whitehead's criteria with five theories of justice, in their application to four main pathways along which health inequalities arise: living conditions, health-related behaviours, (innate) personal characteristics, and health-related selection.

According to Whitehead's criteria, health inequalities that are due to inequalities in living conditions are inequitable, and most of the theories of justice agree. The exceptions are 'luck egalitarianism' (which accepts inequalities in living conditions that result from 'option luck') and 'equality of opportunity' (which accepts inequalities in living conditions that result from differences between people in talent or effort).

Judgements on health inequalities that arise out of inequalities in health-related behaviour range from 'not inequitable' according to 'luck egalitarianism' (which accepts these inequalities as a consequence of 'option luck'), to fully 'inequitable' according to a radical interpretation of 'equality of welfare'. Most theories, including Whitehead's framework, do not completely reject the idea of 'free choice', although it is unclear where the dividing line between 'choice' and 'circumstance' should be drawn.

One important conclusion is that any other approach than 'equality of welfare' will, if consistently applied, consider at least part of health inequalities 'not inequitable'. On the other hand, if one would relax the requirement of consistency and be willing to take an eclectic approach and to borrow from different theories, it would also be possible to find a set of arguments for considering

Table 5.1 Inequitableness of health inequalities according to five theories of justice

Theory of justice	Health inequalities due to inequalities in living conditions	Health inequalities due to health-related behaviour	Health inequalities due to (innate) personal characteristics	Health inequalities due to health-related selection
The concepts and principles of equity in health (Whitehead)	*Inequitable*	*Partly inequitable*	*Not inequitable*	*Partly inequitable*
Equality of welfare/The Health Gap (Marmot)	Inequitable	Inequitable	(Inequitable)	(Inequitable)
Equality of capabilities (Nussbaum/ Venkatapuram)	Inequitable	Partly inequitable	(Inequitable)	(Inequitable)
Equality of resources/ Justice as fairness (Rawls/Daniels)	Inequitable	Partly inequitable	(Inequitable)	(Inequitable)
Equality of resources/ Luck egalitarianism (Dworkin/Segall)	Partly inequitable	Not inequitable	Inequitable	Partly inequitable
(Formal) equality of opportunity	Partly inequitable	Partly inequitable	Not inequitable	Not inequitable

Notes: For comparison, the results of applying Whitehead's principles are given on top. Most theories reserve the label of 'inequitableness' for health inequalities that are (somehow) 'avoidable'. Between brackets: not explicitly discussed by lead authors. For further explanations, see main text.

all health inequalities 'inequitable'. This would be easier if one would take into account the fact that, over the life-course, the four mechanisms distinguished in Table 5.1 do not occur in isolation, but are intertwined.

Health inequalities and social justice: second thoughts

Accumulation of unrelated disadvantage

Some readers will perhaps have noticed that the above considerations are all somewhat narrow in the sense that they focus on health inequalities as a phenomenon separate from other social inequalities, in an attempt to find arguments for the 'inequitableness' (or not) of the specific factors and mechanisms generating health inequalities. This is certainly important, but can we really ignore the broader context of social inequality?

Suppose that there is one set of mechanisms generating inequalities in life expectancy between the low and high educated, and there is another set of mechanisms generating inequalities in income between the low and high educated. Let us assume for the moment—not entirely unreasonably, in view of the evidence presented in the previous chapters—that income inequalities play no key role in generating inequalities in life expectancy. Does it matter morally that the low educated not only have a low income but also live shorter?

In reality, the accumulation of disadvantage in lower socioeconomic groups, whether these are defined in terms of education, occupational class, or income, goes way beyond monetary well-being and length of life. It includes physical and mental functioning, social and psychological well-being, and political participation, to name but a few of the other disadvantages that people in lower socioeconomic groups are exposed to. The factors and mechanisms generating these inequalities are partly overlapping, partly different, may include varying doses of 'choice' and 'circumstance', and may therefore be a mix of more and less unfair mechanisms, but in the end there are huge differences in the lives people lead.

It could be argued that we do have a moral obligation to reduce the clustering of disadvantage. This clustering has been called 'corrosive', because one form of disadvantage may exacerbate another one, for example when being overwhelmed by financial worries reduces the ability of disadvantaged people to supervise their children's homework or to lead a healthy life.[675] According to American political scientist Michael Walzer, a just society is one in which different 'spheres of justice' are kept separated, and in which inequalities in one sphere do not invade another one.[676]

It is beyond the scope of this book to assess the inequitableness of all these other inequalities: that would require a similar type of analysis for each of these other outcomes as the one reported for health inequalities in Table 5.1. But let it suffice to recall that income inequalities are far larger than can reasonably be justified by differences in 'merit' (either in the form of 'talent' or 'effort')—current income inequalities are the result of market forces and 'rent-seeking' behaviour[39]—and that therefore reducing health inequalities can be seen as an attempt to partially redress the effects on well-being of these income inequalities, whether or not there is a causal connection between the two.[iii]

Solidarity

Although considerations of justice probably provide the most powerful normative arguments in favour of policies to reduce health inequalities, other moral considerations can be applied as well. Do our governments, or other collective agencies have a duty to rectify health inequalities, over and above rectifying the inequalities that are clearly inequitable?

Whereas considerations of justice are prominent in the Anglo-Saxon ethical tradition (as exemplified by the work of Rawls, Dworkin, and Nussbaum, who are all Americans), continental

Europe also relies on the concept of 'solidarity', particularly for allocative decisions in health and social services.[677] 'Solidarity' is a term with many meanings, from the recognition that caring for each other is in the common interest, to a non-calculating or truly altruistic commitment to the well-being of others.[678]

'Solidarity does not attempt to offer an alternative for distributive justice, but must be regarded as an important corrective to arrangements of health care practices that are based on a just distribution of goods only'.[677] (p. 18) This complementary nature of 'solidarity' becomes evident when we deal with health inequalities for which there is no consensus that they are inequitable, for example health inequalities generated by inequalities in health-related behaviour. As we have seen above, most theories of justice leave some normative space for free choice, and thus for 'subtracting' inequalities in health due to 'freely chosen' behaviour before declaring health inequalities 'inequitable'. Philosophers working within the Anglo-Saxon liberal tradition cannot do otherwise.

Some forms of solidarity, particularly 'interest solidarity' which is based on the recognition of a common interest, may in effect do the same, because they tend to restrict solidarity to cases wherein a person needs help because of a problem he or she could not avoid. However, other forms of solidarity are less restrictive, leaving more space for the benevolent acceptance of other people's bad choices. Do we not all have our weaknesses, and would we not all like to be helped even when (or particularly when) we do not act in our own self-interest?[679]

Solidarity may therefore cover some aspects of health inequalities that are not easily covered by justice frameworks, particularly health inequalities that are not due to inequalities in material and non-material living conditions. Experiences in European countries with a strong presence of Christian-democratic parties, illustrate that calls for solidarity can indeed play a powerful role in generating commitment to reducing social and health inequalities.[579,680]

However, solidarity inherently is a less powerful basis for action against health inequalities, because it does not give 'rights' to the disadvantaged, as theories of justice can do, and because solidarity with the disadvantaged is ultimately dependent on the voluntary altruism of the advantaged.

Societal costs

Finally, one may want to reduce health inequalities because of the costs to society they generate. Just as cost-of-illness studies have tried to estimate the costs to society of the occurrence of a particular disease, taking into account not only health care costs but also losses to economic productivity and welfare more generally, a few costs-of-health-inequalities studies have tried to estimate the costs to society of health inequalities.[681–684].

This is not a trivial thing to do: while it may seem obvious that the excess health problems of people with lower socioeconomic positions will give rise to societal costs, calculation of the costs of health inequalities requires the identification of an appropriate counterfactual, and it is not immediately obvious what such a counterfactual would look like. A society with no inequalities but the same average rate of health problems? That would imply increasing the rate of health problems among those with higher socioeconomic positions in order to improve the health situation of the disadvantaged.

Instead, attempts to calculate the economic costs of health inequalities have chosen some 'upward levelling' scenario as their counterfactual, that is, a society in which the rate of health problems in lower socioeconomic groups has been made equal to that in higher socioeconomic groups. Depending on the costs included in the calculations these approaches have shown that health inequalities are a costly affair.

For example, one study of the economic costs of health inequalities used a counterfactual scenario in which the lower half of the population would have the same good health as the upper half. For the European Union as a whole, the estimates of inequality-related losses to health as a capital good (leading to less labour productivity) are modest in relative terms (1.4% of GDP) but large in absolute terms (€141 billion). The estimates of inequality-related losses to health as a consumption good, which involves applying the concept of the value of a statistical life, are much higher: €980 billion, or 9.5% of GDP. Also, inequalities-related health losses account for 20% of the total costs of health care, and 15% of the total costs of social security benefits in the European Union as a whole.[681]

There are different ways of interpreting these estimates. One could interpret them as 'the costs of inaction', that is, benefits to society that are forgone because we have not acted to eliminate health inequalities.[684] One could also interpret them as the benefits to society that would accrue if we were willing and able to eliminate health inequalities—but one would then of course also have to take into account the (unknown) costs of reducing health inequalities.[681] In any case, these and other calculations clearly illustrate that health inequalities carry substantial societal costs.

Some conclusions

Is it up to scientists (such as the author of this book) to state that eliminating health inequalities is a requirement of social justice? As has been shown above, different conceptions of social justice are possible, and the choice of one particular conception can only be made on non-scientific, ideological grounds. It is ultimately up to politicians, as representatives of a public that is likely to hold diverging, conflicting, and confused views of social justice, to decide which parts of social inequality in general, and which parts of health inequalities specifically, are inequitable.

But scientists can provide guidance, based on their understanding of what generates health inequalities, and of how these mechanisms relate to different conceptions of justice. From what we have seen above it appears that it is possible to argue that all health inequalities deserve to be eliminated, albeit with varying degrees of moral urgency. Some health inequalities are at least partly inequitable under any conception of social justice, and all health inequalities are at least partly inequitable under at least one conception of social justice (Table 5.1). Honesty obliges me to write that it is also possible to argue the reverse—but if that would have been my point of view, I would not have taken the trouble to write this book.

In choosing their point of view, politicians may want to keep in mind that, in order to obtain a democratic mandate for policies to reduce health inequalities, an eclectic rationale is likely to be more effective than a systematically elaborated rationale based on a single conception of social justice. And when an eclectic set of social justice arguments does not provide a sufficiently convincing argument for eliminating health inequalities, other arguments can be brought forward: the need to avoid an accumulation of disadvantage, the necessity of solidarity with those who are less well off, and the huge societal costs of doing nothing.

Key points

◆ Sociological theories of the origins of social inequality suggest that this is ineradicable. This implies that as long as health is a highly desired good, health inequalities are unlikely to go away completely. However, not all health inequalities are a consequence of social inequality, so there is considerable scope for reducing health inequalities even if social inequality persists.

◆ Current attempts at welfare state reform pay insufficient attention to the necessity of tackling health inequalities, and some welfare state reform initiatives may even aggravate health inequalities. Nevertheless, some aspects of welfare state reform, particularly pension reforms and the move towards a more activating welfare state, offer new opportunities for reducing health inequalities.

◆ It is too simple to say that health inequalities are a matter of 'social injustice killing on a grand scale', but health inequalities are certainly partly unfair, as becomes clear from an analysis of five theories of justice ('equality of welfare', 'capabilities approach', 'luck egalitarianism', 'justice as fairness', and 'equality of opportunity'), under all of which at least some mechanisms underlying health inequalities are considered inequitable. In addition, there are other compelling reasons to want to reduce them, including avoiding accumulation of disadvantage, solidarity with the less well-off, and reducing costs to society.

Chapter 6

Policy implications

6.1 Proposals for tackling health inequalities

Progression on the 'action spectrum'

It is probably fair to say that the first 20 years after the 'rediscovery' of health inequalities around 1980 were spent doing research. Policymakers and politicians were often not yet ready to contemplate reducing health inequalities. This is illustrated most dramatically by the cold reception of the Black report in the United Kingdom,[20] which had been commissioned by a Labour government, but disappeared into a desk drawer after the Conservatives won the 1979 elections. On the other hand, more research was probably needed anyway to better understand why health inequalities were still there.

Even when countries subscribed to the World Health Organization's Health for All policy targets, which were published in 1985 and called for a 25% reduction in health inequalities by the year 2000,[685] concrete actions were often limited to commissioning research. For example, the Netherlands' government funded two five-year research programmes, with the first one devoted to explanatory studies[686] and the second one to intervention studies.[55]

But when the results of these studies began to accumulate, it seemed that the time had come to start developing rational strategies to reduce health inequalities—at least in countries which had reached a more advanced stage on the 'action spectrum'. Reviewing the diffusion of ideas on socioeconomic inequalities in health in different European countries, Margaret Whitehead distinguished several stages: a primordial stage in which socioeconomic inequalities in health are not even measured, then the subsequent stages of 'measurement', 'recognition', 'awareness', and either 'denial/indifference' or 'concern', and then finally, following 'concern' the stages of 'will to take action', 'isolated initiatives', 'more structured developments', and 'comprehensive coordinated policy'.[687]

Analyses using this 'action spectrum' not only showed where European countries were in the early 2000s, but also identified several factors that had promoted or blocked progression. Raising awareness and concern among policymakers appeared to be greatly facilitated by availability of national data on health inequalities. Presence or absence of political will was another obvious and important factor. As we will see below, after more than a decade of blocked progression under Conservative governments, election of a Labour government in 1997 quickly brought the United Kingdom into the most active stage. Also, international agencies like WHO played an important role by legitimizing concerns for health inequalities.[680]

National policy proposals

Around the year 2000 several European countries, including the United Kingdom, the Netherlands, and the Nordic countries, had reached one of the more advanced stages, and as a result their governments installed committees to develop a comprehensive strategy to reduce health inequalities.[680] Table 6.1 gives an overview of the most salient of these policy proposals.

Table 6.1 Entry-points targeted by proposals for tackling health inequalities

Contributing factor	Independent Inquiry (UK, 1998)[688]	Programme Committee (Netherlands, 2001)[55]	National strategy (Norway, 2006)[689]	National Action Plan (Finland, 2008)[690]	European Review (2013)[691]	National Commission (Sweden, 2017)[692]
Childhood	Pre-school education, education for disadvantaged children, social support of parents	Education for disadvantaged children, improve school outcomes for sick children	Pre-school education, school drop-outs, child welfare and health services	Comprehensive schools, health of youth at vocational schools, day-care, child health care	Pregnancy care, parenting skills, income protection for families, child care, education	Maternal and child health care, pre-school education
Material living conditions	Income in-equality, so-cial benefits, employment opportunities, quality of jobs, housing, public transport, road safety	Income inequality, long-term and child poverty, physical workload in manual occupations, disability benefits, health barriers to work	Income inequality, poverty, working conditions, company health services, employment opportunities, homelessness	Poverty, youth and long-term unemployment, homelessness	Occupational risks, em-ployment opportunities, pensions, so-cial protection, air pollution, urban planning	Barriers to enter labour market, working conditions, social benefits, housing conditions
Social and psychological factors	Suicide prevention				Community empowerment, social exclusion	Opportunities for control, influence and participation
Health-related behaviours	Health-promoting schools, walking and cycling, access to healthy diet, healthier lifestyles, smoking in pregnancy	Adapt health promotion for disadvantaged groups, school health promotion, link urban regeneration to health promotion	Reduce inequalities in smoking, diet, physical activity by taxation, healthy school meals, restrictions on tobacco	Workplace health promotion, excessive drinking, smoking, diet, exercise,	(Smoking in pregnancy, exercise and healthy diet in elderly)	Limit access to hazardous products, increase access to healthy products
Health care	Services for elderly, access to care, equitable allocation NHS resources	Financial access to care, reinforce primary care disadvantaged areas, homelessness among mentally ill	Reduce cost sharing, low threshold services, evaluate distributional effects of health care reform, substance abuse services	Improve social work, strengthen primary health care, occupational health care, strengthen mental health care	(Access and quality of care for elderly)	Equal and health promoting health care system

Table 6.1 Continued

Contributing factor	Independent Inquiry (UK, 1998)[688]	Programme Committee (Netherlands, 2001)[55]	National strategy (Norway, 2006)[689]	National Action Plan (Finland, 2008)[690]	European Review (2013)[691]	National Commission (Sweden, 2017)[692]
Other	Health inequalities impact assessment, minority groups	Quantitative targets, evaluation of policies when implemented	Inequality impact assessment, develop indicators, strengthen research, evaluate policies	Immigrant health services, system for monitoring health inequalities, strengthen research	Strengthen local communities, link to sustainable development, strengthen governance	Cross-sectorial policy framework, infrastructure for monitoring and research

The first of these proposals was developed in the United Kingdom, by a small commission chaired by Sir Donald Acheson (1926–2010), former Chief Medical Officer of the United Kingdom. When Labour returned to power in 1997, almost 20 years after the Black report had been shelved, it immediately commissioned this expert report, the Independent Inquiry into Inequalities in Health,[693] and took action with a series of policy initiatives which were further elaborated upon in subsequent years.

The Independent Inquiry covered many of the contributing factors that had been identified at that point in time. It made 39 recommendations, with many sub-clauses, ranging from higher living standards of households in receipt of social security benefits to improvements in school meals, and from improved insulation and heating systems to a more equitable allocation of resources within the National Health Service.[693] Although criticized for being a 'shopping list',[694] it emphasized the importance of investing in the health of families with children and of reducing income inequality and poverty.[695]

A few years later, a government commission in the Netherlands also published its policy proposals, which were based on a series of small-scale intervention studies and were—perhaps for that reason—less wide-ranging than the recommendations of the Independent Inquiry. After evaluating the results of the intervention studies—only some of which showed effectiveness in reducing health inequalities—26 recommendations were made, which were translated into 11 quantitative policy targets. This included an overall policy target to reduce, 'by the year 2020, the difference in healthy life expectancy between people with a low and people with a high socioeconomic status [...] from 12 to 9 years'.[696 (p. 3)]

In the early 2000s, several of the Nordic countries were also active in developing policy proposals to reduce health inequalities. The Swedish National Public Health Commission developed a national health policy with a strong focus on reducing health inequalities. Based on extensive consultation of numerous organizations, the commission formulated 18 health policy objectives.[697] Although quantitative policy targets were later rejected, policy development in Sweden has continued until the present day, and Table 6.1 summarizes the recommendations of a recent Commission for Equity in Health that was appointed by the Swedish Government in 2015.[692]

Norway's parliament adopted a 'National strategy to reduce social inequalities in health' in 2006, partly in response to a Lancet paper showing comparatively large health inequalities,[26] and the Finnish Ministry of Social Affairs and Health adopted a 'National Action Plan to Reduce Health

Inequalities' in 2008. Each had its own emphasis, probably reflecting differences in sensitivity of national policymakers to particular arguments for reducing health inequalities, or differences in opportunities for linking up to other, already established national policies.

For example, the Finnish policy paper, when listing its overall objectives, first spoke about reducing 'social inequalities in work ability and functional capacity', probably because occupational health and rehabilitation were already well-established components of Finland's social and health strategies.[698]

Two important reports from the world health organization

In 2006 the World Health Organization set up the global Commission on Social Determinants of Health, chaired by Michael Marmot. This was a comprehensive, and well-resourced, attempt at developing a policy strategy to reduce health inequalities, based on all the available evidence at that time. The commission, supported by 'Knowledge Networks' and governmental and civil society organizations around the world, published its final report, 'Closing the gap in a generation', in 2008.[653] As illustrated by this report and several other milestones, mentioned elsewhere in this book, Marmot has been uniquely influential in shaping this area, both in terms of research and policy development.

Compared to most of the previous attempts to develop policy proposals, this report stands out not only by its comprehensiveness, but also by its radical stance, as illustrated by strongly phrased statements like 'social justice is a matter of life and death', 'putting right these inequities [...] is a matter of social justice', and—already cited above—'social injustice is killing on a grand scale'.

'The [...] social gradient in health within countries [is] caused by the unequal distribution of power, income, goods, and services, the consequent unfairness in the immediate, visible circumstances of people's lives [...] and their chances of leading a flourishing life. This unequal distribution of health-damaging experiences is not in any sense a "natural" phenomenon but is the result of a toxic combination of poor social policies and programmes, unfair economic arrangements, and bad politics.'

This translated into an emphasis on policy proposals aimed at removing the structural causes of social inequality, and at tackling 'upstream' causes of health inequalities. Its first principle was to 'improve the conditions of daily life—the circumstances in which people are born, grow, live, work, and age', by promoting early child development, better urban planning, fair employment and decent work, universal social protection, and universal health care. Its second principle was to 'tackle the inequitable distribution of power, money, and resources—the structural drivers of those conditions of daily life'.[653] (all citations from preface and executive summary)

The reception of this report has been remarkably favourable, to the extent that many municipal, national, and international organizations have embraced its recommendations and set up their own commissions to adapt them to local circumstances. In 2011, the regional office for Europe of the World Health Organization set up a 'Review of social determinants and the health divide in the WHO European Region' to support the development of its future health policies. The Review was chaired by (now Sir) Michael Marmot, and its report was published in 2013.[691,699,700]

Its main recommendations can be seen in Table 6.1. The radical stance taken by the Global Commission on Social Determinants returns in the recommendations of the European Review, which have a strong emphasis on early child development, social protection, and employment opportunities. References to other contributing factors, such as health-related behaviours and health care, can be found as well, but are hidden below headlines on various structural determinants.[691]

Similarities and dissimilarities

The over-all impression from Table 6.1 is one of considerable overlap between the policy proposals. This is hardly surprising in view of the fact that all these proposals were to a large extent based on a common knowledge base, as published in an international scientific literature to which researchers from the United Kingdom, the Netherlands, and the Nordic countries had all contributed.

However, there are also some important differences. We have already mentioned the relative lack of emphasis on health-related behaviour and health care access in the European Review, which derived from the report of the WHO Commission on Social Determinants of Health. This reluctance to acknowledge the role of smoking and other health-related behaviours in generating health inequalities, and the potential role of health care in ameliorating health inequalities, is not found in the policy proposals from the Netherlands and the Nordic countries, which on the contrary emphasize the importance of tackling inequalities in smoking, excessive alcohol consumption, access to health care etc.

The same applies to the role of health-related selection in generating health inequalities. In the policy proposals from the Netherlands and the Nordic countries policy interventions to counteract health-related selection, for example by improving retention in, and access to, work for people with chronic conditions, are included in the main recommendations, on an equal footing with other policy interventions. The explanation for these differences in emphasis should probably be sought in the political context of debates on the explanation of health inequalities. In the United Kingdom—where many of the ideas on tackling health inequalities in the WHO reports originated—the debate on the causes and remedies of health inequalities is strongly polarized along party-political lines.[226] In the Netherlands and the Nordic countries this is much less the case, which reduces the need for avoiding topics such as health-related behaviours and health-related selection, which have sometimes been used by the political right as an excuse for not addressing the underlying social inequality.[680]

6.2 National attempts at tackling health inequalities

The Netherlands and the Nordic countries

To what extent were all these policy proposals carried out? What happened in European countries was highly variable, and ranged between almost nothing in the Netherlands to full-blown action in the United Kingdom.

Despite careful build-up over a period of 15 years, the strategy developed in the Netherlands was not adopted by the government. The official cabinet reaction to the recommendations when they were presented in November 2001, was positive but because elections were looming decision-making was deferred to the next cabinet. These elections turned out to be uncharacteristically turbulent, culminating in the dramatic murder of populist politician Pim Fortuyn by a far-left political activist in May 2002. A new cabinet was formed after the elections, but fell within three months without making decisions on a strategy to reduce health inequalities, and after new elections had been held in January 2003 a right-wing cabinet banned health inequalities from the political discourse.[696] Municipal governments have sometimes taken action to reduce health inequalities, but for more than 10 years the national government emphasized personal responsibility as the main route to health improvement.[i]

Fortunately, developments were less dramatic in the Nordic countries, but despite verbal support for the policy proposals concrete action to reduce health inequalities often remained limited.

In Sweden for example, most of the action—often consisting of new commissions preparing action plans—could be found at local and regional levels.[692]

In Norway, the 'National strategy' adopted in 2006 clearly showed that 'the theme of health inequalities [had] developed from a non-topic to a high-priority topic in public health policy policy-making'.[702] (p. 521) The strategy was ambitious, had a long-term (i.e. 10 year) perspective, and included among its priority areas not only measures to reduce inequalities in health-related behaviours and service use, but also measures to reduce income inequality, increase access to pre-school education, and improve working conditions. Specific aims for the implementation of these measures were specified, the attainment of which had to be monitored using quantitative indicators. An evaluation published in 2013 showed that many measures had indeed been implemented, but doubts were expressed about their effectiveness as health inequalities had not been reduced.[703]

In Finland, an evaluation study of the 'Action Plan' found that most of the proposals had been implemented as planned. Examples include the strengthening of occupational health services, raising tobacco taxes, and a series of new studies on health inequalities. However, it also stated that 'health inequalities have not been noticeably reduced during the Action Plan period; if anything, they have increased'. This was attributed to the fact that 'the measures selected [in the action plan] are not necessarily comprehensive enough for addressing health inequalities, or appropriately aimed, or sufficiently addressing the root causes of health inequalities'. Nevertheless, 'much was learned, understanding of the phenomenon increased, and public awareness increased of the co-operation needed to tackle these problems'.[704] (p. 10)

The English strategy to reduce health inequalities

The country where the most serious attempts were made to implement a national policy to reduce health inequalities was the United Kingdom, and although all four parts of the United Kingdom participated, most of the action happened in England. After the Independent Inquiry published its report in 1998, the Labour government quickly developed an ambitious and comprehensive strategy to reduce health inequalities, which only came to an end when the Conservatives came into power again, following the 2010 elections. For more than 10 years, the English government made reducing health inequalities part of its core political programme. The process of developing this strategy and its main components are summarized in Box 6.1.

Because the English strategy was accompanied by an equally admirable attempt to assess its effectiveness, it is relatively easy to come to a conclusion on whether or not its objectives have been reached.[684] Unfortunately, the official evaluation reports show that, despite more than 10 years of systematic policy action, health inequalities in England have not narrowed. [ii]

Has the English strategy to reduce health inequalities indeed failed? The importance of this question cannot easily be overstated. Not only was the level of political commitment behind the strategy historically and internationally unique, but Labour stayed in power for an exceptional 13 years, and in Western democracies it is difficult to imagine a longer window of opportunity for tackling health inequalities. Also, the policy initiatives built on decades of public health research, and more often than not were based on empirical evidence which had been collected and summarized by leading public health experts. If this did not work, what will?

Why did the English strategy not lead to a measurable reduction of health inequalities?

In-depth analyses showed that all the 'departmental commitments' (Box 6.1) were fulfilled, indicating that all elements of the strategy as originally planned had been implemented, from Sure Start to the creation of sports facilities, from neighbourhood renewal programmes to smoking cessation

Box 6.1 The English strategy to reduce health inequalities

The English strategy to reduce health inequalities was shaped in two steps. The first was in 1999, when the Department of Health issued 'Reducing health inequalities: an action report'. This was the government's response to the Independent Inquiry, and adopted many of its recommendations, rightly claiming that '[t]his is the most comprehensive programme of work to tackle health inequalities ever undertaken in this country'. It listed a range of new government policies including the introduction of a national minimum wage, higher benefits and pensions, and substantially increased spending on education, housing, urban regeneration, and healthcare. It also announced a number of specific initiatives including the 'Sure Start' programme (free childcare, early education, and parent support for low income families), 'Health Action Zones' (local strategies to improve health in deprived areas), and a series of anti-tobacco policies (including free nicotine-replacement therapy for low-income smokers).[705]

The second step followed in 2003 after the publication of the 'Cross-Cutting Review of Health Inequalities', a systematic assessment by government of its progress in tackling health inequalities. This took as its starting-point the two national health inequalities targets, which had suddenly been announced by the Secretary of State for Health in 2001, to narrow the gap in life expectancy between areas and the difference in infant mortality across social classes by 10% in 2010. The Cross-Cutting Review tried to identify the most significant interventions that would support the delivery of these targets, by quantifying the contribution that the interventions would make to reducing inequalities in specific health outcomes [Cross-Cutting Review 2003].

In response to this analysis the Department of Health published a revised strategy in 2003, entitled 'Tackling health inequalities: a Programme for Action'. It had a foreword by Prime Minister, Tony Blair, and set out the government's plans to achieve the two health inequalities targets by 2010. It reiterated the need to tackle the structural 'upstream' determinants of health inequalities, but it had a stronger emphasis on 'downstream' policies than the 1999 Action Report. Key interventions expected to contribute to closing the life expectancy gap were reducing smoking in manual social groups, managing other risks for coronary heart disease and cancer (poor diet and obesity, physical inactivity, hypertension), improving housing quality by tackling cold and dampness, and reducing accidents at home and on the road.[706]

The strategy was structured around the two overall targets, and underpinned by 12 'headline indicators' (specific targets for intermediate outcomes) and 82 'departmental commitments' (specific actions by various governmental departments) which together were expected to ensure the timely delivery of the targets. The departmental commitments included further poverty reduction efforts, improved educational outcomes, expansion of the Sure Start scheme, expansion of smoking cessation services, improvement of primary care facilities in inner cities, and improved access to treatment for cancer and cardiovascular disease. Many of the departmental commitments were explicitly targeted towards low-income groups or deprived areas, and most were quantified in terms of numbers of people to be reached and budgets to be allocated. The total budget exceeded £20 billion.[706]

A remarkable series of reports systematically assessing and reviewing progress in achieving headline indicators and fulfilling departmental commitments followed. The high level of government commitment to reducing health inequalities was matched by an equally remarkable commitment to critically review, revise, and then re-review its policies.[707] Quite clearly, the English strategy to reduce health inequalities was both historically and internationally unique.[680]

Box 6.1 adapted with permission from Mackenbach J.P. 'Can we reduce health inequalities? An analysis of the English strategy (1997–2010).' *Journal of Epidemiology & Community Health*, Volume 65, Issue 7. pp.568–75. © 2011, Published by the BMJ Publishing Group Limited. http://dx.doi.org/10.1136/jech.2010.128280.

support, and from improving access to health care services to reducing 'fuel poverty'. This was a great achievement, but only some of the headline indicators showed reduced inequalities, in terms of smaller relative or absolute inequalities in intermediate outcomes like educational credentials, child poverty, or cardiovascular risk factors. Others, including several that matter for inequalities in life expectancy and infant mortality, such as on primary care, diet, and smoking, suggested stable or even increased inequalities between socioeconomic groups. There was no evidence at all for a reduction of inequalities in infant mortality or life expectancy, as stipulated in the overall targets.[684,708]

On the other hand, more detailed evaluation studies have sometimes found positive effects of the strategy. Interventions to reduce inequalities in smoking have produced small but significant reductions in inequalities in smoking prevalence between deprived and less deprived areas.[711] The Sure Start programme has had beneficial effects on children and their families living in deprived communities.[712] When compared with previous and later trends, the gap in life expectancy between deprived and non-deprived areas developed more favourably and actually diminished during the strategy.[713] However, trends in health inequalities in England were not more favourable than in other countries in a similar stage of awareness of health inequalities.[714]

Factors contributing to relative lack of success

¶Overall, the general consensus is that there were no effects of the strategy on health inequalities at the national level. Why was this strategy not more successful? The reasons have been discussed in several in-depth analyses.[684,708,715–717]

First, the English strategy did not necessarily address the correct entry-points, at least as far as the stated objectives were concerned: it spent resources on entry-points which were largely irrelevant for life expectancy or infant mortality, such as homelessness or fuel poverty, and it ignored relevant entry-points such as working conditions and excessive alcohol consumption.

Second, it often did not use effective policies: it had to rely on policies of unproven effectiveness, and to the extent that policies were evaluated during implementation, many proved to be ineffective in reducing inequalities in health outcomes. It had this in common with all the other policy proposals reviewed in Table 6.1: these were heavily evidence-based, but this 'evidence' was on factors contributing to health inequalities, not on the effectiveness of policies and interventions.

Third, it was not delivered at a large enough scale: despite the fact that the English strategy was the most well-resourced of all the strategies pursued in European countries, the scale required for achieving population-wide impacts was not determined in advance, and where reach was part of the evaluation as in the case of smoking cessation, it proved to be insufficient to substantially reduce inequalities at the population level.

These relative failures were not caused by a lack of determination on the part of the government. Tony Blair's Labour government has been criticized for being indifferent to income inequalities, and for its neoliberal public health philosophy, which emphasized personal responsibility for behaviour change at the expense of attention to underlying determinants. However, for those who are familiar with the situation in other Western European countries, it is clear that with all its weaknesses, this Labour government was probably the most determined European government ever to tackle health inequalities. The ultimate explanation should therefore be sought elsewhere.

First, the suboptimal choice of entry-points reflects the necessity for this (or any) government to match scientific evidence with political opportunity, and the lack of a democratic mandate to

¶ Section 'Factors contributing to relative lack of success' expanded and adapted with permission from Mackenbach J.P. 'Can we reduce health inequalities? An analysis of the English strategy (1997–2010).' *Journal of Epidemiology & Community Health*, Volume 65, Issue 7. pp.568-575. © 2011, Published by the BMJ Publishing Group Limited. http://dx.doi.org/10.1136/jech.2010.128280.

take more radical action. For example, Labour had been elected on the basis of a party programme that simply did not include a radical redistribution of income or wealth.

Second, the choice of inadequate policies reflects the almost complete lack of scientific evidence on effectiveness of interventions and policies to reduce health inequalities. This in turn was due to the relatively short time which had elapsed between the identification of the determinants of health inequalities (mostly in the 1980s and 1990s) and the arrival in power of a government eager to be advised on what it could do to tackle health inequalities.

Third, the insufficient scale of implementation reflects a fundamental discrepancy between the necessary scale of change and the ability of state bureaucracies to change in response to new priorities. This was painfully illustrated by the House of Commons' critique of the slowness of change within the National Health Service. Despite a resource-allocation formula based on need for health care, disadvantaged areas after many years still receive much less than their full needs-based allocations.[717] The scale of change needed to have an impact on health inequalities—a phenomenon that affects tens of millions of people in the United Kingdom—is simply overwhelming.

Returning to the main theme of this book, we are left with the frustrating conclusion that the failure of policies whose explicit aim was to tackle health inequalities at the population level—such as the English strategy—is another reason for the persistence of health inequalities in modern welfare states.

However, as a final conclusion this would do insufficient justice to these and other, less systematic, attempts to reduce health inequalities. Although we do not yet know exactly how to reduce health inequalities, the lessons from the English experience mentioned above have provided a strong basis for developing and implementing strategies that may be more successful in the future.

6.3 **Realistic expectations**

Aim for reducing absolute inequalities in health

Clearly then, we have to manage the expectations on how far health inequalities can realistically be reduced. We do not yet know exactly what works to reduce health inequalities, but what we do know is that it would have to be applied on a massive scale to reduce health inequalities at the population level. To further guide policymakers' thoughts about what is feasible, we will have a final look at what we can learn from the European experience.

Lessons learned from trends in health inequalities

The target to reduce health inequalities by 25%, proposed by the World Health Organization in 1985, was renewed in 1998.[718] Several European countries, such as England, Finland, and Lithuania, have adopted similar national targets for the reduction of socioeconomic inequalities in mortality [719]. It is often thought that these targets have been missed by a wide margin, but whether that is true critically depends on whether one looks at changes in relative or absolute inequalities in health.[499]

Whereas inequalities in self-reported morbidity have not changed much since these targets were set, inequalities in mortality have been quite dynamic, as we have seen earlier (Figure 2.5). A summary picture of what happened to absolute and relative inequalities in mortality since ca 1990 is presented in Figure 6.1, in which countries' changes were plotted in a two-dimensional graph.[720] A country's position in the lower left hand quadrant would indicate, that due to larger absolute and relative mortality declines in the lower socioeconomic groups, both absolute and relative inequalities in mortality have decreased over time. However, such an optimal combination of changes has occurred nowhere among men, and only in Spain among women.[iii]

For men, most countries can be found in the upper left hand quadrant, where absolute inequalities narrow but relative inequalities widen. Austria has performed best, with a reduction of absolute inequalities by around 30% and almost no increase in relative inequalities. Denmark has performed worst, with a small increase in absolute inequalities and a massive increase in relative inequalities. For women, many countries have experienced an increase in absolute inequalities in mortality. Finland, Denmark, and Norway have performed worst, with an increase in absolute inequalities by 30–40% and a more-than-doubling of relative inequalities.

These results show that, in a context of declining mortality, a narrowing of relative inequalities is very rare, but a narrowing of absolute inequalities is not. This is not only empirically true, as shown in Figure 6.1, but it can also be mathematically demonstrated that a narrowing of absolute inequalities occurs under a much wider range of conditions, in terms of combinations of changes to mortality in lower and higher socioeconomic groups, than a narrowing of relative inequalities in mortality.[521]

This implies that policymakers are more likely to achieve their quantitative targets if they aim for reducing absolute instead of relative inequalities. Ironically, the World Health Organization has never specified whether its targets should be measured in absolute or relative terms. As Figure 6.1 shows, not a single country has achieved a 25% reduction of relative inequalities in mortality since the early 1990s, but several have achieved a 25% reduction of absolute inequalities— without noticing, because most monitoring reports and research studies have focused on relative inequalities.

These reductions in absolute inequalities have not been achieved by specific national programmes to reduce health inequalities. Although England and Wales come out favourably in Figure 6.1, so do several countries which did not have a national programme to reduce health inequalities, and Norway and Finland, two other countries which did have a national programme, come out unfavourably.

Analyses by cause of death suggest that these reductions of absolute inequalities in mortality have been achieved as a by-product of population-wide improvements in prevention and treatment. Absolute declines in mortality were often larger in lower than in higher socioeconomic groups (with absolute inequalities narrowing as a result) for ischemic heart disease, smoking-related causes, and causes amenable to medical intervention. Because these mortality declines were due to improvements in ischemic heart disease prevention and treatment, smoking prevention, and health care more generally, the substantial absolute declines from these causes in lower socioeconomic groups show that many European countries have been successful in letting these groups share in the benefits of these improvements, for example, by ensuring equal access to health care.[499]

'Realpolitik'

There is thus a strong case to be made for the 'Realpolitik' of aiming to reduce absolute health inequalities, and for being more relaxed about what happens to relative health inequalities. When overall health improves, as it does in the case of mortality, it is extremely difficult to reduce relative inequalities. This is not only suggested by the near-absence of empirically observed reductions of relative inequalities, but can also be underpinned by theoretical reasons.

A reduction of relative inequalities in morbidity or mortality requires larger relative reductions in lower than in higher socioeconomic groups. It can easily be seen that even achieving an *equal* relative reduction is very hard. This requires that our intervention reaches equal proportions of people at risk of morbidity or mortality in lower and in higher socioeconomic groups, and then saves equal proportions of those reached. These two conditions are already very difficult to fulfil, because lower socioeconomic groups are more difficult to reach and more difficult to treat than higher socioeconomic groups. Allocation of resources according to need would not

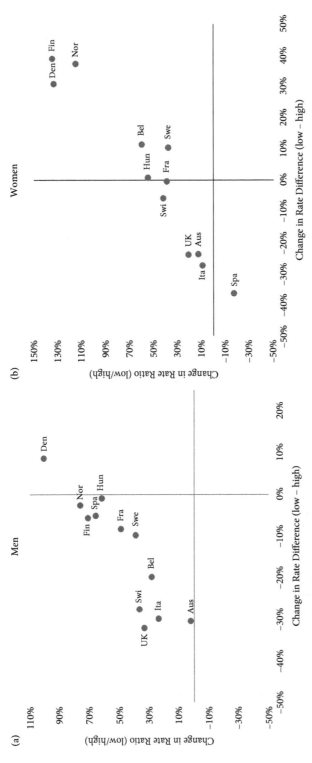

Figure 6.1 Changes in absolute and relative educational inequalities in mortality

Notes: Changes in absolute and relative educational inequalities in all-cause mortality in men and women, based on observations on varying periods between ca. 1988 and ca. 2012, but calibrated to a standard 20 year period. Percentage change in Rate Difference (RD) calculated as: 100×(RD(begin)−RD(end))÷RD(begin). Percentage change in Rate Ratio (RR) calculated as: 100×(RR(begin)−RR(end))÷(RR(begin)−1). All data are age standardized. Western European countries only. Aus = Austria, Bel = Belgium, Den = Denmark, UK = England and Wales, Fin = Finland, Fra = France, Hun = Hungary, Ita = Italy (Turin), Nor = Norway, Spa = Spain (Barcelona), Swe = Sweden, Swi = Switzerland.

Source: dataset constructed in DEMETRIQ/LIFEPATH projects, with harmonized data from national/regional mortality registers.

be enough: achieving equal reductions in morbidity or mortality requires substantially more re-sources to be spent per person at risk in lower than in higher socioeconomic groups.[90]

To achieve a *greater* relative decline in lower socioeconomic groups one would have to do much more than create equal reach and equal effectiveness. One would have to create greater reach and/or greater effectiveness among people with a lower socioeconomic position, and therefore have to spend even more resources per person at risk in lower socioeconomic groups than are necessary to achieve *equal* relative declines. While this is not inherently impossible, it would necessitate a massive shift of resources that has so far not been considered, and is prob-ably not politically feasible. It is therefore more realistic to aim for reducing absolute health inequalities.[90]

Historical evidence on the reduction of inequalities in mortality from infectious diseases such as tuberculosis also supports the view that what we can hope for is a reduction of absolute, not relative inequalities in mortality. European countries' efforts to reduce tuberculosis mortality, and to bring the benefits of tuberculosis prevention and treatment to all sections of the population, have strongly reduced absolute inequalities in tuberculosis mortality, at the expense of rising rela-tive inequalities. The latter are still with us, but now concern a very small absolute number of deaths.[721]

Setting targets after calculating potential impacts

What is a realistic expectation for how far we can reduce health inequalities, in view of what we know about the contribution of various risk factors to health inequalities? Here again, the European experience warns us not to be over-ambitious.

Health inequalities impact assessment

Simple mathematical models have been developed that can help to estimate the impact on health inequalities of changing the distribution of risk factors over socioeconomic groups.[iv] A com-plete elimination of inequalities in risk factors, by bringing the prevalence of risk factors in lower socioeconomic groups down to the level currently seen in the highest socioeconomic group, will obviously result in a reduction of inequalities in morbidity or mortality. However, the potential impact depends on the current gap in exposure to the risk factor between socioeconomic groups, and on the effect of the risk factor on morbidity or mortality. The wider the current gap, and the stronger the effect on morbidity or mortality, the larger the potential reduction of inequalities in morbidity or mortality will be.[722]

This is illustrated in Figure 6.2 for two childhood conditions (manual occupation of father, fi-nancial hardship in childhood), two social and economic conditions in adulthood (low income and few social contacts), and three behavioural risk factors in adulthood (smoking, excessive alcohol consumption, and obesity). All these risk factors, with the exception of excessive alcohol consumption among women, are more frequent among the lower than the higher educated, with gaps in exposure being widest for financial hardship in childhood, low income in adulthood, and smoking. The risk factors also have independent effects on mortality, which were estimated from the literature, with relative risks ranging from 1.05 for manual occupation of father to 2.20 for smoking (both after adjustment for adult educational level).[723]

When all this information is combined with data on current inequalities in life expectancy, it is possible to calculate the potential impact of equalizing the distribution of these risk factors on the gap in life expectancy between people of low and high education. Taking all European coun-tries together, the gap in partial life expectancy between the ages of 35 and 80 years is 5.8 years among men, and 2.4 years among women. Equalizing the distribution of smoking, by reducing

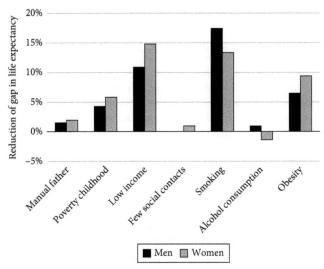

Figure 6.2 Potential impact of equalizing the distribution of risk factors

Notes: Graphs show the estimated percentage reduction of the gap in partial life expectancy (ages 35–80 years) between low and high educated, following a reduction of the prevalence of risk factors among the low educated to the level currently observed among the high educated in the same country. Population-weighted average of 13 European countries around 2010. Results of analysis with health inequalities impact assessment tool, based on the method of population-attributable fractions.[722]

Source: dataset constructed in DEMETRIQ/LIFEPATH projects, with harmonized data from mortality registers and national and international surveys.

the prevalence of smoking among the low educated to that among the high educated, would reduce this gap by 1.0 year (17%) for men, and 0.3 year (13%) for women.[723]

Second comes low income: if we assume that being in the lowest income quintile has an independent effect on mortality with a relative risk of 1.5, equalizing the distribution of having a low income between education groups will reduce the gap in life expectancy by 11% for men, and 15% for women. Third comes obesity, with reductions of 6% and 9%, respectively. Equalizing the distribution of the other risk factors has much smaller effects.[723]

A successful elimination of differences in smoking would reduce inequalities in mortality to a larger extent among men than women, because inequalities in smoking are usually larger among men. Because inequalities in smoking among women are larger-than-average in the Nordic countries, and smaller-than-average in Southern Europe, equalizing the distribution of smoking results in a much greater reduction of the gap in life expectancy in the former than in the latter. The reverse is true for obesity, where inequalities are larger among women than among men, and larger in Southern than in Northern Europe.[724]

While this suggests that reductions of inequalities in mortality (or health inequalities more generally) in the order of 25% by changing the distribution of risk factors are not completely out of reach, particularly if we would address more than one risk factor at the same time, it is also quite clear that a complete elimination of inequalities in exposure to specific risk factors is utopian. We do not currently have the arsenal of effective interventions and policies that would reduce the prevalence of smoking or obesity in lower socioeconomic groups to that in higher socioeconomic groups—in reality, we do not even know for sure how to only partially reduce the gap in smoking or obesity. The same applies to other risk factors, such as low income, social isolation, adverse childhood experiences, etc.

More realistic scenarios take into account current 'best practice', for example by looking at the risk factor distribution seen in the country with the smallest gap. When this is done, the percentage reduction that can be achieved usually goes down considerably, and often stays below 5% per risk factor. In the case of smoking, it is possible to be even more specific, and to estimate the reduction of inequalities in mortality should the price of tobacco be raised to the currently highest price in the EU (i.e. the price in Ireland). The largest reductions would then be seen in Southern, Central-Eastern, and Eastern European countries, where an estimated 3–5% reduction would be achieved in such a scenario.[262]

In contrast to raising the price of tobacco, where one single action, that is, signing a decree to raise tobacco taxes, will affect all smokers and smokers-to-be, many other policies and interventions will only effectively change the health of millions of people if they are adopted by hundreds of organizations, thousands of localities, tens of thousands of professionals, or even millions of individuals. These calculations therefore clearly illustrate the inevitability of modest aims for reducing health inequalities by changing the distribution of risk factors: a 25% reduction is probably out of reach, and a 5–10% reduction of health inequalities in a period of 10–20 years would already be a surprisingly large achievement.

It is easier to 'go with the flow' when average exposures go down, and to make sure that the benefits are somewhat larger in absolute terms in lower socioeconomic groups. Because starting levels are higher in lower socioeconomic groups, this does not require faster declines of morbidity or mortality in relative terms, and should therefore be feasible. It can also be done, if good care is taken, within mainstream policies and programmes, which are usually more generously funded than policies and programmes specifically intended to reduce inequalities.

The evidence-base

As mentioned in passing, the evidence-base on the effectiveness of policies in reducing health inequalities is still very thin. Since the Acheson report (1999) which had to make do with almost nothing [693] (see section 6.2 'National attempts at tackling health inequalities'), it has certainly grown, but recent overviews of the evidence led by British political scientist Clare Bambra still lament the lack of good empirical studies investigating the differential effects of relevant policies and interventions.[725–728]

A recent 'umbrella review' (i.e. a systematic overview of systematic reviews) looked at evidence for the effectiveness of 'social protection policies', mainly income maintenance and active labour market policies. Although lower quality reviews did find some evidence for inequalities reducing effects of these policies, the umbrella review concluded that 'the more rigorously conducted reviews found no significant health effects of any social protection policy'.[725]

An umbrella review of various types of health care reform found that introduction of private insurance and out-of-pocket payments as well as the marketization and privatization of services are likely to have negative equity effects, that is, to increase inequality in health care use. This review judged the evidence base on the equity effects of reforms intended to improve service delivery, particularly managed care programmes or integrated partnerships between health and social services, to be 'inconclusive' [726].

Other umbrella reviews found more mixed evidence. Changes to the psychosocial work environment, such as increasing employee control, increasing task variety, and changes in the organization of shift work, were found to have beneficial health effects overall, with some indications for positive equity effects.[727]

Finally, one umbrella review covered a wide range of public health policies. Although the quality of the evidence was again characterized as mostly poor, several examples were found of policies that may be effective in reducing health inequalities, such as taxes on unhealthy food and drinks, water fluoridation, regulating traffic speed, and population-wide cancer screening programmes. However, most of the more rigorous evaluation studies have been conducted in the United States, and it is unclear whether the results are transferable to other high-income countries. There were also policies for which there is evidence of increasing health inequalities, for example, introduction of 20 mph zones and some health education programmes.[728]

At this point in time, it is therefore impossible to identify with confidence the types of policies that will, or will not, reduce health inequalities. This even applies to some of the most extensively investigated areas, such as tobacco control. Although there is a limited degree of consensus, based on systematic reviews, that raising tobacco taxes and offering smoking cessation support may be effective in reducing health inequalities, the evidence is far from unambiguous.[535,729,730] This has been interpreted as indicating that the effects depend on the way the policy is implemented—for example, if restrictions on smoking around schools are not communicated in the right way, they may lead to rebellious behaviour and then have adverse effects.[731]

This dependence of the distributional impacts on the way policies and interventions are delivered could well be a more general phenomenon that would help to explain some of the inconsistencies in the evidence-base, and may help to develop more effective policies and interventions in the future.

Proportionate universalism

One approach to reducing health inequalities that has recently been advocated is 'proportionate universalism', defined as 'universal action with a scale and intensity that is proportionate to the level of disadvantage'. This approach cleverly combines two approaches to social policy that have often been seen as being in competition with each other: 'universalism' (i.e. application of interventions and policies in such a way that all members of society can benefit from them) and 'selectivism' (i.e. targeting of interventions and policies to those in greatest need). The idea behind proportionate universalism is that it will help to reduce health inequalities along the whole social gradient, not only between the worst and the best off.[684,732]

This idea certainly deserves to be further developed—but what would it mean in practice? Whether proportionate universalism will effectively flatten the gradient will depend on how 'disadvantage' or 'need' is taken into account. Allocating resources proportional to current levels of morbidity or mortality by socioeconomic group will not be sufficient, because outcomes of interventions are usually worse in lower socioeconomic groups.[442] To reverse this, it will be necessary to operationalize need in more radical terms, that is, as whatever would be necessary to achieve larger declines of morbidity or mortality in lower than in higher socioeconomic groups.

Here one would again have to decide whether one aims—pragmatically—for larger absolute declines, or—more radically—for larger relative declines in lower socioeconomic groups. In the first case, the policy, if effective, will reduce absolute inequalities only, whereas in the second case the policy will also reduce relative inequalities. As argued above, the latter requires a substantially larger redistribution of health care and other welfare resources from higher to lower socioeconomic groups than has been realized in even the most advanced European welfare states.[499]

6.4 **Final reflections**

Sobering conclusions

The role of personal beliefs

In the preface to this book, I warned the reader that some of the its conclusions would be sobering. On the other hand, I also promised some good news. In these final pages I will tie a few knots in the book's story-lines, and at the same time give some personal reflections on its main conclusions.

This book was written around a central question: why do health inequalities persist in modern welfare states? I have been intrigued by this question ever since I discovered, in the late 1990s, that health inequalities are not smaller in countries with advanced welfare states.[26] I also soon discovered that reasonable explanations of this paradox were often considered heretical by colleagues in social epidemiology, who more often than not consider health inequalities to be a direct reflection of social inequality, and who feel attracted to this research area precisely because they are deeply concerned with social inequality.

My personal interest in the area also comes from a deep conviction that our societies are far too unequal, and that we must do more to reduce inequalities, including the health inequalities that we see wherever we look. I also feel attracted to this research area because it allows me to combine scientific research with pursuing valuable social goals. But allow me to make these personal beliefs, and how they were formed, somewhat more explicit.

I am only a half-Marxist, and while I recognize the pernicious nature of power relations, I prefer Lenski's middle road which allows for more complex explanations of social inequality. Living in the Netherlands—a country with a long history of seeking political compromise—probably makes me less inclined to take radical viewpoints, and has made me aware of the fact that the political left has not had a monopoly in building generous welfare states. I am also one of the many Europeans born around the middle of the twentieth century who, thanks to educational expansion and based on their above-average cognitive abilities, were able to escape from the socioeconomic conditions of their childhood. Living through different social classes has made me acutely aware of the existence of social inequality—but also of the existence of social mobility.

These personal circumstances have undoubtedly influenced my interpretation of the available evidence, and have perhaps made it easier for me not to ignore the inconsistencies in the research findings, but to use them instead to build a better understanding of how health inequalities are generated—even if this would lead to a more complex story. This has led to a few sobering conclusions. Let me briefly restate them one-by-one.

Unwelcome evidence

The review of the existing evidence on the explanation of health inequalities that was carried out in Chapter 3, showed that some of the most crucial questions have not yet been answered satisfactorily. We know that the explanation of health inequalities involves three basic mechanisms: direct causation, reverse causation, and confounding (due to selection on personal characteristics during social mobility). This was already known when I started to work in this area in the late 1980s, but after decades of research we still do not know what the relative importance of each of these mechanisms is. If we are to believe the new evidence from quasi-experimental and genetic studies, direct causation is less important than previously thought. Although this may feel sobering, it does help to partly understand why welfare arrangements aimed at reducing socioeconomic disadvantage have not eliminated health inequalities.

More generally, the macro-level analyses reported in Chapter 4 show that health inequalities are driven by several partly autonomous forces—remodelling and persistence of social inequality, in interaction with a rapidly changing health landscape—which have counteracted the beneficial effects of the European welfare state. Social and health inequalities have been a 'moving target' to which the welfare state has not yet adjusted its focus. Some of these forces are difficult to counteract, and others we may not even want to counteract. Three factors appear to play a role:

First, the nature of social inequality has changed in such a way that new mechanisms linking social inequality to health inequalities have arisen. Education has become a more important stratification variable, which has strengthened the association between socioeconomic position and cognitive ability and other personal characteristics important for health. European societies have also become more 'fluid', which has created more opportunities for social selection on the basis of health and health determinants. Some of this may be remediable, at least in theory, but the underlying processes are either inevitable or in everyone's interest.

Second, population health has dramatically improved in many countries, but these improvements are almost always smaller in relative terms in lower socioeconomic groups. Also, when population health deteriorates, it takes time before the new hazards can effectively be tackled collectively, and in the meantime those with higher education or income will usually be better able to protect themselves. It is difficult to imagine how these differences could ever be eliminated, and to the extent that social and health progress is dependent on forerunners leading the way we should be careful not to block this mechanism.

Third, despite the welfare state, people in lower socioeconomic groups still have less access to both material and non-material resources that are important for their health, and as a result, there are social inequalities in practically all health determinants. We identified six groups of contributing factors (genetics, childhood environment, material living conditions, social and psychological factors, health-related behaviour, health care) that could provide entry-points for policy action.

Here are the inequalities that we may want to counteract, but our analysis in Chapter 5 of why social inequality is so persistent warns against optimism about what can be achieved. Even without assuming that health inequalities ultimately arise from perennial class conflict, the simple notion that human beings are often driven by self-interest should make us sceptical about the possibility of eliminating inequalities in opportunities for good health.

Lack of optimism about what can be achieved is also what recent attempts to reduce health inequalities, reviewed in Chapter 6, inspire. Although research in this area has now progressed to a stage in which we can more confidently than in the past identify entry-points for action, we know very little about what works to reduce health inequalities, as shown by the mixed results of systematic reviews of intervention studies. Here is another reason for the persistence of health inequalities: we simply do not yet know what works.

Unfortunately, the most ambitious and well-resourced strategy to reduce health inequalities ever (i.e. the English strategy (1997–2010)) has not had a measurable impact on health inequalities at the population level. Many factors have contributed to its lack of effectiveness, but the most important are that it did not have effective interventions at its disposal, and where it did these were not applied at the scale necessary for improving the health of tens of millions of people. These are important policy lessons—hard lessons, but also a precious gift of Britain to the world.

Another sobering finding is that the history of policy-making on health inequalities shows that this has been strongly dependent on political will. This is probably inevitable when the problem is phrased in terms that invite ideological dissensus ('health inequity', 'social injustice'). This facilitates strong policy action when there is a temporary democratic mandate, that is, an election victory for left-wing parties, but will block policymaking in another political climate.

Support for left-wing parties is variable, and it seems unlikely that this support will rise substantially in the near future. Political scientists have shown that more and more of those who would benefit from reducing social inequality no longer vote for left-wing parties that support redistribution of resources, but now vote for culturally conservative parties [733-735]. This is aptly illustrated by the election of Donald Trump as US president in 2017, thanks to the votes of millions of lower educated Americans who risk losing the health care insurance his predecessor Barack Obama fought for. How can we ever hope to reduce social and health inequalities if those who would benefit the most do not vote for the parties supporting such policies?

New inspiration

Why reduce health inequalities?

Now that we have cleared this away, let's ask ourselves again why health inequalities should be reduced, what we know about their explanation, and what can be done to reduce health inequalities. We must do better, but how?

First of all, reducing health inequalities is still extremely important. Although, as discussed in Chapter 5, health inequalities cannot simply and integrally be called a form of social injustice, there are several other compelling reasons to reduce health inequalities. Avoiding accumulation of social disadvantage, solidarity with the less well-off, and the necessity of reducing costs to society are three of those reasons. These are to some extent independent of whether health inequalities result from direct causation, reverse causation, or confounding. Furthermore, if one takes an eclectic approach to theories of justice, one can find arguments for all health inequalities to be inequitable, albeit with different levels of moral urgency.

If policymaking on health inequalities is to become less dependent on political will at the left side of the political spectrum, a pragmatic and eclectic argumentation may work best in creating the broader democratic mandate that is needed for the scale of action required for reducing health inequalities. Although social inequality and health inequalities are to some extent linked, other mechanisms also play a role, and counteracting the effects of ill-health on socioeconomic position or compensating the effects of genetic or cognitive disadvantage are equally legitimate objectives of public policy as reducing the extent of social inequality in society.

When formulating policy objectives, policymakers need to take into account that when overall health improves, there is much more scope for reducing absolute than for reducing relative inequalities in health. One of the pieces of good news in this book is that several European countries have managed to reduce absolute inequalities in health, by achieving larger absolute declines in health problems in lower than in higher socioeconomic groups. It is not only defensible philosophically, but also more productive in practice to formulate policy objectives in terms of a reduction of absolute health inequalities, and to take a more relaxed attitude with regard to relative health inequalities as long as absolute health inequalities go down.

How to reduce health inequalities?

The European experience shows that this can be achieved by ensuring that policies and interventions that effectively improve population health, have a good reach in lower socioeconomic groups, so that, even if relative reductions in health problems will often be smaller in lower socioeconomic groups, absolute reductions can still be larger because of their higher starting levels. This will require substantial efforts, but if these efforts are made an integral part of 'mainstream' health and social policies it will be less difficult to find the necessary resources.

Although knowledge on effectiveness of policies and interventions to reduce health inequalities remains limited, plausible entry-points are many, and have been included in many proposals for action as reviewed in Chapter 6. The adoption of a life-course perspective in the research on health inequalities has shown how important exposures in childhood are in generating health inequalities in later life. This has inspired a strong emphasis on measures improving childhood development in many proposed strategies for reducing health inequalities. This has obvious merit, but it is not the panacea that some people believe it is, if only because interventions in childhood now will only lead to reduced health inequalities at adult ages many decades into the future. Because these interventions may also promote upward social mobility, some of the beneficial effects may even paradoxically strengthen health inequalities at adult ages.

Inequalities in material living conditions are still an important driver of health inequalities in many countries around the world, which implies that more can be done in terms of conventional welfare policies to reduce health inequalities, such as progressive income taxation, social security safety nets, social housing policies and removing financial barriers to health care access. Within Europe this applies particularly to some Central and Eastern European countries, which still lack a highly developed welfare state and have extremely unequal living conditions.

The persistence of health inequalities is not an argument for reducing the welfare state in countries where it is already highly developed. On the contrary, as was argued in Chapter 5, without the welfare state health inequalities would probably be larger than they currently are. Current initiatives to reform the welfare state, for example, by putting more emphasis on getting people into paid work, create new arguments for reducing health inequalities, and may lead to powerful synergies between welfare state reform and policies to reduce health inequalities. That the effectiveness of welfare state reform partly depends on whether or not health inequalities can be reduced, is also clear in the field of pension reform, where current inequities will be exacerbated when statutory pension age is raised uniformly without the necessary increases in disability-free life expectancy for lower socioeconomic groups.

However, the persistence of large health inequalities in even the most universal and generous welfare states of Europe shows that welfare policies are not enough. As even more radical redistribution measures than have been pursued in the Nordic countries are likely to be democratically unfeasible (and would also not eliminate health inequalities) something else is needed. The only way to substantially reduce health inequalities in the medium term is to reduce inequalities in exposure to 'downstream' risk factors, such as specific working and housing conditions and health-related behaviours.

Not so trivial

The European evidence shows clearly that the magnitude of inequalities in mortality in a country is strongly dependent on the magnitude of inequalities in smoking. Our repeated demonstration of this finding has sometimes annoyed other researchers in this area. One reason is that smoking, as compared to more complex exposures such as psychosocial stress, seems such a trivial factor. Another reason is that emphasizing smoking (and other health-related behaviours) creates a risk of 'blaming the victim', that is, suggesting that the worse health status of lower socioeconomic groups is their own fault.[736]

However, smoking is neither trivial nor a matter of free choice. Personally, I find the global history of the use of cigarettes, the semi-criminal conduct of the tobacco industry, and the role of genetics in creating susceptibility to nicotine addiction both fascinating and a cause of immense concern.[737] In a sense, smoking can be seen as John Snow's 'pump handle': although the causes of cholera were much more complex that the simple act of drinking water from an infected pump, removing its handle worked miracles.[738]

Whether we like it or not, smoking, excessive alcohol consumption, and other behaviourally mediated risk factors need to be specifically targeted by policy if we are serious about reducing health inequalities. Experience with health promotion programmes suggests that a reduction of these inequalities cannot be achieved by 'demand-side' policies alone, such as health education interventions, but also require 'supply-side' policies, which reduce exposure to health-damaging products and create health-promoting environments for the population as a whole.

The European experience also shows that health care can play an important role in alleviating health inequalities. Over the past decades, health care expansion has helped to narrow absolute inequalities in mortality, thanks to a combination of increased effectiveness of health care interventions and reasonably equal access to good quality health care regardless of socioeconomic position. Although this can be regarded as 'symptom treatment', because it does not take away the direct, let alone the ultimate, causes of health inequalities, it is certainly most useful. With the expectation of new methods of prevention and treatment to arrive in the future, the importance of preserving equal access even if health care costs continue to rise, can thus hardly be overestimated.

Because evidence for the effectiveness of policies and interventions for reducing health inequalities is still very thin, policy-making in this area can only be tentative, that is, conducted on a trial-and-error basis with serious evaluations accompanying all policy implementations. If conducted properly, such evaluation studies will also contribute to better insight into the causes of health inequalities. In view of the massive scale of the problem, and the limited possibilities for any single country to make big steps forward, international collaboration is required to increase learning speed.[680]

Coda

Perhaps the biggest piece of good news, extensively documented in Chapter 2, is that the scope for reducing health inequalities is so enormous. Variations between countries in the magnitude of health inequalities are stunning: on some measures, the magnitude of inequalities in mortality varies by a factor of 20.[273] Changes in the magnitude of health inequalities over time are no less impressive, again suggesting that they are less fixed than their persistence suggests.[504] It must therefore be possible to reduce health inequalities—and they must be reduced. Even the Netherlands can be made flatter.

Key points

- In several European countries, strategies for reducing health inequalities have been developed, based on the fruits of several decades of research into health inequalities. Despite some differences in emphasis, these strategies largely identify similar entry points for policy, and provide a good basis for further policy development.

- Several European countries have also made serious efforts to implement a strategy to reduce health inequalities, but none of these efforts has been effective in terms of actually reducing health inequalities at the population level, probably because of a combination of insufficient scale and a reliance on interventions and policies of unproven effectiveness. This even applies to the well-developed and well-resourced English strategy (1997–2010).

- Time-trend analyses and numerical exercises both suggest that a reduction of relative inequalities in health, by changing the distribution of health determinants, is unlikely to be easy. Reduction of absolute inequalities in health, by ensuring that all socioeconomic groups participate in on-going health improvements, is more likely to be feasible.

- This chapter ends with a number of, partly personal, reflections on the sobering conclusions of 30 years of research, but also highlights some new inspirations for continued efforts to reduce health inequalities.

Appendix

Detailed results underlying Table 4.1

A. Men

Determinant	Control variables	Effect on all-cause mortality		Interaction
		Stratified by education		
		Low	High	Significance
National income	c, p	−0.200	−0.327	p < 0.001
Income inequality	c, p, g	0.013	−0.008	p < 0.001
Level of democracy	c, p, g	0.025	−0.047	p = 0.001
Health care expenditure	c, p, g	−0.043	−0.053	p = 0.002

B. Women

Determinant	Control variables	Effect on all-cause mortality		Interaction
		Stratified by education		
		Low	High	Significance
National income	c, p	−0.190	−0.290	p = 0.001
Income inequality	c, p, g	0.006	−0.023	p < 0.001
Level of democracy	c, p, g	0.000	−0.071	p = 0.001
Health care expenditure	c, p, g	−0.024	−0.034	p = 0.002

Notes: c = country dummies, p = period dummies, g = lnGDP. Analysis with natural logarithm of age-standardized mortality rates as dependent variable. Source: analyses on dataset constructed in DEMETRIQ/LIFEPATH projects, with harmonized data from mortality registers and national and international surveys.

Notes

Chapter 1

i. In contrast to income inequalities, wealth inequalities in the Netherlands are not among the lowest in Europe (see ref. 574).

Chapter 2

i. Moreover, one advantage is often used to generate another, so that gains and losses accumulate over the life-course and even over generations, and tend to cluster together in the same people who, on top of that, mainly meet with others in the same category of (dis)advantage. It is therefore unlikely that one can fully capture the health effects of the stratification of society by measuring, with all other things kept constant, what the health effects are of giving people an extra unit of education or income. We will come back to the implications of this insight in section 3.2 'Education, occupation, income and health'.

ii. I apologize for the use of the terms 'low' and 'high', which could be perceived as being somewhat pejorative. However, it is difficult to find a more sympathetic alternative that is not unduly long.

iii. In at least one case, cross-sectional data have been shown to overestimate inequalities in mortality (see ref. 74), so we need to be careful when comparing inequalities in mortality between countries with cross-sectional and countries with longitudinal data.

iv. In the analyses presented in this book we use a variety of data sources to measure inequalities in self-assessed health or disability: national health interview surveys (which often date back to the 1970s, but required 'ex post' harmonization before the data could be used) and international surveys like the European Social Survey (ESS), the European Survey of Income and Living Conditions (EU-SILC), and the Study of Health Aging and Retirement (SHARE) (which cover a more recent period only, but were harmonized 'ex ante').

v. All morbidity and mortality data used in this book were directly age-standardized using the European Standard Population (see ref. 81).

vi. We leave aside the issue of whether health inequalities should be measured in terms of 'attainment' (actually observed rates of morbidity or mortality) or 'shortfall' (difference between observed rates of morbidity and mortality, and some maximum or ideal rate) (see ref. 88). This distinction matters for relative measures of inequality only—absolute measures will not change when we switch from the more common rates of 'attainment' to rates of 'shortfall'. For example, when studying trends in inequalities in mortality, we often see the Rate Ratio of the mortality rate (in deaths per 100,000 person-years) go up, but when we look at the Rate Ratio of not-dying (in survivors per 100,000 person-years) instead, we would see the Rate Ratio go down, whereas the Rate Difference is the same for rates of 'attainment' and 'shortfall'. In practice, patterns of changes over time or differences between countries calculated with relative 'shortfall' measures are often similar to those based on absolute 'attainment' measures.

vii. The values for the Population Attributable Fraction for mortality by education and occupational class among men aged 35–64 in 2005–9 are: Finland 45% and 49%; Denmark 42% and 38%; England and Wales 33% and 31%; France 44% and 30%; Switzerland 36% and 26%; Italy (Turin) 39% and 35%; Lithuania 54% and 50%; Estonia 53% and 45%.

viii. It is tricky, though, to refer to these phenomena in terms of 'speed'. It is only in absolute terms that mortality rises faster with age among the low educated. When we apply the rules of the demographic 'laws of mortality', in which the rise of mortality is expressed in relative terms, we find that mortality rises faster with age among the high educated.

ix. Measures of life span variation can also be used to calculate the contribution of variations linked to socioeconomic position to the total amount of variation in age-at-death in the population. We have calculated that educational inequalities in life span make up around 10% of the total variation in life span within the population—sometimes a bit less (as in Sweden and in Southern Europa), sometimes a bit more (as in Central and Eastern Europe) (see ref. 122).

x. As explained in footnote vi, it may be useful to measure health inequalities not only on the basis of a comparison between low and high socioeconomic groups of their levels of 'attainment' (e.g. mortality rates), but also on the basis of their levels of 'shortfall' as compared to an ideal or maximum value (e.g. survival rates) (see ref. 88). The 'shortfall' perspective is not always intuitive, but it can be useful when we consider inequalities in life expectancy (or healthy life expectancy), as in the case of Figure 2.7. For partial life expectancy between the ages of 35 and 80 years there is a plausible upper value, that is, 45 years, which allows us to calculate the shortfall of each educational group with respect to this maximum value. For example, because the partial life expectancies of low and high educated men in England and Wales in the early 2010s were 40.1 and 42.1 years, respectively, their shortfalls are 4.9 and 2.9 years, which gives us a 'shortfall absolute difference' of 2.0 years and a 'shortfall relative difference' of 1.7. Over time, the shortfall absolute difference in England and Wales has narrowed somewhat (as can also be seen in Figure 2.7, because the shortfall absolute difference equals the 'attainment' absolute difference, that is, the conventional gap in life expectancy), but the shortfall rate ratio has increased considerably, as it has in many other European countries.

xi. Some of the arguments that are being used against relative measures are mathematical in nature. When ratios of mortality go up, ratios of the reverse outcome (survival) will go down, and vice versa, leading to diametrically opposed conclusions (see ref. 89). Suppose that in country X the mortality rate declines from 100 to 50 among the rich, and from 200 to 120 among the poor. Some will regret that inequalities have gone up, because the Rate Ratio has increased from 2.0 (200/100) to 2.4 (120/50). Others will rejoice that inequalities have gone down, because the Rate Difference has fallen from 100 (200–100) to 70 (120–50). Things get even more complicated when we realize that the flip-side of mortality is survival. In this example, suppose that rich and poor groups both have 1000 members. While the Rate Ratio of mortality goes up from 2.0 to 2.4, the Rate Ratio of survival goes down from 1.12 (900/800) to 1.08 (950/880). Are inequalities going up or down? This ambiguity of relative measures does not apply to absolute inequalities, because these are insensitive to such reversals. In the example quoted above, the Rate Differences for mortality and survival are identical, except for a change of sign (100=200–100=800–900 and 70=120–50=880–950). On the other hand, one could also mount mathematical arguments against absolute measures of inequality. When overall mortality levels fall, absolute inequalities in mortality will fall as well, without any changes in the socioeconomic distribution of risk or protective factors for mortality (see ref. 90).

xii. In the table we only mention the Average Intergroup Difference, but this actually represents a family of flexible measures of health inequalities that are also denoted as 'Index of Dissimilarity' and 'Index of Disparity' (see ref. 83). What these measures have in common is that they do not require a hierarchical ordering of socioeconomic groups and/or the identification of a reference group of high socioeconomic position ('non-exposed').

xiii. The calculation of the RII and SII goes as follows. First, each socioeconomic group is given a value on an interval scale, by calculating the average proportion of the population with a lower socioeconomic position (this is called its 'rank'). For example, when the highest educational group contains 30% of the population, its 'rank' will be (1.0 − (0.3/2)) = 0.85. Then, the morbidity or mortality rate of each socioeconomic group is regressed on this 'rank' value. The parameters estimated in this regression analysis then give the SII and the RII: SII = −β, RII = α/α+β (see ref. 48). Recently, more advanced calculation methods have been proposed by Moreno et al. (see ref. 94). There are actually two versions of the RII. The original version, proposed by Pamuk (see ref. 12), calculates the RII by dividing the SII by the average rate of morbidity or mortality in the population. The interpretation of this RII is not in terms of a Rate Ratio comparing the most to the least disadvantaged, but in terms of the relative range of variation around the average rate for the whole population. The version of the RII described above and used in this book (and by most researchers of health inequalities) is a modification proposed by Kunst and Mackenbach (see ref. 48), which has therefore sometimes been called the 'Kunst-Mackenbach index of inequality' (see refs. 95 and 87). Although the RII and SII are useful measures, it is important to note that they do not adjust for changes in composition of lower and higher educated groups, for example, for the fact that the lower educated are likely to have become more homogeneous with regard to various forms of personal and social disadvantage. As a result, the RII and SII are still sensitive to changes in the educational distribution of the population.

xiv. Although the computed values for the CI do not have an intuitive interpretation, it has been shown that multiplication by 75 gives the percentage of the health variable that would need to be redistributed from the richer half to the poorer half of the population to arrive at a distribution with an index value of zero (see ref. 96).

Chapter 3

i. For economists/econometrists, 'health-related selection' falls under the heading of 'simultaneity': due to a loop of causality between socioeconomic position and health, the presumed dependent variable actually affects the independent variable, potentially leading to 'simultaneity bias' (https://en.wikipedia.org/wiki/Endogeneity_econometrics).

ii. Epidemiologists label such situations 'confounding', whereas economists call the bias resulting from not controlling for such confounders 'omitted variable bias'. ('Simultaneity bias', mentioned in the previous paragraph, and 'omitted variable bias' are the two important causes of what economists/econometricians call 'endogeneity', a technical term referring to the problem that the independent variable is correlated with the error term in a regression analysis (https://en.wikipedia.org/wiki/Endogeneity_econometrics). Social epidemiologists, in recognition of the mechanism through which these personal attributes get sorted across socioeconomic groups, sometimes use the term 'indirect selection' (see ref. 230).

iii. Other terms for 'mediators' are 'intermediate variables', 'mediating variables', and 'intervening variables'.

iv. This implies that, strictly speaking, a third variable can be considered a mediator of the effect of socioeconomic position on health if, and only if, (i) a person's socioeconomic position causally influences his or her exposure to the third variable, and (ii) exposure to the third variable causally influences his or her health outcome. In other words, assessment of mediation requires evaluation of two causal relationships. While such strict requirements may be essential for scientific explanation, the first of the two requirements can often be relaxed in a context of policy support. Even if socioeconomic differences in exposure to unfavourable working conditions, smoking behaviour, and lack of access to health care are coincidental—for example, brought about by confounding variables such as other sociodemographic characteristics or personal attributes like cognitive ability—it would still be policy-relevant to know that these differences explain some of the higher mortality rates of lower socioeconomic groups. However, in such a situation it would be better to avoid using the stricter term 'mediator', and use a more neutral term like 'contributory factor' instead.

v. However, although these aims often coincide, there is a subtle difference between the requirements of scientific explanation and the requirements of policy support. In the latter case, it is less important to have certainty about whether differences in exposure to specific health determinants between socioeconomic groups are caused by people's socioeconomic position. As long as we do have certainty about the causal effect of the determinants on health, and even if the differences in exposure between socioeconomic groups are coincidental, reducing them will help to reduce health inequalities. For example, as long as we know for sure that smoking causes lung cancer, we can reasonably assume that reducing smoking among the lower educated will reduce their higher risks of lung cancer, even if we do not know whether their higher rates of smoking are actually caused by their lower level of education. Of course, if their higher rates of smoking are actually caused by their lower level of education, it may be more difficult to lower their rates of smoking, and this would then have to be taken into account in developing an effective intervention programme.

vi. Various technical terms are used to denote 'moderation', its analysis, and its interpretation. Whereas 'moderation' is a term commonly used in social sciences, epidemiologists more commonly use the equivalent term 'effect modification' or more fully 'effect measure modification'. 'Moderation' is also sometimes called 'effect heterogeneity'. In quantitative analyses, 'moderation' translates to 'statistical interaction' (on a relative or absolute scale).

vii. In health economics, a different but conceptually similar approach to mediation analysis is sometimes used. This approach is based on the so-called Oaxaca-Blinder decomposition method which was originally developed in labour economics in the 1970s. A modification of this method, proposed by Wagstaff et al., allows the 'decomposition' of health inequalities, as measured by the 'concentration index', into the contribution of differences in the distribution of various explanatory variables and a residual or 'unexplained' portion (see ref. 266). In the social sciences, another technique to study mediation is 'structural equation modelling'. Specific techniques that may be useful for mediation analysis include 'path analysis' (in which the putative causal 'paths' between several variables can be modelled in linked regression equations) and 'latent growth modelling' (in which repeated measures of the dependent variable can be modelled as a function of several explanatory variables). The main added value of these techniques is that they allow the estimation of more complex relationships than those between a single independent variable, a single dependent variable, and a set of unrelated mediators (see ref. 267).

viii. Two relatively straightforward conditions for unbiased results are that (i) there is no uncontrolled socioeconomic position-outcome confounding, and (ii) there is no uncontrolled mediator-outcome confounding. In addition to these relatively straightforward conditions there are two other conditions which are less self-evident: (iii) there is no socioeconomic position-mediator interaction on the outcome (i.e. the effect of the mediator on the health outcome does not differ between socioeconomic groups), and (iv) there is no mediator-outcome confounding affected by socioeconomic position (i.e., confounders of the mediator-outcome relationship may not be on the causal pathway between socioeconomic position and the health outcome) (see ref. 254).

ix. Actually, a life-course approach may start even earlier, by asking what the role is of maternal and paternal (and even grandmaternal or grandpaternal) health and exposure to health determinants.

x. Because the original model assumed a constant delay of one or two decades between smoking uptake among men and women, a refinement of the model has been proposed which decouples the trends of men and women, thereby allowing for the possibility of a shorter or longer delay, depending on, for example, the degree of gender equality in a country (see ref. 464).

xi. Such cultural differences can also be found in preferences with respect to body size. This applies in particular to women who are more subject to these aesthetic standards than men (see ref. 132). The interaction between cultural differences and sex-specific aesthetic norms may also explain why overweight among women shows a stronger correlation with socioeconomic status than among men (section 3.3 'Six groups of contributing factors').

xii. Others have—on a more critical note—proposed that cognitive ability could be another of these resources and perhaps even be THE 'fundamental cause' of health inequalities. In contrast to the way the theory was originally conceptualized, cognitive ability represents a personal resource that is partly innate, and does not represent a resource in the environment, the access to which is determined by people's position in the socioeconomic hierarchy (see ref. 102).

Chapter 4

i. The adjustment for the size of socioeconomic groups as applied in the calculation of the Relative Index of Inequality does not take away this effect: the RII goes up, like the Rate Ratio does, when the proportion of low educated goes down.

ii. Not everybody agrees. Michael Marmot claims that 'lack of health care cannot be a cause of disease', just like Ichiro Kawachi has argued that 'lack of aspirin is not the cause of fever' (see ref. 47). Both statements are of course true, but they do not logically imply that health care, if present, cannot reduce or magnify health inequalities, dependent on its effectiveness and the existence or not of inequalities in access or quality of health care. Lack of health care can thus be a cause of larger health inequalities in one country than another.

iii. For each country characteristic we applied the following rules to determine whether a relevant interaction effect was present: (1) in an analysis stratified by level of education, the country characteristic needed to have a statistically significant (p<.05) association with the health outcome among the low or high educated or both, and (2) in a pooled analysis the interaction between the country characteristic and low education needed to be statistically significant (p<.05), and (3) the direction of the interaction effect (i.e. whether the effect among the low educated was stronger than that among the high educated, or vice versa) needed to be consistent with the results of the stratified analysis. Numerical results underlying summary Table 4.1 can be found in the appendix table presented after the Notes.

iv. For self-assessed health (but not for GALI limitations) there is a cross-sectional relationship with national income, but this relationship disappears in a more rigorously controlled country- and period-fixed effects analysis. In a similar country- and period-fixed effects analysis as that for lnGDP and mortality reported in Table 4.1, we found no statistically significant effects of lnGDP on self-assessed among low or high educated men or women in stratified analyses, nor did we find statistically significant interaction effects between lnGDP and education in pooled analyses.

v. In a similar country- and period-fixed effects analysis controlling for lnGDP as that for level of democracy and mortality reported in Table 4.1, we found inconsistent effects on mortality of the cumulative number of years of left party government since 1990. In stratified analyses there was a statistically significant downward effect of left party government on mortality among low educated men, but not on mortality among high educated men. However, in pooled analyses, we found a statistically significant interaction effect between left party government and education among men suggesting that left party government increases mortality among low educated men. There were no statistically significant effects on mortality among women.

vi. It is important to note that, although the underlying data on health determinants and health outcomes have all been collected at the individual level, these analyses were actually performed at the aggregate or population level. In these analyses we related the rate of mortality or self-reported morbidity in each aggregate cell in our data set to the prevalence of material deprivation, smoking or obesity in the same aggregate cell, with cells defined by level of education (three groups), country (17 countries), and time (variable number of time-points, ranging between 2 and 10). In other words, these are 'ecological' analyses of which the results should be interpreted with caution, but against the background of our knowledge of the strong individual-level relationships between material deprivation, smoking, and obesity on the one hand and mortality and self-reported morbidity on the other.

vii. These results are based on the 'difference method' for mediation analysis, which we discussed in more detail in Chapter 3. Because of the limitations of this method, the results should be interpreted with caution.

viii. We note in passing that the absence of a correlation between (inequalities in) material deprivation and (inequalities in) smoking and other health-related behaviours also contradicts the idea that larger inequalities in health-related behaviour in advanced welfare states reflect a universal desire for social distinction that can no longer be based on material assets.

ix. They are also remarkably consistent with individual-level studies which have found a Relative Risk of mortality for smokers as compared to non-smokers of between two and three (see refs. 587 and 588).

x. The European Social Survey includes measures of cultural values (such as security seeking, conformity, traditionalism, universalism, self-direction, hedonism, etc.), which were analysed according to the same format as in Figure 4.2, that is, by distinguishing three birth and five European regions, and calculating absolute differences in prevalence of value orientations between educational groups. While there are important differences in all value orientations between educational groups, the magnitude of these inequalities was larger in Northern Europe than in most other European regions for several cultural value orientations (security seeking, traditionalism, self-direction, hedonism).

Chapter 5

i. Studies among baboons and other nonhuman primates have shown that the induction of stress-related health problems among subordinate animals involves the same physiological stress responses (elevated cortisol levels, immunosuppression, hypertension, …) as those seen in humans (see ref. 618). The remarkable similarity between social inequalities among nonhuman primates and humans has often been ironically commented upon—as in the case of a comparison between social hierarchies among baboons in Kenya and social hierarchies among Whitehall civil servants—but it raises deeper questions than those of immunology or endocrinology. If social hierarchies are so common among nonhuman species, and produce health inequalities similar to those seen among ourselves, how can we ever hope to get rid of them?

ii. I will mostly be using the term 'inequitable(ness)', instead of the simpler 'unfair(ness)', because in some approaches a distinction between the two is made. For example, in Margaret Whitehead's principles, an 'inequity' is a health inequality that is both 'avoidable' and 'unfair' (see ref. 654), and in John Rawls's 'Justice as fairness' the concept of 'fairness' has a very specific meaning referring to fair dealings between people in which they do not take advantage of each other (see ref. 655).

iii. Those who benefit from all the advantages, health or otherwise, accruing to people with a higher socioeconomic position would also do well to realize that their own talents and efforts are not the only factors involved in generating these advantages. On the contrary, without the collective talents and efforts of others in society, including previous generations, it would be impossible for individual talent or effort to generate a high level of education or income, and to avoid the health risks of smoking or survive a myocardial infarction.

Chapter 6

i. A recent report by the Scientific Council for Government Policy complains that 35 years of policymaking have not reduced health inequalities in the Netherlands, and proposes to abandon explicit policy goals to reduce health inequalities. Instead, the government should be concerned only with improving the health situation of lower socioeconomic groups, regardless of what happens to health inequalities (see ref. 701). By giving too much credit to Dutch national policymakers (who have in reality done very little to reduce health inequalities), this report threatens to further undermine the support for policies to reduce health inequalities.

ii. Other parts of the United Kingdom, such as Scotland, also developed and implemented strategies to reduce health inequalities (see ref. 709). The achievements were reviewed in 2013, and the review concluded that 'absolute health inequalities have remained high and relative health inequalities have continued to increase' (see ref. 710).

iii. A more complex three-dimensional typology, taking into account changes in relative inequalities, absolute inequalities, and average mortality rates has been proposed by Tony Blakely (see ref. 211).

iv. See Box 4.3 for explanation of this method, which has been more fully documented in ref. 722.

References

1. **Schultz H.** Social differences in mortality in the eighteenth century: An analysis of Berlin church registers. *International Review of Social History* 1991; **36**(2): 232–48.
2. **Perrenoud A.** L'inégalité sociale devant la mort à Genève au XVIIe siècle. *Population (édition Francaise)* 1975; **30**(1): 221–43.
3. **Antonovsky A.** Social class, life expectancy and overall mortality. *Milbank Memorial Fund Quarterly* 1967; **45**(2): 31–73.
4. **Kunitz SJ, Engerman SL.** The ranks of death: Secular trends in income and mortality. *Health Transition Review* 1992; **2**(Suppl.): 29–46.
5. **Hollingsworth TH.** The demography of the British Peerage. *Population Studies* 1964; **18**(Suppl.): 1–68.
6. **Wrigley EA, Schofield R.** The population history of England 1541–1871. Cambridge: Cambridge University Press; 1989.
7. **Cipolla CM, Zanetti DE.** Peste et mortalité différentielle. Annales de démographie historique techniques et méthodes; actes du colloque de Florence, 1er–3 octobre 1971. Florence: Mouton; 1972. pp. 197–202.
8. **Ackerknecht EH.** Rudolf Virchow. Doctor, statesman, anthropologist. Madison (WI): University of Wisconsin Press; 1953.
9. **Coleman W.** Death is a social disease: Public health and political economy in early industrial France. Madison (WI): University of Wisconsin Press; 1982.
10. **Chave SPW.** The origins and development of public health. In: Holland WW, Detels R, Knox EG, eds. Oxford Textbook of Public Health Oxford: Oxford University Press; 1984.
11. **Mackenbach JP.** Politics is nothing but medicine at a larger scale: Reflections on public health's biggest idea. *Journal of Epidemiology and Community Health* 2009; **63**(3): 181–4.
12. **Pamuk ER.** Social class inequality in mortality from 1921 to 1972 in England and Wales. *Population Studies (Cambridge)* 1985; **39**(1): 17–31.
13. **Van Kersbergen K, Vis B.** Comparative welfare state politics. Development, opportunities, and reform. Cambridge etc: Cambridge University Press; 2014.
14. **Mackenbach JP.** The persistence of health inequalities in modern welfare states: The explanation of a paradox. *Social Science and Medicine* 2012; **75**(4): 761–9.
15. **Gøsta EA.** The three worlds of welfare capitalism. London: Polity; 1990.
16. **Ferrera M.** The 'Southern model'of welfare in social Europe. *Journal of European Social Policy* 1996; **6**(1): 17–37.
17. **Hemerijck A.** Changing welfare states. Oxford etc: Oxford University Press; 2013.
18. **Bambra C.** Going beyond the three worlds of welfare capitalism: Regime theory and public health research. *Journal of Epidemiology and Community Health* 2007; **61**(12): 1098–1102.
19. **Lau-IJzerman A, Habbema JDF, van der Maas PJ, van den Bos T, Drewes JBJ, Verbeek-Heida PM.** Vergelijkend buurtonderzoek Amsterdam. Amsterdam: Gemeentelijke Geneeskundige Dienst, 1981.
20. **Inequalities in Health:** Report of a research working group (the Black report). London Department of Health and Social Services; 1980.
21. **Marmot MG, Adelstein AM, Robinson N, Rose GA.** Changing social-class distribution of heart disease. *British Medical Journal* 1978; **2**(6145): 1109–12.
22. **Marmot MG, Rose G, Shipley M, Hamilton PJ.** Employment grade and coronary heart disease in British civil servants. *Journal of Epidemiology and Community Health* 1978; **32**(4): 244–9.

23. **Bambra C.** Health inequalities and welfare state regimes: Theoretical insights on a public health 'puzzle'. *Journal of Epidemiology and Community Health* 2011; **65**(9): 740–5.

24. **Adema W, Fron P, Ladaique M.** Is the European welfare state really more expensive? Paris: Organization for Economic Cooperation and Development, 2011.

25. **Vagerö D, Lundberg O.** Health inequalities in Britain and Sweden. *The Lancet* 1989; **334**(8653): 35–6.

26. **Mackenbach JP, Kunst AE, Cavelaars AE, Groenhof F, Geurts JJ.** Socioeconomic inequalities in morbidity and mortality in western Europe. *Lancet* 1997; **349**(9066): 1655–9.

27. **Beckfield J, Krieger N.** Epi+ demos+ cracy: Linking political systems and priorities to the magnitude of health inequities—evidence, gaps, and a research agenda. *Epidemiologic Reviews* 2009; **31**(1): 152–77.

28. **Muntaner C, Borrell C, Ng E, et al.** Politics, welfare regimes, and population health: Controversies and evidence. *Sociology of Health and Illness* 2011; **33**(6): 946–64.

29. **Brennenstuhl S, Quesnel-Vallée A, McDonough P.** Welfare regimes, population health and health inequalities: A research synthesis. *Journal of Epidemiology and Community Health* 2012; **66**: 397–409.

30. **Bergqvist K, Yngwe MA, Lundberg O.** Understanding the role of welfare state characteristics for health and inequalities—an analytical review. *BMC Public Health* 2013; **13**: 1234.

31. **Marx I, Nolan B, Olivera Angulo J.** The welfare state and anti-poverty policy in rich countries. In: Atkinson AB, Bourguignon F, eds. Handbook of Income Distribution. Amsterdam etc.: Elsevier; 2014: 2063–140.

32. **Lundberg O, Yngwe MÅ, Stjärne MK, et al.** The role of welfare state principles and generosity in social policy programmes for public health: An international comparative study. *The Lancet* 2008; **372**(9650): 1633–40.

33. **Parsons T.** The social system. Glencoe (Ill.): Free Press; 1951.

34. **Davis K, Moore WE.** Some principles of stratification. *American Sociological Review* 1945; **10**(2): 242–9.

35. **Marx K.** Capital: A critique of political economy, 3 vols. London: Lawrence and Wishart 1894 [1972].

36. **Milanovic B.** Global inequality: A new approach for the age of globalization. Cambridge (Mass.) etc.: Belknap Press; 2016.

37. **Piketty T.** Capital in the twenty-first century. Cambridge (Mass.): Harvard University Press; 2014.

38. **Scheidel W.** The Great Leveller: Violence and the global history of inequality from the stone age to the present. Oxford etc: Oxford University Press; 2017.

39. **Stiglitz JE.** The price of inequality: How today's divided society endangers our future. New York etc.: WW Norton and Company; 2012.

40. **Wilkinson RG.** Income distribution and life expectancy. *Bmj* 1992; **304**(6820): 165–8.

41. **Wilkinson RG, Pickett K.** The spirit level: Why more equal societies almost always do better. London: Allen Lane; 2009.

42. **Hu Y, van Lenthe FJ, Mackenbach JP.** Income inequality, life expectancy and cause-specific mortality in 43 European countries, 1987–2008: A fixed effects study. *European Journal of Epidemiology* 2015; **30**(8): 615–25.

43. **Whitehead M.** The concepts and principles of equity and health. *Health Promotion International* 1991; **6**(3): 217–28.

44. **Braveman P, Gruskin S.** Defining equity in health. *Journal of Epidemiology and Community Health* 2003; **57**(4): 254–8.

45. **Rosanvallon P.** The society of equals. Cambridge (Mass.) etc: Harvard University Press; 2013.

46. **Bartley M.** Health inequality: An introduction to concepts, theories and methods. 2 ed. Cambridge etc: Polity Press; 2017.

47. **Marmot M.** The health gap: The challenge of an unequal world: Bloomsbury Publishing; 2015.

48. **Mackenbach JP, Kunst AE.** Measuring the magnitude of socio-economic inequalities in health: An overview of available measures illustrated with two examples from Europe. *Social Science and Medicine* 1997; **44**(6): 757–71.

49. **Grusky DB**. The Past, Present, and Future of Social Inequality. In: Grusky DB, Ku MC, Szelényi S, editors. Social stratification: Class, race, and gender in sociological perspective. Boulder CO: Westview Press; 2001.

50. **Krieger N, Williams DR, Moss NE**. Measuring social class in US public health research: concepts, methodologies, and guidelines. *Annual Review of Public Health* 1997; **18**(1): 341–78.

51. **Galobardes B, Lynch J, Smith GD**. Measuring socioeconomic position in health research. *Br Med Bull* 2007; **81–82**: 21–37.

52. **Glymour MM, Avendano M, Kawachi I**. Socioeconomic status and health. In: Berkman LF, Kawachi I, Glymour MM, editors. Social epidemiology (second edition). Oxford etc.: Oxford University Press; 2014. p. 17–62.

53. **Schumpeter J**. Aufsatze zur Soziologie. Tubingen: Mohr/Siebeck; 1953.

54. **Lenski GE**. Power and privilege: A theory of social stratification. Chapel Hill and London: University of North Carolina Press; 1966.

55. **Savage M**. Social class in the 21st century. A Pelican introduction. Harmondsworth: Penguin Random House UK; 2015.

56. **Galobardes B, Shaw M, Lawlor DA, Lynch JW, Smith GD**. Indicators of socioeconomic position (part 1). *Journal of Epidemiology & Community Health* 2006; **60**(1): 7–12.

57. **Young MD**. The rise of the meritocracy. London: Thames and Hudson; 1958.

58. **Mirowsky J, Ross CE**. Education, personal control, lifestyle and health: A human capital hypothesis. *Research on Aging* 1998; **20**(4): 415–49.

59. **Erikson R, Goldthorpe JH**. The constant flux: A study of class mobility in industrial societies. Oxford etc: Oxford University Press; 1992.

60. **Martikainen P, Mäkelä P, Koskinen S, Valkonen T**. Income differences in mortality: a register-based follow-up study of three million men and women. *International Journal of Epidemiology* 2001; **30**(6): 1397–405.

61. **Östergren O**. Growing gaps: the importance of income and family for educational inequalities in mortality among Swedish men and women 1990–2009. *Scandinavian Journal of Public Health* 2015; **43**(6): 563–70.

62. **Mortensen LH, Rehnberg J, Dahl E**, et al. Shape of the association between income and mortality: A cohort study of Denmark, Finland, Norway and Sweden in 1995 and 2003. *BMJ Open* 2016; **6**(12): e010974.

63. **Collins PH**. Intersectionality's definitional dilemmas. *Annual Review of Sociology* 2015; **41**: 1–20.

64. **Gkiouleka A, Huijts T, Beckfield J, Bambra C**. Understanding the micro and macro politics of health: Inequalities, intersectionality and institutions—A research agenda. *Social Science and Medicine* 2018; **200**: 92–8.

65. **Rechel B, Mladovsky P, Ingleby D, Mackenbach JP, McKee M**. Migration and health in an increasingly diverse Europe. *The Lancet* 2013; **381**(9873): 1235–45.

66. **Smith GD, Chaturvedi N, Harding S, Nazroo J, Williams R**. Ethnic inequalities in health: A review of UK epidemiological evidence. *Critical Public Health* 2000; **10**(4): 375–408.

67. **Boulogne R, Jougla E, Breem Y, Kunst AE, Rey G**. Mortality differences between the foreign-born and locally-born population in France (2004–2007). *Social Science and Medicine* 2012; **74**(8): 1213–23.

68. **Bos V, Kunst AE, Keij-Deerenberg IM, Garssen J, Mackenbach JP**. Ethnic inequalities in age- and cause-specific mortality in The Netherlands. *International Journal of Epidemiology* 2004; **33**(5): 1112–19.

69. **Rafnsson SB, Bhopal RS, Agyemang C**, et al. Sizable variations in circulatory disease mortality by region and country of birth in six European countries. *European Journal of Public Health* 2013; **23**(4): 594–605.

70. **Ikram UZ, Mackenbach JP, Harding S**, et al. All-cause and cause-specific mortality of different migrant populations in Europe. *European Journal of Epidemiology* 2016; **31**(7): 655–65.

71. **Bos V, Kunst AE, Garssen J, Mackenbach JP.** Socioeconomic inequalities in mortality within ethnic groups in the Netherlands, 1995–2000. *Journal of Epidemiology and Community Health* 2005; **59**(4): 329–35.

72. **Zufferey J.** Investigating the migrant mortality advantage at the intersections of social stratification in Switzerland: The role of vulnerability. *Demographic Research* 2016; **34**: 899–926.

73. **Agyemang C, van Oeffelen AAM, Bots ML, Stronks K, Vaartjes I.** Socioeconomic inequalities in acute myocardial infarction incidence in migrant groups: Has the epidemic arrived? Analysis of nation-wide data. *Heart* 2014; **100**: 239–46.

74. **Shkolnikov VM, Jasilionis D, Andreev EM, Jdanov DA, Stankuniene V, Ambrozaitiene D.** Linked versus unlinked estimates of mortality and length of life by education and marital status: Evidence from the first record linkage study in Lithuania. *Social Science and Medicine* 2007; **64**(7): 1392–1406.

75. **Berger N, Van Oyen H, Cambois E, et al.** Assessing the validity of the Global Activity Limitation Indicator in fourteen European countries. *BMC Medical Research Methodology* 2015; **15**: 1.

76. **Johnston DW, Propper C, Shields MA.** Comparing subjective and objective measures of health: Evidence from hypertension for the income/health gradient. *Journal of Health Economics* 2009; **28**(3): 540–52.

77. **Cawley J, Choi A.** Health disparities across education: The role of differential reporting error. Cambridge MA: National Bureau of Economic Research, 2015.

78. **Bago d'Uva T, O'Donnell O, Van Doorslaer E.** Differential health reporting by education level and its impact on the measurement of health inequalities among older Europeans. *International Journal of Epidemiology* 2008; **37**(6): 1375–83.

79. **Dowd JB, Todd M.** Does self-reported health bias the measurement of health inequalities in US adults? Evidence using anchoring vignettes from the Health and Retirement Study. *Journals of Gerontology Series B: Psychological Sciences and Social Sciences* 2011; **66**(4): 478–89.

80. **Peracchi F, Rossetti C.** Heterogeneity in health responses and anchoring vignettes. *Empirical Economics* 2012; **42**(2): 513–38.

81. **Ahmad OB, Boschi-Pinto C, Lopez AD, Murray CJL, Lozano R, Inoue M.** Age standardization of rates: A new WHO standard. Geneva: World Health Organization, 2001.

82. **Kakwani N, Wagstaff A, Van Doorslaer E.** Socioeconomic inequalities in health: Measurement, computation, and statistical inference. *Journal of Econometrics* 1997; **77**(1): 87–103.

83. **Harper S, Lynch J, Meersman SC, Breen N, Davis WW, Reichman ME.** An overview of methods for monitoring social disparities in cancer with an example using trends in lung cancer incidence by area-socioeconomic position and race-ethnicity, 1992–2004. *American Journal of Epidemiology* 2008; **167**(8): 889–99.

84. **Wagstaff A, Paci P, Van Doorslaer E.** On the measurement of inequalities in health. *Social Science and Medicine* 1991; **33**(5): 545–57.

85. **Regidor E.** Measures of health inequalities: Part 1. *Journal of Epidemiology and Community Health* 2004; **58**(10): 858–61.

86. **Regidor E.** Measures of health inequalities: Part 2. *Journal of Epidemiology and Community Health* 2004; **58**(11): 900–3.

87. **Hosseinpoor AR, Nambiar D, Schlotheuber A, Reidpath D, Ross Z.** Health Equity Assessment Toolkit (HEAT): Software for exploring and comparing health inequalities in countries. *BMC Medical Research Methodology* 2016; **16**(1): 141.

88. **Kjellsson G, Gerdtham U-G, Petrie D.** Lies, damned lies, and health inequality measurements: Understanding the value judgments. *Epidemiology* 2015; **26**(5): 673–80.

89. **Scanlan JP.** Guest editorial: Can we actually measure health disparities? *Chance* 2006; **19**(2): 47–51.

90. **Mackenbach JP.** Should we aim to reduce relative or absolute inequalities in mortality? *European Journal of Public Health* 2015; **25**(2): 185.

91. Harper S, King NB, Meersman SC, Reichman ME, Breen N, Lynch J. Implicit value judgments in the measurement of health inequalities. *The Milbank Quarterly* 2010; **88**(1): 4–29.

92. Shkolnikov VM, Andreev EM, Jdanov DA, et al. Increasing absolute mortality disparities by education in Finland, Norway and Sweden, 1971–2000. *Journal of Epidemiology and Community Health* 2012; **66**: 372–8.

93. Graham H. Tackling inequalities in health in England: Remedying health disadvantages, narrowing health gaps or reducing health gradients? *Journal of Social Policy* 2004; **33**(1): 115–31.

94. Moreno-Betancur M, Latouche A, Menvielle G, Kunst AE, Rey G. Relative index of inequality and slope index of inequality: A structured regression framework for estimation. *Epidemiology* 2015; **26**(4): 518–27.

95. Hayes LJ, Berry G. Sampling variability of the Kunst-Mackenbach relative index of inequality. *Journal of Epidemiology and Community Health* 2002; **56**(10): 762–5.

96. Koolman X, Van Doorslaer E. On the interpretation of a concentration index of inequality. *Health Economics* 2004; **13**(7): 649–56.

97. Regidor E, Kunst AE, Rodriguez-Artalejo F, Mackenbach JP. Small socio-economic differences in mortality in Spanish older people. *Eur J Public Health* 2012; **22**(1): 80–5.

98. Marinacci C, Grippo F, Pappagallo M, et al. Social inequalities in total and cause-specific mortality of a sample of the Italian population, from 1999 to 2007. *Eur J Public Health* 2013; **23**(4): 582–7.

99. Erikson R, Torssander J. Clerics die, doctors survive: A note on death risks among highly educated professionals. *Scandinavian Journal of Public Health* 2009; **37**(3): 227–31.

100. Marmot MG. Understanding social inequalities in health. *Perspectives in Biology and Medicine* 2003; **46**(3): S9–S23.

101. Adler NE, Boyce T, Chesney MA, et al. Socioeconomic status and health: The challenge of the gradient. *American Psychologist* 1994; **49**(1): 15–24.

102. Gottfredson LS. Intelligence: Is it the epidemiologists' elusive 'fundamental cause' of social class inequalities in health? *Journal of Personality and Social Psychology* 2004; **86**(1): 174–99.

103. Wilkinson RG. Health, hierarchy, and social anxiety. *Annals of the New York Academy of Sciences* 1999; **896**(1): 48–63.

104. Kunst AE, Groenhof F, Mackenbach JP. Occupational class and cause specific mortality in middle aged men in 11 European countries: Comparison of population based studies. *British Medical Journal* 1998; **316**(7145): 1636–42.

105. Toch-Marquardt M, Menvielle G, Eikemo TA, et al. Occupational class inequalities in all-cause and cause-specific mortality among middle-aged men in 14 European populations during the early 2000s. *PLoS One* 2014; **9**(9): e108072.

106. Jørgensen T, Mortensen LH, Nybo Andersen A-M. Social inequality in fetal and perinatal mortality in the Nordic countries. *Scandinavian Journal of Public Health* 2008; **36**(6): 635–49.

107. Pillas D, Marmot M, Naicker K, Goldblatt P, Morrison J, Pikhart H. Social inequalities in early childhood health and development: A European-wide systematic review. *Pediatric Research* 2014; **76**(5): 418.

108. Köhler L. Children's health in Europe-challenges for the next decades. *Health Promotion International* 2017: 1–9.

109. Oakley L, Maconochie N, Doyle P, Dattani N, Moser K. Multivariate analysis of infant death in England and Wales in 2005–6, with focus on socio-economic status and deprivation. *Health Statistics Quarterly* 2009; **42**(1): 22–39.

110. Wickham S, Anwar E, Barr B, Law C, Taylor-Robinson D. Poverty and child health in the UK: Using evidence for action. *Archives of Disease in Childhood* 2016; **101**: 759–66.

111. Ostberg V. Social class differences in child mortality, Sweden 1981–1986. *Journal of Epidemiology and Community Health* 1992; **46**(5): 480–4.

112. **Currie C, Molcho M, Boyce W, Holstein B, Torsheim T, Richter M.** Researching health inequalities in adolescents: The development of the Health Behaviour in School-Aged Children (HBSC) family affluence scale. *Social Science and Medicine* 2008; **66**(6): 1429–36.

113. **Elgar FJ, Pförtner T-K, Moor I, De Clercq B, Stevens GWJM, Currie C.** Socioeconomic inequalities in adolescent health 2002–2010: A time-series analysis of 34 countries participating in the health behaviour in school-aged children study. *The Lancet* 2015; **385**(9982): 2088–95.

114. **Cavelaars AEJM, Kunst AE, Geurts JJM, et al.** Persistent variations in average height between countries and between socio-economic groups: An overview of 10 European countries. *Annals of Human Biology* 2000; **27**(4): 407–21.

115. **Meredith HV.** Body size of infants and children around the world in relation to socioeconomic status. *Advances in Child Development and Behavior* 1984; **18**: 81–145.

116. **Li L, Manor O, Power C.** Are inequalities in height narrowing? Comparing effects of social class on height in two generations. *Archives of Disease in Childhood* 2004; **89**(11): 1018–23.

117. **Galobardes B, McCormack VA, McCarron P, et al.** Social inequalities in height: persisting differences today depend upon height of the parents. *PLoS One* 2012; **7**(1): e29118.

118. **Gompertz B.** XXIV. On the nature of the function expressive of the law of human mortality, and on a new mode of determining the value of life contingencies. In a letter to Francis Baily, Esq. FRS andc. *PhilosophicalTtransactions of the Royal Society of London* 1825; **115**: 513–83.

119. **Huisman M, Kunst AE, Andersen O, et al.** Socioeconomic inequalities in mortality among elderly people in 11 European populations. *Journal of Epidemiology and Community Health* 2004; **58**(6): 468–75.

120. **Perlman RL.** Socioeconomic inequalities in ageing and health. *The Lancet* 2008; **372**: S34-S9.

121. **Adams JM, White M.** Biological ageing: A fundamental, biological link between socio-economic status and health? *The European Journal of Public Health* 2004; **14**(3): 331–4.

122. **van Raalte AA, Kunst AE, Deboosere P, et al.** More variation in lifespan in lower educated groups: Evidence from 10 European countries. *International Journal of Epidemiology* 2011; **40**(6): 1703–14.

123. **Mackenbach JP, Kunst AE, Groenhof F, et al.** Socioeconomic inequalities in mortality among women and among men: An international study. *Am J Public Health* 1999; **89**(12): 1800–6.

124. **Gove WR.** Sex, marital status, and mortality. *American Journal of Sociology* 1973; **79**(1): 45–67.

125. **Umberson D.** Gender, marital status and the social control of health behavior. *Social Science and Medicine* 1992; **34**(8): 907–17.

126. **Kravdal Ø.** Large and growing social inequality in mortality in Norway: The combined importance of marital status and own and spouse's ediucation. *Population and Development Review* 2017; **43**(4): 645–65.

127. **Arber S, Thomas H.** From women's health to a gender analysis of health. In: Cockerham WC, ed. The Blackwell Companion to Medical Sociology. Oxford etc: Blackwell; 2001: 94–113.

128. **Lahelma E, Martikainen P, Rahkonen O, Silventoinen K.** Gender differences in ill-health in Finland: Patterns, magnitude and change. *Social Science and Medicine* 1999; **48**(1): 7–19.

129. **Dalstra JAA, Kunst AE, Borrell C, et al.** Socioeconomic differences in the prevalence of common chronic diseases: An overview of eight European countries. *International Journal of Epidemiology* 2005; **34**(2): 316–26.

130. **Bergmann RL, Edenharter G, Bergmann KE, Lau S, Wahn U.** Socioeconomic status is a risk factor for allergy in parents but not in their children. *Clinical and Experimental Allergy* 2000; **30**(12): 1740–5.

131. **Chen JT, Krieger N, Van Den Eeden SK, Quesenberry CP.** Different slopes for different folks: Socioeconomic and racial/ethnic disparities in asthma and hay fever among 173,859 US men and women. *Environmental Health Perspectives* 2002; **110**(Suppl 2): 211.

132. **Sobal J, Stunkard AJ.** Socioeconomic status and obesity: A review of the literature. *Psychol Bull* 1989; **105**(2): 260–75.

133. **Wardle J, Griffith J.** Socioeconomic status and weight control practices in British adults. *Journal of Epidemiology and Community Health* 2001; **55**(3): 185–90.

134. **Gard MCE, Freeman CP.** The dismantling of a myth: A review of eating disorders and socioeconomic status. *International Journal of Eating Disorders* 1996; **20**(1): 1–12.

135. **Stirbu I, Looman C, Nijhof GJ, Reulings PG, Mackenbach JP.** Income inequalities in case death of ischaemic heart disease in the Netherlands: A national record-linked study. *Journal of Epidemiology and Community Health* 2012; **66**(12): 1159–66.

136. **Davies CA, Leyland AH.** Trends and inequalities in short-term acute myocardial infarction case fatality in Scotland, 1988–2004. *Population Health Metrics* 2010; **8**(1): 33.

137. **Kirchberger I, Meisinger C, Golüke H,** et al. Long-term survival among older patients with myocardial infarction differs by educational level: Results from the MONICA/KORA myocardial infarction registry. *International Journal for Equity in Health* 2014; **13**(1): 19.

138. **Dalton SO, Schüz J, Engholm G,** et al. Social inequality in incidence of and survival from cancer in a population-based study in Denmark, 1994–2003: Summary of findings. *European Journal of Cancer* 2008; **44**(14): 2074–85.

139. **Aarts MJ, Lemmens VEPP, Louwman MWJ, Kunst AE, Coebergh JWW.** Socioeconomic status and changing inequalities in colorectal cancer? A review of the associations with risk, treatment and outcome. *European Journal of Cancer* 2010; **46**(15): 2681–95.

140. **Rachet B, Ellis L, Maringe C,** et al. Socioeconomic inequalities in cancer survival in England after the NHS cancer plan. *British Journal of Cancer* 2010; **103**(4): 446–53.

141. **Idorn LW, Wulf HC.** Socioeconomic status and cutaneous malignant melanoma in Northern Europe. *British Journal of Dermatology* 2014; **170**(4): 787–93.

142. **Van der Heyden JH, Schaap MM, Kunst AE,** et al. Socioeconomic inequalities in lung cancer mortality in 16 European populations. *Lung Cancer* 2009; **63**(3): 322–30.

143. **Gadeyne S, Menvielle G, Kulhanova I,** et al. The turn of the gradient? Educational differences in breast cancer mortality in 18 European populations during the 2000s. *International Journal of Cancer* 2017; **141**(1): 33–44.

144. **Kulik MC, Menvielle G, Eikemo TA,** et al. Educational inequalities in three smoking-related causes of death in 18 European populations. *Nicotine Tobacco Research* 2014; **16**(5): 507–18.

145. **Stickley A, Leinsalu M, Kunst AE,** et al. Socioeconomic inequalities in homicide mortality: A population-based comparative study of 12 European countries. *European Journal of Epidemiology* 2012; **27**(11): 877–84.

146. **Mackenbach JP, Kulhánová I, Bopp M,** et al. Inequalities in alcohol-related mortality in 17 European countries: A retrospective analysis of mortality registers. *PLoS medicine* 2015; **12**(12): e1001909.

147. **Nagavci B, de Gelder R, Martikainen P,** et al. Inequalities in tuberculosis mortality: Long-term trends in 11 European countries. *International Journal of Tuberculosis and Lung Disease* 2016; **20** (5): 574–81.

148. **Lorant V, de Gelder R, Kapadia D, Mackenbach JP.** Suicide socioeconomic inequalities in Europe: The widening gradient. . *British Journal of Psychiatry* 2018; 212: 356–61.

149. **Roskam AJ, Kunst AE, Van Oyen H,** et al. Comparative appraisal of educational inequalities in overweight and obesity among adults in 19 European countries. *International Journal of Epidemiology* 2010; **39**(2): 392–404.

150. **Vandenheede H, Deboosere P, Espelt A,** et al. Educational inequalities in diabetes mortality across Europe in the 2000s: The interaction with gender. *International journal of public health* 2015; **60**(4): 401–10.

151. **Stirbu I, Kunst AE, Bopp M,** et al. Educational inequalities in avoidable mortality in Europe. *Journal of Epidemiology and Community Health* 2010; **64**(10): 913–20.

152. **Marmot MG, McDowall ME.** Mortality decline and widening social inequalities. *Lancet* 1986; **2**(8501): 274–6.

153. **Avendano M, Kunst AE, Huisman M**, et al. Socioeconomic status and ischaemic heart disease mortality in 10 western European populations during the 1990s. *Heart* 2006; **92**(4): 461–7.

154. **Kunst AE, Groenhof F, Andersen O**, et al. Occupational class and ischemic heart disease mortality in the United States and 11 European countries. *American Journal of Public Health* 1999; **89**(1): 47–53.

155. **Mackenbach JP, Cavelaars AE, Kunst AE, Groenhof F.** Socioeconomic inequalities in cardiovascular disease mortality: An international study. *European Heart Journal* 2000; **21**(14): 1141–51.

156. **Borrell C, Plasencia A, Huisman M**, et al. Education level inequalities and transportation injury mortality in the middle aged and elderly in European settings. *Injury Prevention* 2005; **11**(3): 138–42.

157. **Lorant V, Kunst AE, Huisman M, Costa G, Mackenbach JP.** Socio-economic inequalities in suicide: A European comparative study. *British Journal of Psychiatry* 2005; **187**: 49–54.

158. **Fryers T, Melzer D, Jenkins R.** Social inequalities and the common mental disorders. *Social Psychiatry and Psychiatric Epidemiology* 2003; **38**(5): 229–37.

159. **Lorant V, Deliège D, Eaton W, Robert A, Philippot P, Ansseau M.** Socioeconomic inequalities in depression: A meta-analysis. *American Journal of Epidemiology* 2003; **157**(2): 98–112.

160. **Reiss F.** Socioeconomic inequalities and mental health problems in children and adolescents: A systematic review. *Social Science and Medicine* 2013; **90**: 24–31.

161. **Fisher M, Baum F.** The social determinants of mental health: Implications for research and health promotion. *Australian and New Zealand Journal of Psychiatry* 2010; **44**(12): 1057–63.

162. **Wahlbeck K, Westman J, Nordentoft M, Gissler M, Laursen TM.** Outcomes of Nordic mental health systems: Life expectancy of patients with mental disorders. *British Journal of Psychiatry* 2011; **199**(6): 453–8.

163. **Hemminki E, Merikukka M, Gissler M**, et al. Antidepressant use and violent crimes among young people: A longitudinal examination of the Finnish 1987 birth cohort. *Journal Epidemiology Community Health* 2017; **71**: 12–8.

164. **Piff PK, Stancato DM, Côté S, Mendoza-Denton R, Keltner D.** Higher social class predicts increased unethical behavior. *Proceedings of the National Academy of Sciences* 2012; **109**(11): 4086–91.

165. **Wilkinson R.** Why is violence more common where inequality is greater? *Annals of the New York Academy of Sciences* 2004; **1036**(1): 1–12.

166. **Murtin F, Mackenbach JP, Jasilionis D, Mira d'Ercole M.** Inequalities in longevity by education in OECD countries: Insights from new OECD estimates. Paris: OECD Publishing, 2017.

167. **Majer IM, Nusselder WJ, Mackenbach JP, Kunst AE.** Socioeconomic inequalities in life and health expectancies around official retirement age in 10 Western-European countries. *Journal of Epidemiology and Community Health* 2011; **65**(11): 972–9.

168. **Maki N, Martikainen P, Eikemo T**, et al. Educational differences in disability-free life expectancy: A comparative study of long-standing activity limitation in eight European countries. *Social Science and Medicine* 2013; **94**: 1–8.

169. **OECD.** Pensions at a Glance 2017. Paris: Organization for Economic Cooperation and Development, 2017.

170. **Krieger N, Rehkopf DH, Chen JT, Waterman PD, Marcelli E, Kennedy M.** The fall and rise of US inequities in premature mortality: 1960–2002. *PLoS Medicine* 2008; **5**(2): e46.

171. **Strand BH, Steingrímsdóttir ÓA, Grøholt E-K, Ariansen I, Graff-Iversen S, Næss Ø.** Trends in educational inequalities in cause specific mortality in Norway from 1960 to 2010: A turning point for educational inequalities in cause specific mortality of Norwegian men after the millennium? *BMC Public Health* 2014; **14**(1): 1208.

172. **Menvielle G, Chastang J-F, Luce D, Leclerc A.** Changing social disparities and mortality in France (1968–1996): Cause of death analysis by educational level. *Epidemiology and Public Health/Revue d'Epidémiologie et de Santé Publique* 2007; **55**(2): 97–105.

173. **Stringhini S, Spadea T, Stroscia M**, et al. Decreasing educational differences in mortality over 40 years: Evidence from the Turin Longitudinal Study (Italy). *Journal of Epidemiology and Community Health* 2015; **69**: 1208–16.

174. **de Gelder R, Menvielle G, Costa G**, et al. Long-term trends in socioeconomic inequalities in mortality in 6 European countries. *International Journal of Public Health* 2017; **62**(1): 127–41.

175. **Mackenbach JP, Rubio Valverde J, Artnik B**, et al. Recent trends in health inequalities in 27 European countries. *Proceedings of the National Academy of Sciences* 2018; **115**(5): 6440–5.

176. **Mackenbach JP, Karanikolos M, Lopez Bernal J, Mckee M.** Why did life expectancy in Central and Eastern Europe suddenly improve in the 1990s? An analysis by cause of death. *Scandinavian Journal of Public Health* 2015; **43**(8): 796–801.

177. **Steingrimsdottir OA, Naess O, Moe JO**, et al. Trends in life expectancy by education in Norway 1961–2009. *European Journal of Epidemiology* 2012; **27**(3): 163–71.

178. **Palosuo H, Koskinen S, Lahelma E**, et al. Trends in socioeconomic health differences 1980–2005. Helsinki: Ministry of Social Affairs and Health; 2009.

179. **Bronnum-Hansen H, Baadsgaard M.** Widening social inequality in life expectancy in Denmark. A register-based study on social composition and mortality trends for the Danish population. *BMC Public Health* 2012; **12**: 994.

180. **Kunst AE, Bos V, Lahelma E**, et al. Trends in socioeconomic inequalities in self-assessed health in 10 European countries. *International Journal of Epidemiology* 2004; **34**(2): 295–305.

181. **Hu Y, van Lenthe FJ, Borsboom GJ**, et al. Trends in socioeconomic inequalities in self-assessed health in 17 European countries between 1990 and 2010. *Journal of Epidemiology and Community Health* 2016.

182. **Mackenbach JP, Cavelaars AEJM, Kunst AE, Groenhof F.** Socioeconomic inequalities in cardiovascular disease mortality. An international study. *European heart journal* 2000; **21**(14): 1141–51.

183. **Avendano M, Aro AR, Mackenbach JP.** Socio-economic disparities in physical health in 10 European countries. In: Boersch-Supan A, Brugiavini A, Juerges H, Mackenbach JP, Siegrist J,W. eds. Health, ageing and retirement in Europe: First results of the Survey of Health, Ageing and Retirement in Europe. Morlenbach: Strauss; 2005: 102–7.

184. **Hairi FM, Mackenbach JP, Andersen-Ranberg K, Avendano M.** Does socio-economic status predict grip strength in older Europeans? Results from the SHARE study in non-institutionalised men and women aged 50+. *Journal of Epidemiology and Community Health* 2010; **64**(9): 829–37.

185. **Stringhini S, Carmeli C, Jokela M**, et al. Socioeconomic status, non-communicable disease risk factors, and walking speed in older adults: Multi-cohort population based study. *British Medical Journal* 2018; **360**: k1046.

186. **Lasser KE, Himmelstein DU, Woolhandler S.** Access to care, health status, and health disparities in the United States and Canada: Results of a cross-national population-based survey. *American Journal of Public Health* 2006; **96**(7): 1300–7.

187. **Baker M, Currie J, Schwandt H.** Mortality inequality in Canada and the US: Divergent or Convergent Trends? Cambridge MA: National Bureau of Economic Research, 2017.

188. **Chetty R, Stepner M, Abraham S**, et al. The association between income and life expectancy in the United States, 2001–2014. *JAMA* 2016; **315**(16): 1750–66.

189. **Dwyer-Lindgren L, Bertozzi-Villa A, Stubbs RW**, et al. Inequalities in life expectancy among US counties, 1980 to 2014: Temporal trends and key drivers. *JAMA Internal Medicine* 2017; **177**(7): 1003–11.

190. **Murray CJL, Kulkarni S, Ezzati M.** Eight Americas: New perspectives on US health disparities. *American Journal of Preventive Medicine* 2005; **29**(5): 4–10.

191. **Currie J, Schwandt H.** Mortality inequality: The good news from a county-level approach. *Journal of Economic Perspectives* 2016; **30**(2): 29–52.

192. **Currie J, Schwandt H.** Inequality in mortality decreased among the young while increasing for older adults, 1990–2010. *Science* 2016; **352**(6286): 708–12.

193. **Pappas G, Queen S, Hadden W, Fisher G.** The increasing disparity in mortality between socioeconomic groups in the United States, 1960 and 1986. *New England Journal of Medicine* 1993; **329**(2): 103–9.

194. **Montez JK, Zajacova A.** Why is life expectancy declining among low-educated women in the United States? *Am J Public Health* 2014; **104**(10): e5–7.

195. **Case A, Deaton A.** Rising morbidity and mortality in midlife among white non-Hispanic Americans in the 21st century. *Proc Natl Acad Sci U S A* 2015; **112**(49): 15078–83.

196. **Case A, Deaton A.** Mortality and morbidity in the 21st century. *Brookings Papers on Economic Activity* 2017: 23–4.

197. **Mackenbach JP, Kulhanova I, Bopp M,** et al. Inequalities in alcohol-related mortality in 17 European countries: A retrospective analysis of mortality Registers. *PLoS Med* 2015; **12**(12): e1001909.

198. **Banks J, Marmot M, Oldfield Z, Smith JP.** Disease and disadvantage in the United States and in England. *JAMA* 2006; **295**(17): 2037–45.

199. **Avendano M, Glymour MM, Banks J, Mackenbach JP.** Health disadvantage in US adults aged 50 to 74 years: A comparison of the health of rich and poor Americans with that of Europeans. *American Journal of Public Health* 2009; **99**(3): 540–8.

200. **Van Hedel K, Avendano M, Berkman LF,** et al. The contribution of national disparities to international differences in mortality between the United States and 7 European countries. *American Journal of Public Health* 2015; **105**(4): e112–e9.

201. **Turrell G, Mathers CD.** Socioeconomic status and health in Australia. *The Medical Journal of Australia* 2000; **172**(9): 434–8.

202. **Turrell G, Stanley L, De Looper M, Oldenburg B.** Health inequalities in Australia: Morbidity, health behaviours, risk factors and health service use. Canberra: Queensland University of Technology and the Australian Institute of Health and Welfare, 2006.

203. **Draper G, Oldenburg B, Turrell G.** Health inequalities in Australia: Mortality. Canberra: Queensland University of Technology and the Australian Institute of Health and Welfare 2004.

204. **Howden-Chapman P, Tobias M.** Social inequalities in health: New Zealand 1999. Wellington Ministry of Health, 2000.

205. **Blakely T, Woodward A, Salmond C.** Anonymous linkage of New Zealand mortality and census data. *Australian and New Zealand Journal of Public Health* 2000; **24**(1): 92–5.

206. **Fawcett J, Blakely T.** Cancer is overtaking cardiovascular disease as the main driver of socioeconomic inequalities in mortality: New Zealand (1981–99). *Journal of Epidemiology and Community Health* 2007; **61**(1): 59–66.

207. **Teng AM, Atkinson J, Disney G, Wilson N, Blakely T.** Changing socioeconomic inequalities in cancer incidence and mortality: Cohort study with 54 million person-years follow-up 1981–2011. *International Journal of Cancer* 2017; **140**(6): 1306–16.

208. **Blakely T, Tobias M, Atkinson J.** Inequalities in mortality during and after restructuring of the New Zealand economy: Repeated cohort studies. *British Medical Journal* 2008; **336**(7640): 371–5.

209. **Teng A, Atkinson J, Disney G, Wilson N, Blakely T.** Changing smoking-mortality association over time and across social groups: National census-mortality cohort studies from 1981 to 2011. *Scientific Reports* 2017; **7**(1): 11465.

210. **Wilson N, Blakely T, Tobias M.** What potential has tobacco control for reducing health inequalities? The New Zealand situation. *International Journal for Equity in Health* 2006; **5**(1): 14.

211. **Blakely T, Disney G, Atkinson J, Teng A, Mackenbach JP.** A typology for charting socioeconomic mortality gradients: "Go Southwest". *Epidemiology* 2017; **28**(4): 594–603.

212. **Wamala S, Blakely T, Atkinson J.** Trends in absolute socioeconomic inequalities in mortality in Sweden and New Zealand: A 20-year gender perspective. *BMC Public Health* 2006; **6**(1): 164.

213. Fawcett J, Blakely T, Kunst A. Are mortality differences and trends by education any better or worse in New Zealand? A comparison study with Norway, Denmark and Finland, 1980–1990s. *European Journal of Epidemiology* 2005; **20**(8): 683–91.

214. Aspalter C. The East Asian welfare model. *International Journal of Social Welfare* 2006; **15**(4): 290–301.

215. Khang Y-H, Lee S-i. Health inequalities policy in Korea: Current status and future challenges. *Journal of Korean Medical Science* 2012; **27**(Suppl): S33–S40.

216. Khang Y-H, Kim HR. Relationship of education, occupation, and income with mortality in a representative longitudinal study of South Korea. *European Journal of Epidemiology* 2005; **20**(3): 217–20.

217. Khang Y-H, Lynch JW, Kaplan GA. Health inequalities in Korea: Age-and sex-specific educational differences in the 10 leading causes of death. *International Journal of Epidemiology* 2004; **33**(2): 299–308.

218. Khang Y-H, Lynch JW, Yang S, et al. The contribution of material, psychosocial, and behavioral factors in explaining educational and occupational mortality inequalities in a nationally representative sample of South Koreans: Relative and absolute perspectives. *Social Science and Medicine* 2009; **68**(5): 858–66.

219. Tanaka H, Nusselder WJ, Bopp M, et al. Mortality inequalities by occupational class among men in Japan, South Korea, and 8 European countries: A comparative study of national register-based data, 1990–2015. *Journal of Epidemiology and Community Health* 2019; in press.

220. Kagamimori S, Gaina A, Nasermoaddeli A. Socioeconomic status and health in the Japanese population. *Social Science and Medicine* 2009; **68**(12): 2152–60.

221. Wada K, Kondo N, Gilmour S, et al. Trends in cause specific mortality across occupations in Japanese men of working age during period of economic stagnation, 1980–2005: Retrospective cohort study. *British Medical Journal* 2012; **344**: e1191.

222. Tanaka H, Toyokawa S, Tamiya N, Takahashi H, Noguchi H, Kobayashi Y. Changes in mortality inequalities across occupations in Japan: A national register based study of absolute and relative measures, 1980–2010. *BMJ Open* 2017; **7**(9): e015764.

223. Martikainen P, Lahelma E, Marmot M, Sekine M, Nishi N, Kagamimori S. A comparison of socioeconomic differences in physical functioning and perceived health among male and female employees in Britain, Finland and Japan. *Social Science and Medicine* 2004; **59**(6): 1287–95.

224. Lahelma E, Pietiläinen O, Ferrie J, et al. Changes over time in absolute and relative socioeconomic differences in smoking: A comparison of cohort studies from Britain, Finland, and Japan. *Nicotine and Tobacco Research* 2016; **18**(8): 1697–1704.

225. Lahelma E, Lallukka T, Laaksonen M, et al. Social class differences in health behaviours among employees from Britain, Finland and Japan: The influence of psychosocial factors. *Health and Place* 2010; **16**(1): 61–70.

226. Macintyre S. The Black Report and beyond: What are the issues? *Social Science and Medicine* 1997; **44**(6): 723–45.

227. Whitehead M. The concepts and principles of equity and health. *International Journal of Health Services: Planning, Administration, Evaluation* 1992; **22**(3): 429–45.

228. Manor O, Matthews S, Power C. Health selection: The role of inter-and intra-generational mobility on social inequalities in health. *Social Science and Medicine* 2003; **57**(11): 2217–27.

229. Rothman KJ, Greenland S, Lash TL. Modern epidemiology. Third edition. Philadelphia etc.: Lippincott Williams and Wilkins, 2008.

230. West P. Rethinking the health selection explanation for health inequalities. *Social Science and Medicine* 1991; **32**(4): 373–84.

231. Baron RM, Kenny DA. The moderator–mediator variable distinction in social psychological research: Conceptual, strategic, and statistical considerations. *Journal of Personality and Social Psychology* 1986; **51**(6): 1173.

232. **Heraclides A, Brunner E.** Social mobility and social accumulation across the life course in relation to adult overweight and obesity: The Whitehall II Study. *Journal of Epidemiology and Community Health* 2010: jech. 2009.087692.

233. **Makela P.** Alcohol-related mortality as a function of socio-economic status. *Addiction* 1999; **94**(6): 867–86.

234. **Lounsbury JW, Sundstrom E, Loveland JM,** et al. Intelligence, 'big five' personality traits, and work drive as predictors of course grade. *Person Indiv Diff* 2003; **35**: 1231–9.

235. **Judge TA, Higgins CA, Thoreson CJ,** et al. The big five personality traits, general mental ability, and career success across the lifespan. *Person Psychol* 1999; **52**: 621–52.

236. **Mackenbach JP.** New trends in health inequalities research: Now it's personal. *Lancet* 2010; **376**(9744): 854–5.

237. **Mackenbach JP.** Genetics and health inequalities: Hypotheses and controversies. *Journal of Epidemiology and Community Health* 2005; **59**(4): 268–73.

238. **Kawachi I, Adler NE, Dow WH.** Money, schooling, and health: Mechanisms and causal evidence. *Ann N Y Acad Sci* 2010; **1186**: 56–68.

239. **Petticrew M, Cummins S, Ferrell C,** et al. Natural experiments: An underused tool for public health? *Public Health* 2005; **119**(9): 751–7.

240. **Whitehead M, Petticrew M, Graham H, Macintyre SJ, Bambra C, Egan M.** Evidence for public health policy on inequalities: 2: Assembling the evidence jigsaw. *Journal of Epidemiology and Community Health* 2004; **58**(10): 817–21.

241. **Hu Y, van Lenthe FJ, Hoffmann R, van Hedel K, Mackenbach JP.** Assessing the impact of natural policy experiments on socioeconomic inequalities in health: How to apply commonly used quantitative analytical methods? *BMC Med Res Methodol* 2017; **17**(1): 68.

242. **Snyder SE, Evans WN.** The effect of income on mortality: Evidence from the social security notch. *The Review of Economics and Statistics* 2006; **88**(3): 482–95.

243. **Apouey B, Clark AE.** Winning Big but feeling no better? The effect of lottery prizes on physical and mental health. Bonn: Institute for the Study of Labor (IZA), 2010.

244. **Lager AC, Torssander J.** Causal effect of education on mortality in a quasi-experiment on 1.2 million Swedes. *Proc Natl Acad Sci U S A* 2012; **109**(22): 8461–6.

245. **Kaufman JS, Cooper RS.** Seeking causal explanations in social epidemiology. *American Journal of Epidemiology* 1999; **150**(2): 113–20.

246. **Oakes JM.** Invited commentary: Paths and pathologies of social epidemiology. *American Journal of Epidemiology* 2013; **178**(6): 850–1.

247. **Glymour MM, Osypuk TL, Rehkopf DH.** Invited commentary: Off-roading with social epidemiology—exploration, causation, translation. *American Journal of Epidemiology* 2013; **178**(6): 858–63.

248. **Krieger N, Davey Smith G.** The tale wagged by the DAG: Broadening the scope of causal inference and explanation for epidemiology. *International Journal of Epidemiology* 2016; **45**(6): 1787–1808.

249. **Krieger N, Smith GD.** Re: "Seeking causal explanations in social epidemiology". *American Journal of Epidemiology* 2000; **151**(8): 831–2.

250. **Goldthorpe JH.** Sociology as a population science. Cambridge etc: Cambridge University Press; 2016.

251. **Hill AB.** Environment and disease: Association or accusation? *Proceedings of the Royal Society of Medicine* 1965; **58**: 295–300.

252. **Dahlgren G, Whitehead M.** Policies and strategies to promote social equity in health. *Stockholm: Institute for future studies* 1991.

253. **Whitehead M, Dahlgren G.** Concepts and principles for tackling social inequities in health: Levelling up Part 1. *World Health Organization: Studies on social and economic determinants of population health* 2006; **2**.

254. **VanderWeele T.** Explanation in causal inference: Methods for mediation and interaction: Oxford University Press; 2015.

255. **Diderichsen F, Evans T, Whitehead M.** The social basis of disparities in health. *Challenging inequities in health: From ethics to action* 2001; **1**: 12–23.

256. **Diderichsen F.** Policies for health equity: An ethical and epidemiological framework and targets for a new national health policy in Sweden. *Health Care Priority Setting* 2003: 57.

257. **Makela P, Paljarvi T.** Do consequences of a given pattern of drinking vary by socioeconomic status? A mortality and hospitalisation follow-up for alcohol-related causes of the Finnish Drinking Habits Surveys. *Journal of Epidemiology and Community Health* 2008; **62**(8): 728–33.

258. **Christensen HN, Diderichsen F, Hvidtfeldt UA**, et al. Joint effect of alcohol consumption and educational level on alcohol-related medical events. *Epidemiology* 2017; **28**(6): 872–9.

259. **Rod NH, Lange T, Andersen I, Marott JL, Diderichsen F.** Additive interaction in survival analysis: Use of the additive hazards model. *Epidemiology* 2012; **23**(5): 733–7.

260. **Hoffmann R, Eikemo TA, Kulhánová I**, et al. The potential impact of a social redistribution of specific risk factors on socioeconomic inequalities in mortality: Illustration of a method based on population attributable fractions. *Journal of Epidemiology and Community Health* 2012: jech-2011-200886.

261. **Mackenbach JP, Kulhanova I, Menvielle G**, et al. Trends in inequalities in premature mortality: A study of 3.2 million deaths in 13 European countries. *J Epidemiol Community Health* 2015;**69**:207–217.

262. **Kulik MC, Hoffmann R, Judge K**, et al. Smoking and the potential for reduction of inequalities in mortality in Europe. *European Journal of Epidemiology* 2013; **28**(12): 959–71.

263. **Hoffmann R, Eikemo TA, Kulhánová I**, et al. Obesity and the potential reduction of social inequalities in mortality: Evidence from 21 European populations. *The European Journal of Public Health* 2015; **25**(5): 849–56.

264. **Kulhánová I, Menvielle G, Hoffmann R**, et al. The role of three lifestyle risk factors in reducing educational differences in ischaemic heart disease mortality in Europe. *The European Journal of Public Health* 2016; **27**(2): 203–10.

265. **Richiardi L, Bellocco R, Zugna D.** Mediation analysis in epidemiology: Methods, interpretation and bias. *International Journal of Epidemiology* 2013; **42**(5): 1511–19.

266. **Wagstaff A, Van Doorslaer E, Watanabe N.** On decomposing the causes of health sector inequalities with an application to malnutrition inequalities in Vietnam. *Journal of Econometrics* 2003; **112**(1): 207–23.

267. **Ditlevsen S, Christensen U, Lynch J, Damsgaard MT, Keiding N.** The mediation proportion: A structural equation approach for estimating the proportion of exposure effect on outcome explained by an intermediate variable. *Epidemiology* 2005; **16**(1): 114–20.

268. **Groeniger JO, Kamphuis CB, Mackenbach JP, van Lenthe FJ.** Repeatedly measured material and behavioral factors changed the explanation of socioeconomic inequalities in all-cause mortality. *Journal of Clinical Epidemiology* 2017; **91**: 137–45.

269. **VanderWeele TJ, Vansteelandt S.** Conceptual issues concerning mediation, interventions and composition. *Statistics and its Interface* 2009; **2**(4): 457–68.

270. **Kaufman JS.** Methods in social epidemiology: John Wiley and Sons; 2017.

271. **Oakes JM, Naimi AI.** Mediation, interaction, interference for social epidemiology. *International Journal of Epidemiology* 2016; **45**(6): 1912–14.

272. **Naimi AI, Schnitzer ME, Moodie EE, Bodnar LM.** Mediation analysis for health disparities research. *American Journal of Epidemiology* 2016; **184**(4): 315–24.

273. **Mackenbach JP, Stirbu I, Roskam AJ**, et al. Socioeconomic inequalities in health in 22 European countries. *The New England Journal of Medicine* 2008; **358**(23): 2468–81.

274. **Smith JP.** The impact of childhood health on adult labor market outcomes. *The Review of Economics and Statistics* 2009; **91**(3): 478–89.

275. **Deary IJ, Strand S, Smith P, Fernandes C.** Intelligence and educational achievement. *Intelligence* 2007; **35**(1): 13–21.

276. **Plomin R, Deary IJ.** Genetics and intelligence differences: Five special findings. *Molecular Psychiatry* 2015; **20**(1): 98.

277. **Conley D, Fletcher J.** The Genome Factor: What the social genomics revolution reveals about ourselves, our history, and the future: Princeton University Press; 2017.

278. **Deary IJ, Johnson W, Houlihan LM.** Genetic foundations of human intelligence. *Human Genetics* 2009; **126**(1): 215–32.

279. **Marioni RE, Davies G, Hayward C,** et al. Molecular genetic contributions to socioeconomic status and intelligence. *Intelligence* 2014; **44**: 26–32.

280. **Hill WD, Arslan RC, Xia C,** et al. Genomic analysis of family data reveals additional genetic effects on intelligence and personality. *Molecular Psychiatry* 2018: 1.

281. **Yang J, Lee SH, Goddard ME, Visscher PM.** Genome-wide complex trait analysis (GCTA): Methods, data analyses, and interpretations. Genome-wide association studies and genomic prediction: Springer; 2013: 215–36.

282. **Kumar SK, Feldman MW, Rehkopf DH, Tuljapurkar S.** Limitations of GCTA as a solution to the missing heritability problem. *Proceedings of the National Academy of Sciences* 2016; **113**(1): E61–E70.

283. **DiPrete TA, Burik CAP, Koellinger PD.** Genetic instrumental variable regression: Explaining socioeconomic and health outcomes in nonexperimental data. *Proceedings of the National Academy of Sciences* 2018; **115**: E4970–E9.

284. **Belsky DW, Moffitt TE, Corcoran DL,** et al. The genetics of success: How single-nucleotide polymorphisms associated with educational attainment relate to life-course development. *Psychological Science* 2016; **27**(7): 957–72.

285. **Krapohl E, Plomin R.** Genetic link between family socioeconomic status and children's educational achievement estimated from genome-wide SNPs. *Molecular Psychiatry* 2016; **21**(3): 437.

286. **Rietveld CA, Medland SE, Derringer J,** et al. GWAS of 126,559 individuals identifies genetic variants associated with educational attainment. *Science* 2013: 1235488.

287. **Lee JJ, Wedow R, Okbay A,** et al. Gene discovery and polygenic prediction from a genome-wide association study of educational attainment in 1.1-million individuals. *Nature Genetics* 2018; epub ahead of print.

288. **Belsky DW, Domingue BW, Wedow R,** et al. Genetic analysis of social-class mobility in five longitudinal studies. *Proceedings of the National Academy of Sciences* 2018; **115**(31): E7275–E84.

289. **Spinath FM, Bleidorn W.** The new look of behavioral genetics in social inequality: Gene-environment interplay and life chances. *Journal of Personality* 2017; **85**(1): 5–9.

290. **Heath AC, Berg K, Eaves LJ,** et al. Education policy and the heritability of educational attainment. *Nature* 1985; **314**(6013): 734–6.

291. **Colodro-Conde L, Rijsdijk F, Tornero-Gómez MJ, Sánchez-Romera JF, Ordoñana JR.** Equality in educational policy and the heritability of educational attainment. *PloS one* 2015; **10**(11): e0143796.

292. **Sundet JM, Tambs K, Magnus P, Berg K.** On the question of secular trends in the heritability of intelligence test scores: A study of Norwegian twins. *Intelligence* 1988; **12**(1): 47–59.

293. **Branigan AR, McCallum KJ, Freese J.** Variation in the heritability of educational attainment: An international meta-analysis. *Social Forces* 2013; **92**(1): 109–40.

294. **Galama T, Lleras-Muney A, van Kippersluis H.** The effect of education on health and mortality: A review of experimental and quasi-experimental evidence. Cambridge, MA: National Bureau of Economic Research, 2018.

295. **Cutler DM, Lleras-Muney A, Vogl T.** Socioeconomic status and health: Dimensions and mechanisms: National Bureau of Economic Research, 2008.

296. **Davies NM, Dickson M, Smith GD, van den Berg GJ, Windmeijer F.** The causal effects of education on health outcomes in the UK Biobank. *Nature Human Behaviour* 2018: In press.

297. **Marmot MG, Stansfeld S, Patel C**, et al. Health inequalities among British civil servants: The Whitehall II study. *The Lancet* 1991; **337**(8754): 1387–93.

298. **Ravesteijn B, van Kippersluis H, van Doorslaer E.** The contribution of occupation to health inequality. In: Rosa Dias P, O'Donnell O. eds. Health and inequality (Research on Economic Inequality, Volume 21). Bingley: Emerald Group Publishing; 2013: 311–32.

299. **Miech RA, Hauser RM.** Socioeconomic status and health at midlife: A comparison of educational attainment with occupation-based indicators. *Annals of Epidemiology* 2001; **11**(2): 75–84.

300. **Winkleby MA, Jatulis DE, Frank E, Fortmann SP.** Socioeconomic status and health: How education, income, and occupation contribute to risk factors for cardiovascular disease. *American Journal of Public Health* 1992; **82**(6): 816–20.

301. **Geyer S, Hemström Ö, Peter R, Vågerö D.** Education, income, and occupational class cannot be used interchangeably in social epidemiology: Empirical evidence against a common practice. *Journal of Epidemiology and Community Health* 2006; **60**(9): 804–10.

302. **Smith GD, Hart C, Hole D**, et al. Education and occupational social class: Which is the more important indicator of mortality risk? *Journal of Epidemiology and Community Health* 1998; **52**(3): 153–60.

303. **Devaux M, Sassi F.** The labour market impacts of obesity, smoking, alcohol use and related chronic diseases. Paris: OECD Publishing, 2015.

304. **Bartley M, Plewis I.** Increasing social mobility: An effective policy to reduce health inequalities. *Journal of the Royal Statistical Society: Series A (Statistics in Society)* 2007; **170**(2): 469–81.

305. **Blane D, Harding S, Rosato M.** Does social mobility affect the size of the socioeconomic mortality differential? Evidence from the Office for National Statistics Longitudinal Study. *Journal of the Royal Statistical Society: Series A (Statistics in Society)* 1999; **162**(1): 59–70.

306. **Claussen B, Smits J, Naess O, Smith GD.** Intragenerational mobility and mortality in Oslo: Social selection versus social causation. *Social Science and Medicine* 2005; **61**(12): 2513–20.

307. **Boyle PJ, Norman P, Popham F.** Social mobility: Evidence that it can widen health inequalities. *Social Science and Medicine* 2009; **68**(10): 1835–42.

308. **Kunst AE, Leon DA, Groenhof F, Mackenbach JP.** Occupational class and cause specific mortality in middle aged men in 11 European countries: Comparison of population based studies. Commentary: Unequal inequalities across Europe. *Bmj* 1998; **316**(7145): 1636–42.

309. **Marmot MG, Shipley MJ.** Do socioeconomic differences in mortality persist after retirement? 25 year follow up of civil servants from the first Whitehall study. *Bmj* 1996; **313**(7066): 1177–80.

310. **Doorslaer Ev, Koolman X.** Explaining the differences in income-related health inequalities across European countries. *Health Economics* 2004; **13**(7): 609–28.

311. **Mackenbach JP, Martikainen P, Looman CW, Dalstra JA, Kunst AE, Lahelma E.** The shape of the relationship between income and self-assessed health: An international study. *International Journal of Epidemiology* 2004; **34**(2): 286–93.

312. **Backlund E, Sorlie PD, Johnson NJ.** A comparison of the relationships of education and income with mortality: The national longitudinal mortality study. *Social Science and Medicine* 1999; **49**(10): 1373–84.

313. **Lahelma E, Martikainen P, Laaksonen M, Aittomäki A.** Pathways between socioeconomic determinants of health. *Journal of Epidemiology and Community Health* 2004; **58**(4): 327–32.

314. **O'Donnell O, Van Doorslaer E, Van Ourti T.** Health and inequality. Handbook of Income Distribution: Elsevier; 2015: 1419–533.

315. **Smith JP.** Healthy bodies and thick wallets: The dual relation between health and economic status. *Journal of Economic Perspectives* 1999; **13**(2): 145–66.

316. **Hill WD, Hagenaars SP, Marioni RE**, et al. Molecular genetic contributions to social deprivation and household income in UK Biobank. *Current Biology* 2016; **26**(22): 3083–9.

317. **Cooper K, Stewart K.** Does money affect children's outcomes?: A systematic review. York: Joseph Rowntree Foundation; 2013.

318. **Cooper K, Stewart K.** Does money in adulthood affect adult outcomes? York: Joseph Rowntree Foundation, 2015.

319. **Cesarini D, Lindqvist E, Östling R, Wallace B.** Wealth, health, and child development: Evidence from administrative data on Swedish lottery players. *The Quarterly Journal of Economics* 2016; **131**(2): 687–738.

320. **Ben-Shlomo Y, Kuh D.** A life course approach to chronic disease epidemiology: Conceptual models, empirical challenges and interdisciplinary perspectives. Oxford University Press; 2002.

321. **Smith GD, Hart C, Blane D, Gillis C, Hawthorne V.** Lifetime socioeconomic position and mortality: Prospective observational study. *Bmj* 1997; **314**(7080): 547–52.

322. **Power C, Kuh D.** Lifecourse development of unequal health. In: Siegrist J, Marmot MG, eds. Social inequalities in health: New evidence and policy implications. Oxford: Oxford University Press; 2006: 27–53.

323. **Mheen Hvd, Stronks K, Mackenbach JP.** A lifecourse perspective on socioeconomic inequalities in health: The influence of childhood socioeconomic position and selection processes. *Sociology of Health and Illness* 1998; **20**: 754–77.

324. **Barker DJ.** The fetal and infant origins of adult disease. *British Medical Journal* 1990; **301**(6761): 1111.

325. **Hayward MD, Gorman BK.** The long arm of childhood: The influence of early-life social conditions on men's mortality. *Demography* 2004; **41**(1): 87–107.

326. **Keating DP, Hertzman C**, eds. Developmental health and the wealth of nations: Social, biological and educational dynamics. New York: Guildford; 1999.

327. **Fraser S**, ed. The bell curve wars: Race, intelligence, and the future of America. New York: Basic Books; 1995.

328. **Polderman TJC, Benyamin B, De Leeuw CA**, et al. Meta-analysis of the heritability of human traits based on fifty years of twin studies. *Nature Genetics* 2015; **47**(7): 702–9.

329. **Holtzman NA.** Genetics and social class. *Journal of Epidemiology and Community Health* 2002; **56**(7): 529–35.

330. **Shanahan MJ, Boardman JD.** Genetics and behavior in the life course: A promising frontier. In: Elder GH, Giele JZ, eds. The craft of life course research. New York: Guildford Press; 2009: 215–35.

331. **Plomin R, DeFries JC, Loehlin JC.** Genotype-environment interaction and correlation in the analysis of human behavior. *Psychological Bulletin* 1977; **84**(2): 309–22.

332. **Belsky DW, Moffitt TE, Caspi A.** Genetics in population health science: Strategies and opportunities. *American Journal of Public Health* 2013; **103**(S1): S73–S83.

333. **Turkheimer E, Haley A, Waldron M, d'Onofrio B, Gottesman II.** Socioeconomic status modifies heritability of IQ in young children. *Psychological Science* 2003; **14**(6): 623–8.

334. **Thayer ZM, Kuzawa CW.** Biological memories of past environments: Epigenetic pathways to health disparities. *Epigenetics* 2011; **6**(7): 798–803.

335. **van Dongen J, Bonder MJ, Dekkers KF**, et al. DNA methylation signatures of educational attainment. *npj Science of Learning* 2018; **3**(1): 7.

336. **Mortensen LH, Diderichsen F, Arntzen A**, et al. Social inequality in fetal growth: A comparative study of Denmark, Finland, Norway and Sweden in the period 1981–2000. *Journal of Epidemiology and Community Health* 2008; **62**(4): 325–31.

337. **Silva LM, Jansen PW, Steegers EAP**, et al. Mother's educational level and fetal growth: The genesis of health inequalities. *International Journal of Epidemiology* 2010; **39**(5): 1250–61.

338. **Jansen PW, Tiemeier H, Looman CWN**, et al. Explaining educational inequalities in birthweight: The Generation R Study. *Paediatric and Perinatal Epidemiology* 2009; **23**(3): 216–28.

339. **Bradley RH, Corwyn RF.** Socioeconomic status and child development. *Annual Review of Psychology* 2002; **53**(1): 371–99.

340. **Currie J.** Healthy, wealthy, and wise: Socioeconomic status, poor health in childhood, and human capital development. *Journal of Economic Literature* 2009; **47**(1): 87–122.

341. **Hackman DA, Farah MJ.** Socioeconomic status and the developing brain. *Trends in Cognitive Sciences* 2009; **13**(2): 65–73.

342. **Galobardes B, Lynch JW, Davey Smith G.** Childhood socioeconomic circumstances and cause-specific mortality in adulthood: Systematic review and interpretation. *Epidemiologic Reviews* 2004; **26**(1): 7–21.

343. **Power C, Kuh D, Morton S.** From developmental origins of adult disease to life course research on adult disease and aging: Insights from birth cohort studies. *Annual Review of Public Health* 2013; **34**: 7–28.

344. **Graham H, Power C.** Childhood disadvantage and adult health: A lifecourse framework: Health Development Agency London; 2004.

345. **Van De Mheen H, Stronks K, Van Den Bos J, Mackenbach JP.** The contribution of childhood environment to the explanation of socio-economic inequalities in health in adult life: A retrospective study. *Social Science and Medicine* 1997; **44**(1): 13–24.

346. **Lawson GM, Hook CJ, Hackman DA,** et al. Socioeconomic status and neurocognitive development: Executive function. In: Griffin JA, Freund LS, McCardle P, eds. Executive function in preschool children: integrating measurement, neurodevelopment, and translational research American Psychological Association Press; 2016: 259–78.

347. **Brito NH, Noble KG.** Socioeconomic status and structural brain development. *Frontiers in Neuroscience* 2014; **8**: 276.

348. **Hackman DA, Farah MJ, Meaney MJ.** Socioeconomic status and the brain: Mechanistic insights from human and animal research. *Nature Reviews Neuroscience* 2010; **11**(9): 651–9.

349. **Conger RD, Donnellan MB.** An interactionist perspective on the socioeconomic context of human development. *Annual Review of Psychology* 2007; **58**: 175–99.

350. **Landecker H, Panofsky A.** From social structure to gene regulation, and back: a critical introduction to environmental epigenetics for sociology. *Annual Review of Sociology* 2013; **39**.

351. **Stringhini S, Polidoro S, Sacerdote C,** et al. Life-course socioeconomic status and DNA methylation of genes regulating inflammation. *International Journal of Epidemiology* 2015; **44**(4): 1320–30.

352. **Needham BL, Smith JA, Zhao W,** et al. Life course socioeconomic status and DNA methylation in genes related to stress reactivity and inflammation: The multi-ethnic study of atherosclerosis. *Epigenetics* 2015; **10**(10): 958–69.

353. **Giesinger I, Goldblatt P, Howden-Chapman P, Marmot M, Kuh D, Brunner E.** Association of socioeconomic position with smoking and mortality: The contribution of early life circumstances in the 1946 birth cohort. *Journal of Epidemiology and Community Health* 2014; **68**(3): 275–9.

354. **Gottfredson LS.** Mainstream science on intelligence: An editorial with 52 signatories, history, and bibliography. *Intelligence* 1997; **24**(1): 13–23.

355. **Neisser U, Boodoo G, Bouchard Jr TJ,** et al. Intelligence: Knowns and unknowns. *American Psychologist* 1996; **51**(2): 77–101.

356. **Nettle D.** Intelligence and class mobility in the British population. *British Journal of Psychology* 2003; **94**(4): 551–61.

357. **Batty GD, Gale CR, Tynelius P, Deary IJ, Rasmussen F.** IQ in early adulthood, socioeconomic position, and unintentional injury mortality by middle age: A cohort study of more than 1 million Swedish men. *American Journal of Epidemiology* 2009; **169**(5): 606–15.

358. **Judge TA, Higgins CA, Thoresen CJ, Barrick MR.** The big five personality traits, general mental ability, and career success across the life span. *Personnel Psychology* 1999; **52**(3): 621–52.

359. **Hart CL, Taylor MD, Smith GD,** et al. Childhood IQ and cardiovascular disease in adulthood: Prospective observational study linking the Scottish Mental Survey 1932 and the Midspan studies. *Social Science and Medicine* 2004; **59**(10): 2131–8.

360. **Deary IJ, Weiss A, Batty GD**. Intelligence and personality as predictors of illness and death: How researchers in differential psychology and chronic disease epidemiology are collaborating to understand and address health inequalities. *Psychological Science in the Public Interest* 2010; **11**(2): 53–79.

361. **Batty GD, Wennerstad KM, Smith GD**, et al. IQ in early adulthood and mortality by middle age: Cohort study of 1 million Swedish men. *Epidemiology* 2009; **20**: 100–9.

362. **Singh-Manoux A, Ferrie JE, Lynch JW, Marmot M**. The role of cognitive ability (intelligence) in explaining the association between socioeconomic position and health: Evidence from the Whitehall II prospective cohort study. *American Journal of Epidemiology* 2005; **161**(9): 831–9.

363. **Calvin CM, Deary IJ, Fenton C**, et al. Intelligence in youth and all-cause-mortality: Systematic review with meta-analysis. *International Journal of Epidemiology* 2010; **40**(3): 626–44.

364. **Batty GD, Der G, Macintyre S, Deary IJ**. Does IQ explain socioeconomic inequalities in health? Evidence from a population based cohort study in the west of Scotland. *Bmj* 2006; **332**(7541): 580–4.

365. **Bijwaard GE, van Kippersluis H, Veenman J**. Education and health: The role of cognitive ability. *Journal of Health Economics* 2015; **42**: 29–43.

366. **Chapman BP, Fiscella K, Kawachi I, Duberstein PR**. Personality, socioeconomic status, and all-cause mortality in the United States. *American Journal of Epidemiology* 2009; **171**(1): 83–92.

367. **Nabi H, Kivimäki M, Marmot MG**, et al. Does personality explain social inequalities in mortality? The French GAZEL cohort study. *International Journal of Epidemiology* 2008; **37**(3): 591–602.

368. **Morris JN, Donkin AJM, Wonderling D, Wilkinson P, Dowler EA**. A minimum income for healthy living. *Journal of Epidemiology and Community Health* 2000; **54**(12): 885–9.

369. **McDonough P, Berglund P**. Histories of poverty and self-rated health trajectories. *Journal of Health and Social Behavior* 2003: 198–214.

370. **Fritzell J, Rehnberg J, Hertzman JB, Blomgren J**. Absolute or relative? A comparative analysis of the relationship between poverty and mortality. *International Journal of Public Health* 2015; **60**(1): 101–10.

371. **van Oort FV, van Lenthe FJ, Mackenbach JP**. Material, psychosocial, and behavioural factors in the explanation of educational inequalities in mortality in The Netherlands. *Journal of Epidemiology and Community Health* 2005; **59**(3): 214–20.

372. **Skalická V, Van Lenthe F, Bambra C, Krokstad S, Mackenbach J**. Material, psychosocial, behavioural and biomedical factors in the explanation of relative socio-economic inequalities in mortality: Evidence from the HUNT study. *International Journal of Epidemiology* 2009; **38**(5): 1272–84.

373. **Aldabe B, Anderson R, Lyly-Yrjänäinen M**, et al. Contribution of material, occupational, and psychosocial factors in the explanation of social inequalities in health in 28 countries in Europe. *Journal of Epidemiology and Community Health* 2010; **65**(12): 1123–31.

374. **Lynch JW, Kaplan GA, Salonen JT**. Why do poor people behave poorly? Variation in adult health behaviours and psychosocial characteristics by stages of the socioeconomic lifecourse. *Social Science and Medicine* 1997; **44**(6): 809–19.

375. **Marsh A, McKay S**. Poor smokers. London: Policy Studies Institute; 1994.

376. **Montano D**. Chemical and biological work-related risks across occupations in Europe: A review. *Journal of Occupational Medicine and Toxicology* 2014; **9**(1): 28.

377. **Wahrendorf M, Dragano N, Siegrist J**. Social position, work stress, and retirement intentions: A study with older employees from 11 European countries. *European Sociological Review* 2012; **29**(4): 792–802.

378. **Hoven H, Siegrist J**. Work characteristics, socioeconomic position and health: A systematic review of mediation and moderation effects in prospective studies. *Occup Environ Med* 2013; **70**(9): 663–9.

379. **Benach J, Vives A, Amable M, Vanroelen C, Tarafa G, Muntaner C**. Precarious employment: Understanding an emerging social determinant of health. *Annual Review of Public Health* 2014; **35**: 229–53.

380. **Milner A, Page A, LaMontagne AD.** Long-term unemployment and suicide: A systematic review and meta-analysis. *PloS one* 2013; **8**(1): e51333.

381. **Dupre ME, George LK, Liu G, Peterson ED.** The cumulative effect of unemployment on risks for acute myocardial infarction. *Archives of Internal Medicine* 2012; **172**(22): 1731–7.

382. **Vågerö D, Garcy AM.** Does unemployment cause long-term mortality? Selection and causation after the 1992–6 deep Swedish recession. *European Journal of Public Health* 2016; **26**(5): 778–83.

383. **Dunn JR.** Housing and health inequalities: Review and prospects for research. *Housing Studies* 2000; **15**(3): 341–66.

384. **Pickett KE, Pearl M.** Multilevel analyses of neighbourhood socioeconomic context and health outcomes: A critical review. *Journal of Epidemiology and Community Health* 2001; **55**(2): 111–22.

385. **Bernard P, Charafeddine R, Frohlich KL, Daniel M, Kestens Y, Potvin L.** Health inequalities and place: A theoretical conception of neighbourhood. *Social Science and Medicine* 2007; **65**(9): 1839–52.

386. **van Lenthe FJ, Brug J, Mackenbach JP.** Neighbourhood inequalities in physical inactivity: The role of neighbourhood attractiveness, proximity to local facilities and safety in the Netherlands. *Social Science and Medicine* 2005; **60**(4): 763–75.

387. **Wheeler BW, Ben-Shlomo Y.** Environmental equity, air quality, socioeconomic status, and respiratory health: A linkage analysis of routine data from the Health Survey for England. *Journal of Epidemiology and Community Health* 2005; **59**(11): 948–54.

388. **Brulle RJ, Pellow DN.** Environmental justice: Human health and environmental inequalities. *Annual Review Public Health* 2006; **27**: 103–24.

389. **Siegrist J, Marmot M.** Health inequalities and the psychosocial environment—two scientific challenges. *Social Science and Medicine* 2004; **58**(8): 1463–73.

390. **Stansfeld SA.** Social support and social cohesion. In: Marmot M, Wilkinson RG, eds. Social determinants of health. 2 ed. Oxford: Oxford University Press; 2006: 148–71.

391. **Kristenson M.** Socio-economic position and health: The role of coping. In: Siegrist J, Marmot M, eds. Social inequalities in health: New evidence and policy implications. Oxford: Oxford University Press; 2006: 127–51.

392. **Marmot MG, Bosma H, Hemingway H, Brunner E, Stansfeld S.** Contribution of job control and other risk factors to social variations in coronary heart disease incidence. *The Lancet* 1997; **350**(9073): 235–9.

393. **Bosma H, Schrijvers C, Mackenbach JP.** Socioeconomic inequalities in mortality and importance of perceived control: cohort study. *British Medical Journal* 1999; **319**(7223): 1469–70.

394. **Droomers M, Schrijvers CT, Mackenbach JP.** Why do lower educated people continue smoking? Explanations from the longitudinal GLOBE study. *Health psychology: Official Journal of the Division of Health Psychology, American Psychological Association* 2002; **21**(3): 263–72.

395. **Droomers M, Schrijvers CT, Mackenbach JP.** Educational differences in starting excessive alcohol consumption: Explanations from the longitudinal GLOBE study. *Social Science and Medicine* 2004; **58**(10): 2023–33.

396. **Droomers M, Schrijvers CT, Stronks K, van de Mheen D, Mackenbach JP.** Educational differences in excessive alcohol consumption: The role of psychosocial and material stressors. *Preventive Medicine* 1999; **29**(1): 1–10.

397. **Droomers M, Schrijvers CT, van de Mheen H, Mackenbach JP.** Educational differences in leisure-time physical inactivity: A descriptive and explanatory study. *Social Science and Medicine* 1998; **47**(11): 1665–76.

398. **Steptoe A.** Psychobiological processes linking socio-economic position to health. In: Siegrist J, Marmot M, eds. Social inequalities in health: New evidence and policy implications. Oxford: Oxford University Press; 2006: 101–26.

399. **Brunner E.** Stress and the biology of inequality. *Bmj* 1997; **314**(7092): 1472–6.

400. Brunner E, Marmot M. Social organization, stress, and health. In: Marmot M, Wilkinson RG, eds. Social determinants of health. 2 ed. Oxford: Oxford University Press; 2006: 6–30.

401. Egan M, Tannahill C, Petticrew M, Thomas S. Psychosocial risk factors in home and community settings and their associations with population health and health inequalities: A systematic meta-review. *BMC Public Health* 2008; **8**(1): 239.

402. Matthews KA, Gallo LC, Taylor SE. Are psychosocial factors mediators of socioeconomic status and health connections? *Annals of the New York Academy of Sciences* 2010; **1186**(1): 146–73.

403. Vrooman JC, Gijsberts MIL, Boelhouwer J, editors. Verschil in Nederland. Sociaal en Cultureel Rapport 2014. The Hague: Sociaal en Cultureel Planbureau; 2014.

404. Hiscock R, Bauld L, Amos A, Fidler JA, Munafò M. Socioeconomic status and smoking: A review. *Annals of the New York Academy of Sciences* 2012; **1248**(1): 107–23.

405. Bloomfield K, Grittner U, Kramer S, Gmel G. Social inequalities in alcohol consumption and alcohol-related problems in the study countries of the EU: Concerted action 'Gender, Culture and Alcohol Problems: A Multi-national Study'. *Alcohol and alcoholism* 2006; **41**(suppl_1): i26–i36.

406. De Irala-Estevez J, Groth M, Johansson L, Oltersdorf U, Prättälä R, Martínez-González MA. A systematic review of socio-economic differences in food habits in Europe: Consumption of fruit and vegetables. *European Journal of Clinical Nutrition* 2000; **54**(9): 706.

407. Sanchez-Villegas A, Martinez JA, Prättälä R, Toledo E, Roos G, Martinez-Gonzalez MA. A systematic review of socioeconomic differences in food habits in Europe: Consumption of cheese and milk. *European Journal of Clinical Nutrition* 2003; **57**(8): 917.

408. Petrovic D, de Mestral C, Bochud M, et al. The contribution of health behaviors to socioeconomic inequalities in health: A systematic review. *Preventive Medicine* 2018; **113**: 15–31.

409. Giskes K, Kunst AE, Benach J, et al. Trends in smoking behaviour between 1985 and 2000 in nine European countries by education. *Journal of Epidemiology and Community Health* 2005; **59**(5): 395–401.

410. Schrijvers CT, Stronks K, van de Mheen HD, Mackenbach JP. Explaining educational differences in mortality: The role of behavioral and material factors. *American Journal of Public Health* 1999; **89**(4): 535–40.

411. Stringhini S, Sabia S, Shipley M, et al. Association of socioeconomic position with health behaviors and mortality. *Jama* 2010; **303**(12): 1159–66.

412. Gregoraci G, Van Lenthe FJ, Artnik B, et al. Contribution of smoking to socioeconomic inequalities in mortality: A study of 14 European countries, 1990–2004. *Tobacco Control* 2016: tobaccocontrol-2015-052766.

413. Cavelaars AE, Kunst AE, Geurts JJ, et al. Educational differences in smoking: International comparison. *British Medical Journal* 2000; **320**(7242): 1102–7.

414. Huisman M, Kunst AE, Mackenbach JP. Educational inequalities in smoking among men and women aged 16 years and older in 11 European countries. *Tobacco Control* 2005; **14**(2): 106–13.

415. Lopez-Azpiazu I, Sanchez-Villegas A, Johansson L, et al. Disparities in food habits in Europe: Systematic review of educational and occupational differences in the intake of fat. *Journal of Human Nutrition and Dietetics* 2003; **16**(5): 349–64.

416. Prättälä RS, Groth MV, Oltersdorf US, Roos GM, Sekula W, Tuomainen HM. Use of butter and cheese in 10 European countries: A case of contrasting educational differences. *The European Journal of Public Health* 2003; **13**(2): 124–32.

417. Beenackers MA, Kamphuis CBM, Giskes K, et al. Socioeconomic inequalities in occupational, leisure-time, and transport related physical activity among European adults: A systematic review. *International Journal of Behavioral Nutrition and Physical Activity* 2012; **9**(1): 116.

418. Demarest S, Van Oyen H, Roskam A-J, et al. Educational inequalities in leisure-time physical activity in 15 European countries. *The European Journal of Public Health* 2013; **24**(2): 199–204.

419. **Roskam A-JR, Kunst AE, Van Oyen H**, et al. Comparative appraisal of educational inequalities in overweight and obesity among adults in 19 European countries. *International Journal of Epidemiology* 2009; **39**(2): 392–404.

420. **Hart CL, Gruer L, Watt GCM.** Cause specific mortality, social position, and obesity among women who had never smoked: 28 year cohort study. *Bmj* 2011; **342**: d3785.

421. **Stringhini S, Dugravot A, Shipley M**, et al. Health behaviours, socioeconomic status, and mortality: Further analyses of the British Whitehall II and the French GAZEL prospective cohorts. *PLoS Medicine* 2011; **8**(2): e1000419.

422. **Room R, Babor T, Rehm J.** Alcohol and public health. *The Lancet* 2005; **365**(9458): 519–30.

423. **Grittner U, Kuntsche S, Gmel G, Bloomfield K.** Alcohol consumption and social inequality at the individual and country levels—results from an international study. *European Journal of Public Health* 2012; **23**(2): 332–9.

424. **Devaux M, Sassi F.** Alcohol consumption and harmful drinking: Trends and social disparities across OECD countries. Paris, 2015.

425. **Grittner U, Kuntsche S, Graham K, Bloomfield K.** Social inequalities and gender differences in the experience of alcohol-related problems. *Alcohol and Alcoholism* 2012; **47**(5): 597–605.

426. **Pampel FC, Krueger PM, Denney JT.** Socioeconomic disparities in health behaviors. *Annual Review of Sociology* 2010; **36**: 349–70.

427. **Deandrea S, Molina-Barceló A, Uluturk A**, et al. Presence, characteristics and equity of access to breast cancer screening programmes in 27 European countries in 2010 and 2014. Results from an international survey. *Preventive Medicine* 2016; **91**: 250–63.

428. **Palència L, Espelt A, Rodríguez-Sanz M**, et al. Socio-economic inequalities in breast and cervical cancer screening practices in Europe: Influence of the type of screening program. *International Journal of Epidemiology* 2010; **39**(3): 757–65.

429. **Spadea T, Bellini S, Kunst A, Stirbu I, Costa G.** The impact of interventions to improve attendance in female cancer screening among lower socioeconomic groups: A review. *Preventive Medicine* 2010; **50**(4): 159–64.

430. **Doorslaer Ev, Wagstaff A, Rutten F.** Equity in the finance and delivery of health care: An international perspective. Oxford etc: Oxford University Press; 1992.

431. **Van Doorslaer E, Wagstaff A, Van der Burg H**, et al. Equity in the delivery of health care in Europe and the US. *Journal of Health Economics* 2000; **19**(5): 553–83.

432. **Van Doorslaer E, Masseria C, Koolman X, Group OHER.** Inequalities in access to medical care by income in developed countries. *Canadian Medical Association Journal* 2006; **174**(2): 177–83.

433. **Devaux M, De Looper M.** Income-related inequalities in health service utilisation in 19 OECD countries, 2008–2009. Paris: OECD Publishing, 2012.

434. **Stirbu I, Kunst AE, Mielck A, Mackenbach JP.** Inequalities in utilisation of general practitioner and specialist services in 9 European countries. *BMC Health Services Research* 2011; **11**(1): 288.

435. **Carrieri V, Wübker A.** Assessing inequalities in preventive care use in Europe. *Health Policy* 2013; **113**(3): 247–57.

436. **OECD/EU.** Health at a Glance: Europe 2016—State of Health in the EU Cycle. Paris: OECD Publishing, 2016.

437. **Lumme S, Manderbacka K, Keskimäki I.** Trends of relative and absolute socioeconomic equity in access to coronary revascularisations in 1995–2010 in Finland: A register study. *International Journal for Equity in Health* 2017; **16**(1): 37.

438. **Manderbacka K, Arffman M, Leyland A, Mccallum A, Keskimäki I.** Change and persistence in healthcare inequities: Access to elective surgery in Finland in 1992—2003. *Scandinavian Journal of Public Health* 2009; **37**(2): 131–8.

439. **Manderbacka K, Keskimäki I, Reunanen A, Klaukka T.** Equity in the use of antithrombotic drugs, beta-blockers and statins among Finnish coronary patients. *International Journal for Equity in Health* 2008; **7**(1): 16.

440. **Forrest LF, Adams J, Wareham H, Rubin G, White M.** Socioeconomic inequalities in lung cancer treatment: Systematic review and meta-analysis. *PLoS Medicine* 2013; **10**(2): e1001376.

441. **Ricci-Cabello I, Ruiz-Pérez I, Labry-Lima D, Olry A, Márquez-Calderón S.** Do social inequalities exist in terms of the prevention, diagnosis, treatment, control and monitoring of diabetes? A systematic review. *Health and Social Care in the Community* 2010; **18**(6): 572–87.

442. **Woods LM, Rachet B, Coleman MP.** Origins of socio-economic inequalities in cancer survival: A review. *Annals of Oncology* 2005; **17**(1): 5–19.

443. **de Koning JS, Klazinga NS, Koudstaal PJ, Prins A, Borsboom GJJM, Mackenbach JP.** 'The role of 'confounding by indication' in assessing the effect of quality of care on disease outcomes in general practice: Results of a case-control study. *BMC Health Services Research* 2005; **5**(1): 10.

444. **Krieger N.** Embodiment: A conceptual glossary for epidemiology. *Journal of Epidemiology and Community Health* 2005; **59**(5): 350–5.

445. **Blane D, Kelly-Irving M, d'Errico A, Bartley M, Montgomery S.** Social-biological transitions: How does the social become biological? *Longitudinal and Life Course Studies* 2013; **4**(2): 136–46.

446. **Brunner E.** Biology and health inequality. *PLoS biology* 2007; **5**(11): e267.

447. **McEwen BS, Stellar E.** Stress and the individual: Mechanisms leading to disease. *Archives of Internal Medicine* 1993; **153**(18): 2093–101.

448. **Beckie TM.** A systematic review of allostatic load, health, and health disparities. *Biological Research for Nursing* 2012; **14**(4): 311–46.

449. **Seeman TE, McEwen BS, Rowe JW, Singer BH.** Allostatic load as a marker of cumulative biological risk: MacArthur studies of successful aging. *Proceedings of the National Academy of Sciences* 2001; **98**(8): 4770–5.

450. **Seeman T, Epel E, Gruenewald T, Karlamangla A, McEwen BS.** Socio-economic differentials in peripheral biology: Cumulative allostatic load. *Annals of the New York Academy of Sciences* 2010; **1186**(1): 223–39.

451. **Seeman TE, Crimmins E, Huang M-H, et al.** Cumulative biological risk and socio-economic differences in mortality: MacArthur studies of successful aging. *Social Science and Medicine* 2004; **58**(10): 1985–97.

452. **Robertson T, Benzeval M, Whitley E, Popham F.** The role of material, psychosocial and behavioral factors in mediating the association between socioeconomic position and allostatic load (measured by cardiovascular, metabolic and inflammatory markers). *Brain, Behavior, and Immunity* 2015; **45**: 41–9.

453. **Hempel CG.** Aspects of scientific explanation. New York: Free Press 1965.

454. **Rogers EM.** Diffusion of innovations. New York: Free Press; 1962.

455. **Lopez AD, Collishaw NE, Piha T.** A descriptive model of the cigarette epidemic in developed countries. *Tobacco Control* 1994; **3**(3): 242–7.

456. **Bourdieu P.** Distinction: A social critique of the judgement of taste. Cambridge: Harvard University Press; 1984.

457. **Abel T.** Cultural capital and social inequality in health. *Journal of Epidemiology and Community Health* 2008; **62**(7): e13–e.

458. **Victora CG, Vaughan JP, Barros FC, Silva AC, Tomasi E.** Explaining trends in inequities: Evidence from Brazilian child health studies. *The Lancet* 2000; **356**(9235): 1093–8.

459. **Hart JT.** The inverse care law. *The Lancet* 1971; **297**(7696): 405–12.

460. **Lynch JW, Smith GD, Kaplan GA, House JS.** Income inequality and mortality: Importance to health of individual income, psychosocial environment, or material conditions. *BMJ: British Medical Journal* 2000; **320**(7243): 1200–4.

461. **Smith GD, Blane D, Bartley M.** Explanations for socio-economic differentials in mortality: Evidence from Britain and elsewhere. *European Journal of Public Health* 1994; **4**(2): 131–44.

462. **Cassel J.** The contribution of the social environment to host resistance: The Fourth Wade Hampton Frost Lecture. *American Journal of Epidemiology* 1976; **104**(2): 107–23.

463. **Marmot M.** The status syndrome: How your social standing affects your health and life expectancy. London: Bloomsbury; 2004.

464. **Wilkinson RG.** The impact of inequality: How to make sick societies healthier: The New Press; 2005.

465. **Lieberson S.** Making it count: The improvement of social research and theory. Berkeley etc: University of California Press; 1987.

466. **Link BG, Phelan J.** Social conditions as fundamental causes of disease. *Journal of Health and Social Behavior* 1995; **Spec No**: 80–94.

467. **Phelan JC, Link BG, Tehranifar P.** Social conditions as fundamental causes of health inequalities: Theory, evidence, and policy implications. *Journal of Health and Social Behavior* 2010; **51** (Suppl): S28–40.

468. **Doyal L, Pennell I.** The political economy of health. London: Pluto Press; 1979.

469. **Navarro V, Shi L.** The political context of social inequalities and health. *Social Science and Medicine* 2001; **52**(3): 481–91.

470. **Krieger N.** Epidemiology and the people's health: Theory and context. Oxford etc: Oxford University Press; 2011.

471. **Breen R, Luijkx R.** Social mobility in Europe between 1970 and 2000. In: Breen R, ed. Social mobility in Europe. Oxford etc: Oxford University Press; 2004: 37–77.

472. **Breen R, Jonsson JO.** Inequality of opportunity in comparative perspective: Recent research on educational attainment and social mobility. *Annual Review of Sociology* 2005; **31**: 223–43.

473. **Braga M, Checchi D, Meschi E.** Educational policies in a long-run perspective. *Economic Policy* 2013; **28**(73): 45–100.

474. **Breen R.** Education and Social Mobility in the Twentieth Century (Trento lecture). In: College N, ed. Oxford 2017.

475. **Blanden J.** Cross-country rankings in intergenerational mobility: A comparison of approaches from economics and sociology. *Journal of Economic Surveys* 2013; **27**(1): 38–73.

476. **Simons AMW, Groffen DAI, Bosma H.** Socio-economic inequalities in all-cause mortality in Europe: An exploration of the role of heightened social mobility. *European Journal of Public Health* 2013; **23**(6): 1010–12.

477. **Arrow KJ, Bowles S, Durlauf SN.** Meritocracy and economic inequality. Princeton: Princeton University Press; 2000.

478. **Bowles S, Gintis H.** The inheritance of inequality. *Journal of Economic Perspectives* 2002; **16**(3): 3–30.

479. **Deaton A.** The great escape: Health, wealth, and the origins of inequality. Princeton and Oxford: Princeton University Press; 2013.

480. **Giskes K, Kunst AE, Benach J, et al.** Trends in smoking behaviour between 1985 and 2000 in nine European countries by education. *Journal of Epidemiology and Community Health* 2005; **59**(5): 395–401.

481. **Monteiro CA, Moura EC, Conde WL, Popkin BM.** Socioeconomic status and obesity in adult populations of developing countries: A review. *Bulletin of the World Health Organization* 2004; **82**(12): 940–6.

482. **Wouters C.** Informalization: Manners and emotions since 1890. London etc: Sage; 2007.

483. **Otterloo AH, Ogtrop JPHM.** Het regime van veel, vet en zoet: praten met moeders over voeding en gezondheid. Amsterdam: VU Uitgeverij; 1989.

484. **Lamont M, Lareau A.** Cultural capital: Allusions, gaps and glissandos in recent theoretical developments. *Sociological Theory* 1988: 153–68.

485. Kamphuis CBM, Jansen T, Mackenbach JP, van Lenthe FJ. Bourdieu's Cultural Capital in Relation to Food Choices: A Systematic Review of Cultural Capital Indicators and an Empirical Proof of Concept. *PloS One* 2015; **10**(8): e0130695.

486. Wilson TC. The paradox of social class and sports involvement: The roles of cultural and economic capital. *International Review for the Sociology of Sport* 2002; **37**(1): 5–16.

487. Pampel FC. Does reading keep you thin? Leisure activities, cultural tastes, and body weight in comparative perspective. *Sociology of Health and Illness* 2012; **34**(3): 396–411.

488. Chan TW. Social status and cultural consumption. Cambridge etc: Cambridge University Press; 2010.

489. Victora CG, Joseph G, Silva ICM, et al. The Inverse Equity Hypothesis: Analyses of Institutional Deliveries in 286 National Surveys. *American Journal of Public Health* 2018: e1–e8.

490. Titmuss RM. Commitment to welfare. London: George Allen and Unwin; 1968.

491. Wilkinson RG, Pickett K. The inner level: How more equal societies reduce stress, restore sanity and improve everyone's well-being. London etc: Allen Lane; 2018.

492. Layte R, Whelan CT. Who feels inferior? A test of the status anxiety hypothesis of social inequalities in health. *European Sociological Review* 2014; **30**(4): 525–35.

493. Seeman M, Merkin SS, Karlamangla A, Koretz B, Seeman T. Social status and biological dysregulation: The 'status syndrome' and allostatic load. *Social Science and Medicine* 2014; **118**: 143–51.

494. Bosma H, Schrijvers C, Mackenbach JP. Socioeconomic inequalities in mortality and importance of perceived control: Cohort study. *Bmj* 1999; **319**(7223): 1469–70.

495. Phelan JC, Link BG. Controlling disease and creating disparities: A fundamental cause perspective. *The Journals of Gerontology Series B: Psychological Sciences and Social Sciences* 2005; **60**(Special Issue 2): S27–S33.

496. Freese J, Lutfey K. Fundamental causality: Challenges of an animating concept for medical sociology. In: Pescosolido BA, Martin JK, McLeod JD, Rogers A, eds. Handbook of the Sociology of Health, Illness, and Healing A blueprint for the 21st century. New York etc.: Springer; 2011: 67–81.

497. Krieger N. Epidemiology and the web of causation: Has anyone seen the spider? *Social Science and Medicine* 1994; **39**(7): 887–903.

498. Navarro V, Muntaner C, Borrell C, et al. Politics and health outcomes. *The Lancet* 2006; **368**(9540): 1033–7.

499. Mackenbach JP, Kulhánová I, Artnik B, et al. Changes in mortality inequalities over two decades: Register based study of European countries. *British Medical Journal* 2016; **353**: i1732.

500. Mackenbach JP, Hu Y, Artnik B, et al. Trends in inequalities in mortality amenable to health care In 17 European countries. *Health Affairs* 2017; **36**(6): 1110–18.

501. Rubio Valverde J, Nusselder WJ, Mackenbach JP. Educational inequalities in GALI disability in 28 European Countries. Does the choice of survey matter? *International Journal of Public Health* 2019; 64:461–474.

502. Hu Y, van Lenthe FJ, Platt S, et al. The impact of population-based tobacco control policies on smoking among socioeconomic groups in 9 European countries between 1990 and 2007: A fixed effects study. *Nicotine and Tobacco Research* 2017: 1441–9.

503. Hoffmann K, De Gelder R, Hu Y, et al. Trends in educational inequalities in obesity in 15 European countries between 1990 and 2010. *International Journal of Behavioral Nutrition and Physical Activity* 2017; **14**(1): 63.

504. Mackenbach JP, Bopp M, Deboosere P, et al. Determinants of the magnitude of socioeconomic inequalities in mortality: A study of 17 European countries. *Health and Place* 2017; **47**: 44–53.

505. Solt F. Standardizing the world income inequality database. *Social Science Quarterly* 2009; **90**(2): 231–42.

506. Teorell J, Dahlberg S, Holmberg S, Rothstein B, Hartmann F, Svensson R. The quality of government standard dataset, version jan17. In: Institute UoGTQoG, editor. Gothenburg; 2015.

507. Armingeon K, Isler C, Knöpfel L, Weisstanner D, Engler S. Comparative political data set 1960–2014. In: Institute of Political Science UoB, ed. Berne; 2016.

508. Forey B, Hamling J, Hamling J, Thornton A, Lee P. International Smoking Statistics, Web Edition. In: Ltd PNLSaC, ed. Sutton; 2006–16.

509. Currie L, Gilmore AB. Tobacco. In: Mackenbach JP, McKee M, eds. Successes and failures of health policy in Europe: Four decades of divergent trends and converging challenges. Buckingham: Open University Press; 2013: 23–40.

510. Joossens L, Raw M. Progress in tobacco control in 30 European countries, 2005 to 2007. Bern: Swiss Cancer League, 2007.

511. Piantadosi S, Byar DP, Green SB. The ecological fallacy. *American Journal of Epidemiology* 1988; **127**(5): 893–904.

512. OECD. Education at a glance 2017: OECD indicators. Paris: OECD Publishing Press, 2017.

513. Östergren O, Lundberg O, Artnik B, et al. Educational expansion and inequalities in mortality: A fixed-effects analysis using longitudinal data from 18 European populations. *PloS One* 2017; **12**(8): e0182526.

514. Liu Y, Grusky DB. The payoff to skill in the third industrial revolution. *American Journal of Sociology* 2013; **118**(5): 1330–74.

515. Schwartz CR, Mare RD. Trends in educational assortative marriage from 1940 to 2003. *Demography* 2005; **42**(4): 621–46.

516. Mackenbach JP, McKee M, eds. Successes and failures of health policy in Europe over four decades: Diverging trends, converging challenges. Buckingham: Open University Press; 2013.

517. Scanlan JP. The misinterpretation of health inequalities in the United Kingdom. British Society for Populations Studies Conference; 2006: Citeseer; 2006. p. 18–20.

518. Eikemo TA, Skalická V, Avendano M. Variations in relative health inequalities: Are they a mathematical artefact? *International Journal for Equity in Health* 2009; **8**(1): 32.

519. Vagerö D, Erikson R. Socioeconomic inequalities in morbidity and mortality in Western Europe [letter]. *Lancet* 1997; **349**: 516.

520. Houweling TAJ, Kunst AE, Huisman M, Mackenbach JP. Using relative and absolute measures for monitoring health inequalities: Experiences from cross-national analyses on maternal and child health. *International Journal for Equity in Health* 2007; **6**(1): 15.

521. Mackenbach JP, Martikainen P, Menvielle G, de Gelder R. The arithmetic of reducing relative and absolute inequalities in health: A theoretical analysis illustrated with European mortality data. *Journal of Epidemiology and Community Health* 2016; **70**: 730–6.

522. Mackenbach JP, Kulhanova I, Bopp M, et al. Variations in the relation between education and cause-specific mortality in 19 European populations: A test of the 'fundamental causes' theory of social inequalities in health. *Social Science and Medicine* 2015; **127**: 51–62.

523. Menvielle G, Leclerc A, Chastang J-F, Luce D. Social inequalities in breast cancer mortality among French women: Disappearing educational disparities from 1968 to 1996. *British Journal of Cancer* 2005; **94**(1): 152–5.

524. Phelan JC, Link BG, Diez-Roux A, Kawachi I, Levin B. 'Fundamental causes' of social inequalities in mortality: A test of the theory. *Journal of Health and Social Behavior* 2004; **45**(3): 265–85.

525. Chang VW, Lauderdale DS. Fundamental cause theory, technological innovation, and health disparities: The case of cholesterol in the era of statins. *Journal of Health and Social Behavior* 2009; **50**(3): 245–60.

526. Glied S, Lleras-Muney A. Technological innovation and inequality in health. *Demography* 2008; **45**(3): 741–61.

527. Lutfey K, Freese J. Toward some fundamentals of fundamental causality: Socioeconomic status and health in the routine clinic visit for diabetes. *American Journal of Sociology* 2005; **110**(5): 1326–72.

528. Mackenbach JP, Looman CWN, Artnik B, et al. Fundamental causes of inequalities in mortality: A test of the theory in 20 European populations. *Sociology of Health and Illness* 2017; **39**(7): 1117–33.

529. Miech R, Pampel F, Kim J, Rogers RG. The enduring association between education and mortality: The role of widening and narrowing disparities. *American Sociological Review* 2011; **76**(6): 913–34.

530. Preston SH, Glei DA, Wilmoth JR. A new method for estimating smoking-attributable mortality in high-income countries. *International Journal of Epidemiology* 2009; **39**(2): 430–8.

531. Jha P, Peto R, Zatonski W, Boreham J, Jarvis MJ, Lopez AD. Social inequalities in male mortality, and in male mortality from smoking: Indirect estimation from national death rates in England and Wales, Poland, and North America. *Lancet* 2006; **368**(9533): 367–70.

532. Thun M, Peto R, Boreham J, Lopez AD. Stages of the cigarette epidemic on entering its second century. *Tobacco Control* 2012; **21**(2): 96–101.

533. Pampel FC. Cigarette diffusion and sex differences in smoking. *Journal of Health and Social Behavior* 2001; **42**: 388–404.

534. Hill S, Amos A, Clifford D, Platt S. Impact of tobacco control interventions on socioeconomic inequalities in smoking: Review of the evidence. *Tobacco Control* 2014; **23**(e2): e89–e97.

535. Brown T, Platt S, Amos A. Equity impact of population-level interventions and policies to reduce smoking in adults: A systematic review. *Drug and Alcohol Dependence* 2014; **138**: 7–16.

536. Schaap MM, Kunst AE, Leinsalu M, et al. Effect of nationwide tobacco control policies on smoking cessation in high and low educated groups in 18 European countries. *Tobacco Control* 2008; **17**(4): 248–55.

537. Bosdriesz JR, Willemsen MC, Stronks K, Kunst AE. Tobacco control policy and socio-economic inequalities in smoking in 27 European countries. *Drug and Alcohol Dependence* 2016; **165**: 79–86.

538. Hu Y, van Lenthe FJ, Platt S, et al. The impact of tobacco control policies on smoking among socioeconomic groups in nine European countries, 1990–2007. *Nicotine and Tobacco Research* 2016; **19**(12): 1441–9.

539. Macintyre S. Deprivation amplification revisited; or, is it always true that poorer places have poorer access to resources for healthy diets and physical activity? *International Journal of Behavioral Nutrition and Physical Activity* 2007; **4**(1): 32.

540. Giskes K, van Lenthe F, Avendano-Pabon M, Brug J. A systematic review of environmental factors and obesogenic dietary intakes among adults: Are we getting closer to understanding obesogenic environments? *Obesity Reviews* 2011; **12**(5): e95–e106.

541. Cummins S, Macintyre S. Food environments and obesity—neighbourhood or nation? *International Journal of Epidemiology* 2006; **35**(1): 100–4.

542. Mackenbach JD, Lakerveld J, van Lenthe FJ, et al. Exploring why residents of socioeconomically deprived neighbourhoods have less favourable perceptions of their neighbourhood environment than residents of wealthy neighbourhoods. *Obesity Reviews* 2016; **17**: 42–52.

543. Mani A, Mullainathan S, Shafir E, Zhao J. Poverty impedes cognitive function. *Science* 2013; **341**(6149): 976–80.

544. Christakis NA, Fowler JH. The spread of obesity in a large social network over 32 years. *New England Journal of Medicine* 2007; **357**(4): 370–9.

545. Rabinovich L, Brutscher P-B, de Vries H, Tiessen J, Clift J, Reding A. The affordability of alcoholic beverages in the European Union: Understanding the link between alcohol affordability, consumption and harms. Santa Monica etc.: RAND Europe; 2009.

546. Herttua K, Mäkelä P, Martikainen P. Changes in alcohol-related mortality and its socioeconomic differences after a large reduction in alcohol prices: A natural experiment based on register data. *American Journal of Epidemiology* 2008; **168**(10): 1110–18.

547. Herttua K, Mäkelä P, Martikainen P. Minimum prices of alcohol and educational disparities in alcohol-related mortality: A time-series analysis. *European Public Health Conference Abstracts* 2013.

548. Norström T, ed. Alcohol in postwar Europe. Consumption, drinking patterns, consequences and policy responses in 15 European countries. Stockholm: National Institute of Public Health; 2002.

549. Simpura J. Mediterranean mysteries: Mechanisms of declining alcohol consumption. *Addiction* 1998; **93**(9): 1301–4.

550. Gual A, Colom J. Why has alcohol consumption declined in countries of southern Europe? *Addiction* 1997; **92**(s1): s21–s31.

551. Sulkunen P. Drinking in France 1965–1979. An analysis of household consumption data. *Addiction* 1989; **84**(1): 61–72.

552. Karlsson T, Österberg E. Scaling alcohol control policies across Europe. *Drugs: Education, Prevention and Policy* 2007; **14**(6): 499–511.

553. Zatonski WA, Sulkowska U, Manczuk M, et al. Liver cirrhosis mortality in Europe, with special attention to Central and Eastern Europe. *European Addiction Research* 2010; **16**(4): 193–201.

554. Leon DA, Chenet L, Shkolnikov VM, et al. Huge variation in Russian mortality rates 1984–94: Artefact, alcohol, or what? *The Lancet* 1997; **350**(9075): 383–8.

555. Moskalewicz J. Lessons to be learnt from Poland's attempt at moderating its consumption of alcohol. *Addiction* 1993; **88** (Suppl): 135S–42S.

556. Stuckler D, King L, McKee M. Mass privatisation and the post-communist mortality crisis: A cross-national analysis. *The Lancet* 2009; **373**(9661): 399–407.

557. Lai T, Habicht J. Decline in alcohol consumption in Estonia: Combined effects of strengthened alcohol policy and economic downturn. *Alcohol Alcoholism* 2011; **46**(2): 200–3.

558. Bunker JP. The role of medical care in contributing to health improvements within societies. *International Journal of Epidemiology* 2001; **30**(6): 1260–3.

559. Mackenbach J. The contribution of medical care to mortality decline: McKeown revisited. *Journal of Clinical Epidemiology* 1996; **49**(11): 1207–13.

560. Hunink MGM, Goldman L, Tosteson ANA, et al. The recent decline in mortality from coronary heart disease, 1980–1990: the effect of secular trends in risk factors and treatment. *Jorunal of the American Medical Association* 1997; **277**(7): 535–42.

561. Unal B, Critchley JA, Capewell S. Explaining the decline in coronary heart disease mortality in England and Wales between 1981 and 2000. *Circulation* 2004; **109**(9): 1101–7.

562. Laatikainen T, Critchley J, Vartiainen E, Salomaa V, Ketonen M, Capewell S. Explaining the decline in coronary heart disease mortality in Finland between 1982 and 1997. *American Journal of Epidemiology* 2005; **162**(8): 764–73.

563. Bajekal M, Scholes S, Love H, et al. Analysing recent socioeconomic trends in coronary heart disease mortality in England, 2000–2007: A population modelling study. *PLoS Medicine* 2012; **9**(6): e1001237.

564. Scholes S, Bajekal M, Love H, et al. Persistent socioeconomic inequalities in cardiovascular risk factors in England over 1994–2008: A time-trend analysis of repeated cross-sectional data. *BMC Public Health* 2012; **12**: 129.

565. Karim-Kos HE, de Vries E, Soerjomataram I, Lemmens V, Siesling S, Coebergh JWW. Recent trends of cancer in Europe: A combined approach of incidence, survival and mortality for 17 cancer sites since the 1990s. *European Journal of Cancer* 2008; **44**(10): 1345–89.

566. Mackenbach JP, Looman CWN. Life expectancy and national income in Europe, 1900–2008: An update of Preston's analysis. *International Journal of Epidemiology* 2013; **42**(4): 1100–10.

567. Pickett KE, Wilkinson RG. Income inequality and health: A causal review. *Social Science and Medicine* 2015; **128**: 316–26.

568. Mackenbach JP, McKee M. A comparative analysis of health policy performance in 43 European countries. *Eur J Public Health* 2013; **23**(2): 195–201.

569. Mackenbach JP, Hu Y, Looman CWN. Democratization and life expectancy in Europe, 1960–2008. *Social Science and Medicine* 2013; **93**: 166–75.

570. Lundberg O, Yngwe MA, Stjarne MK, et al. The role of welfare state principles and generosity in social policy programmes for public health: An international comparative study. *Lancet* 2008; **372**(9650): 1633–40.

571. van Baal P, Obulqasim P, Brouwer W, Nusselder W, Mackenbach J. The influence of health care spending on life expectancy. Tilburg: Netspar; 2013.

572. Preston SH. The changing relation between mortality and level of economic development. *Population Studies* 1975; **29**(2): 231–48.

573. Wagstaff A. Inequalities in health in developing countries: Swimming against the tide? Washington DC: World Bank Publications, 2002.

574. OECD. Divided we stand: Why inequality keeps rising. Paris: OECD Publishing, 2011.

575. Hoffmann R, Hu Y, De Gelder R, Mackenbach JP. The impact of increasing income inequalities on educational inequalities in mortality: An analysis of six European countries *International Journal for Equity in Health* 2016; **15**: 103.

576. Wilkinson RG. Class mortality differentials, income distribution and trends in poverty 1921–1981. *Journal of Social Policy* 1989; **18**(3): 307–35.

577. Kondo N, Sembajwe G, Kawachi I, van Dam RM, Subramanian SV, Yamagata Z. Income inequality, mortality, and self rated health: meta-analysis of multilevel studies. *British Medical Journal* 2009; **339**: b4471.

578. Kawachi I, Kennedy BP, Lochner K, Prothrow-Stith D. Social capital, income inequality, and mortality. *American Journal of Public Health* 1997; **87**(9): 1491–8.

579. Mackenbach JP, McKee M. Social-democratic government and health policy in Europe: A quantitative analysis. *International Journal of Health Services* 2013; **43**(3): 389–413.

580. Klomp J, de Haan J. Is the political system really related to health? *Social Science and Medicine* 2009; **69**(1): 36–46.

581. Mackenbach JP, Hu Y, Looman CWN. Democratization and life expectancy in Europe, 1960–2008. *Social Science and Medicine* 2013; **93**: 166–75.

582. McKee M, Zwi A, Koupilova I, Sethi D, Leon D. Health policy-making in central and eastern Europe: Lessons from the inaction on injuries? *Health Policy and Planning* 2000; **15**(3): 263–9.

583. Dahl E, van der Wel KA. Educational inequalities in health in European welfare states: A social expenditure approach. *Social Science and Medicine* 2013; **81**: 60–9.

584. OECD. Health at a Glance: Europe 2016—State of health in the EU cycle. Paris: OECD Publishing, 2016.

585. Heijink R, Koolman X, Westert GP. Spending more money, saving more lives? The relationship between avoidable mortality and healthcare spending in 14 countries. *European Journal of Health Economics* 2013; **14**(3): 527–38.

586. Spence DP, Hotchkiss J, Williams CS, Davies PD. Tuberculosis and poverty. *British Medical Journal* 1993; **307**(6907): 759–61.

587. Doll R, Peto R, Boreham J, Sutherland I. Mortality in relation to smoking: 50 years' observations on male British doctors. *British Medical Journal* 2004; **328**(7455): 1519.

588. Thun MJ, Carter BD, Feskanich D, et al. 50-year trends in smoking-related mortality in the United States. *New England Journal of Medicine* 2013; **368**(4): 351–64.

589. Gregoraci G, van Lenthe FJ, Artnik B, et al. Changes in the contribution of smoking to socio-economic inequalities in mortality in 13 European countries. *Tobacco Control* 2017; **26**: 260–8.

590. Vandenheede H, Deboosere P, Espelt A, et al. Educational inequalities in diabetes mortality across Europe in the 2000s: The interaction with gender. *International Journal of Public Health* 2015; **60**(4): 401–10.

591. Hoffmann R, Eikemo TA, Kulhanova I, et al. Obesity and the potential reduction of social inequalities in mortality: Evidence from 21 European populations. *European Journal of Public Health* 2015; **25**(5): 849–56.

592. **Kivimaki M, Shipley MJ, Ferrie JE,** et al. Best-practice interventions to reduce socioeconomic inequalities of coronary heart disease mortality in UK: A prospective occupational cohort study. *Lancet* 2008; **372**(9650): 1648–54.

593. **Nordahl H, Rod NH, Frederiksen BL,** et al. Education and risk of coronary heart disease: Assessment of mediation by behavioral risk factors using the additive hazards model. *European Journal of Epidemiology* 2013; **28**(2): 149–57.

594. **Probst C, Roerecke M, Behrendt S, Rehm J.** Socioeconomic differences in alcohol-attributable mortality compared with all-cause mortality: A systematic review and meta-analysis. *International Journal of Epidemiology* 2014; **43**(4): 1314–27.

595. **Shaw J, Hunt IM, Flynn S,** et al. The role of alcohol and drugs in homicides in England and Wales. *Addiction* 2006; **101**(8): 1117–24.

596. **Rossow I.** Alcohol and homicide: A cross-cultural comparison of the relationship in 14 European countries. *Addiction* 2001; **96**(1s1): 77–92.

597. **Plug I, Hoffmann R, Artnik B,** et al. Socioeconomic inequalities in mortality from conditions amenable to medical interventions: Do they reflect inequalities in access or quality of health care? *BMC Public Health* 2012; **12**(1): 346.

598. **Mackenbach JP.** Nordic paradox, Southern miracle, Eastern disaster: Persistence of inequalities in mortality in Europe. *European Journal of Public Health* 2017; **27**(suppl_4): 14–17.

599. **Norberg M, Malmberg G, Ng N, Broström G.** Who is using snus? Time trends, socioeconomic and geographic characteristics of snus users in the ageing Swedish population. *BMC Public Health* 2011; **11**(1): 929.

600. **Schaap MM, Kunst AE, Leinsalu M,** et al. Female ever-smoking, education, emancipation and economic development in 19 European countries. *Social Science and Medicine* 2009; **68**(7): 1271–8.

601. **Kulhanova I, Bacigalupe A, Eikemo TA,** et al. Why does Spain have smaller inequalities in mortality? An exploration of potential explanations. *Eur J Public Health* 2014; **24**(3): 370–7.

602. **OECD.** Educational opportunity for all: Overcoming inequality throughout the life course. Paris: OECD Publishing, 2017.

603. **Leinsalu M, Stirbu I, Vagero D,** et al. Educational inequalities in mortality in four Eastern European countries: Divergence in trends during the post-communist transition from 1990 to 2000. *Int J Epidemiol* 2009; **38**(2): 512–25.

604. **Judt T.** Postwar: A history of Europe since 1945. New York etc: Penguin; 2006.

605. **Szelényi S.** Social inequality and party membership: Patterns of recruitment into the Hungarian Socialist Workers' Party. *American Sociological Review* 1987: 559–73.

606. **Szalai J.** Inequalities in access to health care in Hungary. *Social Science and Medicine* 1986; **22**(2): 135–40.

607. **Mastilica M.** Health and social inequities in Yugoslavia. *Social Science and Medicine* 1990; **31**(3): 405–12.

608. **Shkolnikov VM, Leon DA, Adamets S, Andreev E, Deev A.** Educational level and adult mortality in Russia: An analysis of routine data 1979 to 1994. *Social Science and Medicine* 1998; **47**(3): 357–69.

609. **Józan P, Radnóti L.** A dohányzás hatása a halandóságra Magyarországon 1970–1990 [The effect of smoking on mortality in Hungary 1970–1990]. Budapest: Központi Statisztikai Hivatal, 2002.

610. **Hegedűs I, Kiss JG.** Alkoholizmus Magyarországon [Alcoholism in Hungary]. In: Andorka R, Buda B, Cseh-Szombathy L, eds. A deviáns viselkedés szociológiája. Budapest: Gondolat; 1974: 338–60.

611. **Józan P.** Main features of epidemiological development in Hungary after the Second World War. *Hungarian Statistical Review* 2008; **86**(Special Number 12).

612. **McKee M, Shkolnikov V.** Understanding the toll of premature death among men in eastern Europe. *British Medical Journal* 2001; **323**(7320): 1051–5.

613. **Jasilionis D, Meslé F, Shkolnikov VM, Vallin J.** Recent life expectancy divergence in Baltic countries. *European Journal of Population/Revue Européenne de Démographie* 2011; **27**(4): 403.

614. **Mackenbach JP.** Persistence of social inequalities in modern welfare states: Explanation of a paradox. *Scandinavian Journal of Public Health* 2017; **45**(2): 113–20.

615. **Marmot M,** Health CoSDo. Achieving health equity: From root causes to fair outcomes. *The Lancet* 2007; **370**(9593): 1153–63.

616. **Anderson C.E. B.** The functions and dysfunctions of hierarchy. *Research in Organizational Behavior* 2010; **30**: 55–89.

617. **Wilson EO.** Sociobiology: The new synthesis. Cambridge (Mass.): Harvard University Press; 2000.

618. **Sapolsky RM.** The influence of social hierarchy on primate health. *Science* 2005; **308**(5722): 648–52.

619. **Bercovitch FB.** Social stratification, social strategies, and reproductive success in primates. *Ethology and Sociobiology* 1991; **12**(4): 315–33.

620. **Moor GE.** Principia Ethica. Cambridge: Cambridge University Press; 1903.

621. **Mare RD.** Five decades of educational assortative mating. *American Sociological Review* 1991; **56**: 15–32.

622. **Mare RD.** A multigenerational view of inequality. *Demography* 2011; **48**(1): 1–23.

623. **Pakulski J, Waters M.** The death of class. London: Sage Publications; 1996.

624. **Sørensen AB.** The structural basis of social inequality. *American Journal of Sociology* 1996; **101**: 1333–65.

625. **Marx K, Engels F.** The German ideology [edited by C. Arthur]. New York: International Publishers; 1847 [1970].

626. **Ames KM.** On the evolution of the human capacity for inequality and/or egalitarianism. In: Price TD, Feinman GM, eds. Pathways to power: New perspectives on the emergence of social inequality. New York etc.: Springer; 2010: 15–44.

627. **Leventhal T, Brooks-Gunn J.** The neighborhoods they live in: The effects of neighborhood residence on child and adolescent outcomes. *Psychological Bulletin* 2000; **126**(2): 309–37.

628. **d'Addio AC.** Intergenerational transmission of disadvantage. Paris: OECD; 2007.

629. **Magee JC, Galinsky AD.** Social hierarchy: The self-reinforcing nature of power and status. *The Academy of Management Annals* 2008; **2**(1): 351–98.

630. **Drennan RD, Peterson CE, Fox JR.** Degrees and kinds of inequality. Pathways to Power: New perspectives on the emergence of social inequality. New York etc: Springer; 2010: 45–76.

631. **Boehm C, Barclay HB, Dentan RK,** et al. Egalitarian behavior and reverse dominance hierarchy [and comments and reply]. *Current Anthropology* 1993; **34**(3): 227–54.

632. **Erdal D, Whiten A, Boehm C, Knauft B.** On human egalitarianism: An evolutionary product of Machiavellian status escalation? *Current Anthropology* 1994; **35** (2): 175–83.

633. **Boix C.** Political order and inequality. Cambridge: Cambridge University Press; 2015.

634. **Weber M.** Economy and society: An outline of interpretive sociology. Edited by G. Roth and C. Wittich. Berkeley: University of California Press; 1922 [1978].

635. **Murphy R.** Social closure: The theory of monopolization and exclusion. Oxford etc.: Oxford University Press; 1988.

636. **DeMaggio P.** Cultural capital and school success. *American Sociological Review* 1982; **47**: 189–201.

637. **Piketty T.** Theories of persistent inequality and intergenerational mobility. In: Atkinson A, Bourguignon F, eds. Handbook of income distribution. Amsterdam etc: Elsevier; 2014.

638. **Huber E, Stephens JD.** Development and crisis of the welfare state: Parties and policies in global markets. Chicago: University of Chicago Press; 2001.

639. **Vågerö D, Illsley R.** Explaining health inequalities: Beyond Black and Barker: A discussion of some issues emerging in the decade following the Black report. *European Sociological Review* 1995; **11**(3): 219–41.

640. **Booske BC, Robert SA, Rohan AM.** Awareness of racial and socioeconomic health disparities in the United States: The national opinion survey on health and health disparities, 2008–2009. *Preventing Chronic Disease* 2011; **8**(4): A73.

641. **Allen NB, Badcock PB.** The social risk hypothesis of depressed mood: Evolutionary, psychosocial, and neurobiological perspectives. *Psychological Bulletin* 2003; **129**(6): 887–913.

642. **Price J, Sloman L, Gardner R, Jr., Gilbert P, Rohde P.** The social competition hypothesis of depression. *The British Journal of Psychiatry: The Journal of Mental Science* 1994; **164**(3): 309–15.

643. **Marx I, Nolan B, Olivera Angulo J.** The welfare state and anti-poverty policy in rich countries, 2014.

644. **Korpi W, Palme J.** The paradox of redistribution and strategies of equality: Welfare state institutions, inequality, and poverty in the Western countries. *American Sociological Review* 1998; **63**: 661–87.

645. **Hemerijck A, Dräbing V, Vis B, Nelson M, Soentken M.** European welfare states in motion. Amsterdam/Lund, 2013.

646. **Esping-Andersen G.** A welfare state for the 21st century: Ageing societies, knowledge-based economies and the sustainability of European welfare states. Lisbon, 2000.

647. **Bovenberg H, Mackenbach J, Mehlkopf R.** A fair and ageing-proof old age pension [Een eerlijk en vergrijzingbestendig ouderdomspensioen]. *Economisch-Statistische Berichten* 2006: 648–51.

648. **Van Kersbergen K, Hemerijck A.** Two decades of change in Europe: The emergence of the social investment state. *Journal of Social Policy* 2012; **41**(3): 475–92.

649. **van den Berg T, Schuring M, Avendano M, Mackenbach J, Burdorf A.** The impact of ill health on exit from paid employment in Europe among older workers. *Occupational and Environmental Medicine* 2010; **67**(12): 845–52.

650. **Schuring M, Burdorf L, Kunst A, Mackenbach J.** The effects of ill health on entering and maintaining paid employment: Evidence in European countries. *Journal of Epidemiology and Community Health* 2007; **61**(7): 597–604.

651. **McAllister A, Nylén L, Backhans M, et al.** Do 'flexicurity'policies work for people with low education and health problems? A comparison of labour market policies and employment rates in Denmark, The Netherlands, Sweden, and the United Kingdom 1990–2010. *International Journal of Health Services* 2015; **45**(4): 679–705.

652. **Backhans MC, Mosedale S, Bruce D, Whitehead M, Burström B.** What is the impact of flexicurity on the chances of entry into employment for people with low education and activity limitations due to health problems? A comparison of 21 European countries using Qualitative Comparative Analysis (QCA). *BMC Public Health* 2016; **16**(1): 842.

653. **Commission on Social Determinants of Health. Closing the gap in a generation.** Health equity through the social determinants of health. Geneva: World Health Organization; 2008.

654. **Whitehead M.** The concepts and principles of equity and health. Copenhagen: World Health Organization Regional Office for Europe, 1990.

655. **Rawls J.** A theory of justice. Cambridge, MA: Harvard University Press; 1971.

656. **Daniels N, Kennedy B, Kawachi I.** Why justice is good for our health: The social determinants of health inequalities. *Daedalus* 1999; **128**(4): 215–51.

657. **Stronks K, Gunning-Schepers LJ.** Should equity in health be target number 1? *The European Journal of Public Health* 1993; **3**(2): 104–11.

658. **Stronks K, Toebes B, Hendriks A, Ikram U, Venkatapuram S.** Social justice and human rights as a framework for addressing social determinants of health. Copenhagen: World Health Organization Regional Office for Europe, 2016.

659. **Venkatapuram S.** Health Justice. Cambridge: Polity Press; 2011.

660. **Rawls J.** Justice as fairness. *The Philosophical Review* 1958; **67**(2): 164–94.

661. **Arneson R.** Egalitarianism. Stanford encyclopedia of philosophy. 2013. 2002 (accessed 31 December 2017).

662. **Arneson R.** Equal opportunity. Stanford encyclopedia of philosophy. 2013. 2002 (accessed 31 December 2017).

663. **Dworkin R.** What is equality? Part 2: Equality of resources. *Philosophy and Public Affairs* 1981; **10**(4): 283–345.

664. **Sen A.** Inequality reexamined. Oxford etc.: Clarendon Press; 1992.

665. **Nussbaum MC.** Creating capabilities. Cambridge, MA: Harvard University Press; 2011.

666. **Dworkin R.** What is equality? Part 1: Equality of welfare. *Philosophy and Public Affairs* 1981; **10**(3): 185–246.

667. **Nozick R.** Anarchy, state, and utopia. Malden etc.: Basic Books; 1974.

668. **Pereira J.** What does equity in health mean? *Journal of Social Policy* 1993; **22**(1): 19–48.

669. **Hausman DM.** What's wrong with health inequalities? *Journal of Political Philosophy* 2007; **15**(1): 46–66.

670. **Daniels N.** Justice, health, and healthcare. *American Journal of Bioethics* 2001; **1**(2): 2–16.

671. **Segall S.** Is health (really) special? Health policy between Rawlsian and luck egalitarian justice. *Journal of Applied Philosophy* 2010; **27**(4): 344–58.

672. **Segall S.** In solidarity with the imprudent: A defense of luck egalitarianism. *Social Theory and Practice* 2007; **33**(2): 177–98.

673. **Scheffler S.** Choice, circumstance, and the value of equality. *Politics, Philosophy and Economics* 2005; **4**(1): 5–28.

674. **Jusot F, Tubeuf S, Trannoy A.** Circumstances and efforts: How important is their correlation for the measurement of inequality of opportunity in health? *Health Economics* 2013; **22**(12): 1470–95.

675. **Wolff J, De-Shalit A.** Disadvantage. Oxford etc.: Oxford University Press; 2007.

676. **Walzer M.** Spheres of justice: A defense of pluralism and equality. New York: Basic Books; 2008.

677. **Ter Meulen R.** Solidarity and justice in health care. A critical analysis of their relationship. *Diametros* 2015; (43): 1–20.

678. **Prainsack B, Buyx A.** Solidarity in contemporary bioethics: Towards a new approach. *Bioethics* 2012; **26**(7): 343–50.

679. **Prainsack B, Buyx A.** Solidarity: Reflections on an emerging concept in bioethics. London: Nuffield Council on Bioethics; 2011.

680. **Mackenbach JP, Bakker MJ.** Tackling socioeconomic inequalities in health: Analysis of European experiences. *The Lancet* 2003; **362**(9393): 1409–14.

681. **Mackenbach JP, Meerding WJ, Kunst AE.** Economic costs of health inequalities in the European Union. *Journal of Epidemiology and Community Health* 2011; **65**(5): 412–9.

682. **Meggiolaro S, Mazzuco S, Cookson R, Suhrcke M.** The economic benefits of reducing health inequalities in 11 European countries. In: Suhrcke M, Cookson R, eds. Discussion paper on economics and health inequalities: Review of social determinants of health and the health divide in the WHO European Region. Copenhagen: WHO Regional Office for Europe; 2016: 44–62.

683. **Schoeni RF, Dow WH, Miller WD, Pamuk ER.** The economic value of improving the health of disadvantaged Americans. *American Journal of Preventive Medicine* 2011; **40**(1): S67–S72.

684. **Marmot MG, Allen J, Goldblatt P,** et al. Fair society, healthy lives: Strategic review of health inequalities in England post-2010. London: The Marmot Review, 2010.

685. **World Health Organization.** Targets for health for all 2000. Copenhagen: WHO Regional Office for Europe; 1985.

686. **Mackenbach JP.** Socioeconomic inequalities in health in The Netherlands: Impact of a five year research programme. *British Medical Journal* 1994; **309**(6967): 1487–91.

687. **Whitehead M.** Diffusion of ideas on social inequalities in health: A European perspective. *The Milbank Quarterly* 1998; **76**(3): 469–92.

688. **Acheson D.** Independent inquiry into inequalities in health report. London: HM Stationery Office; 1998.

689. **Norwegian Ministry of Health and Care Services.** National strategy to reduce social inequalities in health. Report No. 20 (2006–2007) to the Storting. Oslo: Storting, 2007.

690. **Ministry of Social Affairs and Health.** National action plan to reduce health inequalities 2008–2011. Helsinki: Ministry of Social Affairs and Health; 2008.

691. **UCL Institute of Health Equity.** Review of social determinants and the health divide in the WHO European Region. Copenhagen: World Health Organization, 2013.

692. **Lundberg O.** The next step towards more equity in health in Sweden: How can we close the gap in a generation? *Scandinavian Journal of Public Health* 2018; **46**(Suppl.): 19–27.

693. Independent inquiry into inequalities in health (the Acheson report). London: Department of Health; 1998.

694. **Smith GD, Morris JN, Shaw M.** The independent inquiry into inequalities in health is welcome, but its recommendations are too cautious and vague. *British Medical Journal* 1998; **317**(7171): 1465–6.

695. **Acheson D.** Inequalities in health: Report on inequalities in health did give priority for steps to be tackled. *British Medical Journal* 1998; **317**(7173): 1659.

696. **Mackenbach JP, Stronks K.** The development of a strategy for tackling health inequalities in the Netherlands. *International Journal for Equity in Health* 2004; **3**(1): 11.

697. **Ministry of Health and Social Affairs.** Hälsa på lika villkor: Nationella mål för folkhälsan. Slutbetänkande av nationella folkhälsokommittén (Health on equal terms: Final proposal on national targets for public health). Stockholm: Ministry of Health and Social Affairs, 2000.

698. **Ministry of Social Affairs and Health.** National action plan to reduce health inequalities 2008–2011. Helsinki: Ministry of Social Affairs and Health, 2008.

699. **UCL Institute of Health Equity.** Review of social determinants and the health divide in the WHO European Region: Final report. Copenhagen: World Health Organization Regional Office for Europe, 2013.

700. **Marmot M, Allen J, Bell R, Bloomer E, Goldblatt P.** WHO European review of social determinants of health and the health divide. *The Lancet* 2012; **380**(9846): 1011–29.

701. **Broeders D, Das D, Jennissen R, Tiemeijer W, De Visser M.** Van verschil naar potentieel; een realistisch perspectief op de sociaaleconomische gezondheidsverschillen. The Hague: Wetenschappelijke Raad voor het Regeringsbeleid, 2018.

702. **Dahl E, Lie M.** Policies to tackle health inequalities in Norway: From laggard to pioneer? *International Journal of Health Services* 2009; **39**(3): 509–23.

703. **Dahl E, Van de Wel KA.** Nordic health inequalities: Patterns, trends, and policies. In: Smith KE, Hill S, Bambra C, eds. Health inequalities: Critical perspectives. Oxford: Oxford University Press; 2016: 33–49.

704. **Rotko T, Kauppinen T, Mustonen N, Linnanmäki E.** Kuilun kaventajat. Kansallinen terveyserojen kaventamisen toimintaohjelma 2008–2011-loppuraportti. Tampere: THL, 2012.

705. **Department of Health.** Reducing health inequalities: An action report. London: Department of Health; 1999.

706. **Department of Health.** Tackling health inequalities: A Program for Action. London: Department of Health; 2003.

707. **Mackenbach JP.** The English strategy to reduce health inequalities. *The Lancet* 2011; **377**(9782): 1986–8.

708. **Mackenbach JP.** Can we reduce health inequalities? An analysis of the English strategy (1997–2010). *Journal of Epidemiology and Community Health* 2011; **65**(7): 568–75.

709. **Scottish Government.** Equally Well. Report of the ministerial taskforce on health inequalities. Edinburgh: Scottish Government, 2008.

710. **Beeston C, McCartney G, Ford J, et al.** Health inequalities Policy review for the Scottish ministerial task force on health inequalities. Edinburgh: NHS Health Scotland, 2013.

711. **Bauld L, Judge K, Platt S.** Assessing the impact of smoking cessation services on reducing health inequalities in England: Observational study. *Tobacco Control* 2007; **16**(6): 400–4.

712. **Melhuish E, Belsky J, Leyland AH, Barnes JT.** National evaluation of sure start research Effects of fully-established sure start local programmes on 3-year-old children and their families living in England: A quasi-experimental observational study. *Lancet* 2008; **372**(9650): 1641–7.

713. **Barr B, Higgerson J, Whitehead M.** Investigating the impact of the English health inequalities strategy: Time trend analysis. *British Medical Journal* 2017; **358**: j3310.

714. Hu Y, van Lenthe FJ, Judge K, et al. Did the English strategy reduce inequalities in health? A difference-in-difference analysis comparing England with three other European countries. *BMC Public Health* 2016; **16**(1): 865.

715. Mackenbach JP. Has the English strategy to reduce health inequalities failed? *Social Science and Medicine* 2010; **71**(7): 1249–53.

716. Hunter DJ, Popay J, Tannahill C, Whitehead M. Getting to grips with health inequalities at last? *British Medical Journal* 2010; **340**: 323–4.

717. House of Commons Health Committee. Health inequalities. London: House of Commons, 2009.

718. World Health Organization. Health 21: The health for all policy framework for the WHO European Region. Copenhagen: WHO Regional Office for Europe, 1999.

719. Bauld L, Day P, Judge K. Off target: A critical review of setting goals for reducing health inequalities in the United Kingdom. *International Journal of Health Services: Planning, Administration, Evaluation* 2008; **38**(3): 439–54.

720. Barros AJD, Victora CG. Measuring coverage in MNCH: Determining and interpreting inequalities in coverage of maternal, newborn, and child health interventions. *PLoS Medicine* 2013; **10**(5): e1001390.

721. Mackenbach JP. An analysis of the role of health care in reducing socioeconomic inequalities in health: The case of The Netherlands. *International Journal of Health Services* 2003; **33**(3): 523–41.

722. Hoffmann R, Eikemo TA, Kulhanova I, et al. The potential impact of a social redistribution of specific risk factors on socioeconomic inequalities in mortality: Illustration of a method based on population attributable fractions. *Journal of Epidemiology and Community Health* 2013; **67**(1): 56–62.

723. Mackenbach JP, Rubio Valverde J, Bopp B, et al. Determinants of inequalities in life expectancy: an international-comparative study of 8 risk factors. The Lancet Public Health 2019; in press.

724. Eikemo TA, Hoffmann R, Kulik MC, et al. How can inequalities in mortality be reduced? A quantitative analysis of 6 risk factors in 21 European populations. *PLoS One* 2014; **9**(11): e110952.

725. Hillier-Brown F, Thomson K, McGowan V, et al. The effects of social protection policies on health inequalities: Evidence from systematic reviews *Scandinavian Journal of Public Health*. 2019; in press

726. Bambra C, Garthwaite K, Hunter D. All things being equal: Does it matter for equity how you organize and pay for health care? A review of the international evidence. *International Journal of Health Services* 2014; **44**(3): 457–77.

727. Bambra C, Gibson M, Sowden AJ, Wright K, Whitehead M, Petticrew M. Working for health? Evidence from systematic reviews on the effects on health and health inequalities of organisational changes to the psychosocial work environment. *Preventive Medicine* 2009; **48**(5): 454–61.

728. Thomson K, Hillier-Brown F, Todd A, McNamara C, Huijts T, Bambra C. The effects of public health policies on health inequalities in high-income countries: An umbrella review. *BMC Public Health* 2018; **18**: 869.

729. Brown T, Platt S, Amos A. Equity impact of European individual-level smoking cessation interventions to reduce smoking in adults: A systematic review. *European Journal of Public Health* 2014; **24**(4): 551–6.

730. Brown T, Platt S, Amos A. Equity impact of interventions and policies to reduce smoking in youth: Systematic review. *Tobacco Control* 2014; **23**(e2): e98–105.

731. Kunst AE. Sociaal-economische verschillen en roken: Sterke verbanden met implicaties voor tabaksbeleid. *Nederlands Tijdschrift voor Geneeskunde* 2017; **161**: D1530.

732. Carey G, Crammond B, De Leeuw E. Towards health equity: A framework for the application of proportionate universalism. *International Journal for Equity in Health* 2015; **14**(1): 81.

733. Jansen G, Evans G, De Graaf ND. Class voting and Left–Right party positions: A comparative study of 15 Western democracies, 1960–2005. *Social Science Research* 2013; **42**(2): 376–400.

734. Huber JD, Stanig P. Why do the poor support right-wing parties? A cross-national analysis. New York: Columbia University, 2007.

735. **Achterberg P, Houtman D.** Why do so many people vote 'unnaturally'? A cultural explanation for voting behaviour. *European Journal of Political Research* 2006; **45**(1): 75–92.

736. **Crawford R.** You are dangerous to your health: The ideology and politics of victim blaming. *International Journal of Health Services* 1977; **7**(4): 663–80.

737. **Proctor RN.** Golden holocaust: Origins of the cigarette catastrophe and the case for abolition. Berkeley etc: University of California Press; 2011.

738. **Paneth N.** Assessing the contributions of John Snow to epidemiology: 150 years after removal of the broad street pump handle. *Epidemiology* 2004; **15**(5): 514–16.

Index

Tables, figures, and boxes are indicated by *t*, *f*, and *b* following the page number; *vs* indicates a comparison
As the subject of this book is health inequalities, entries have been kept to a minimum under this heading. Readers are advised to look for more specific terms (e.g. policies to reduce health inequalities)

For the benefit of digital users, indexed terms that span two pages (e.g., 52–53) may, on occasion, appear on only one of those pages.